Errors in Imaging

Haris Chrysikopoulos

Errors in Imaging

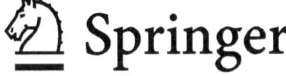 Springer

Haris Chrysikopoulos
CT & MR Division
Eurodiagnosis Imaging Center
Corfu
Greece

ISBN 978-3-030-21102-8   ISBN 978-3-030-21103-5   (eBook)
https://doi.org/10.1007/978-3-030-21103-5

This Springer imprint is published by the registered company Springer Nature Switzerland AG
The registered company address is: Gewerbestrasse 11, 6330 Cham, Switzerland

Dedicated to the younger generation of radiologists

Foreword 1

My career in Radiology so far has spanned 41 years, and I have collaborated and interacted with a large number of physicians. I have spent the past 33 years as the Head of the Imaging Department in a busy private hospital; one of my duties has been, and still is, the supervision and the assessment of performance of junior and senior colleagues. Throughout my career, I have been fascinated and intrigued by the complexities of diagnosing and reporting imaging studies.

Thus, I read with great interest the recent book *Errors in Imaging*, written by Dr. Haris Chrysikopoulos, whom I have personally known since 1992. The author deconvolutes successfully a very complex topic. Furthermore, he shows us that it is possible to disarm errors and biases in medical imaging. He weaves his personal experience and his acumen with a large body of literature from radiology, cognitive psychology, and expertise theory.

When I finished reading the book, I felt proud and happy, since the author started his career in my Department. We worked closely together for several years, and I definitely influenced his thinking to a large extent, as he has confided to me several times. After reading the book, I also realized that, independent of each other, we had drawn similar conclusions about errors in imaging and reporting. I have not written about this topic because I could not devote the time and energy required for such a difficult task. Thus, I am a little jealous of Dr. Chrysikopoulos because he has contributed work of great value.

I wish I had had the good fortune of reading such a book during my first steps as a radiologist. Without a doubt, I would have advanced my diagnostic, communication, and teaching skills at a greater pace to a higher level. I am certain that I would have avoided several misdiagnoses and frustrating incidents of miscommunication with other physicians.

In conclusion, I wholeheartedly recommend this book to all imaging professionals, trainees, and teachers and to all physicians that utilize imaging in the management of their patients.

John Andreou
Adjunct Associate Professor of Radiology
University of Athens Medical School
National and Kapodistrian University of Athens
Athens, Greece

Foreword 2

Errors in imaging, nowadays, is a more complex topic than in previous decades. There are many reasons for this. First, radiologists have gained a leading role in the chain of physicians who build the patient management. Thus, an error may be very important for a remote patient's outcome. Second, evolving technology in all imaging methods introduces new artifacts which need time for us to become familiar with. Primers, in particular, may interpret artifacts as disease. Third, with the wide application of teleradiology, the report tends to provide all inclusive information without isolating the single and most important out of many findings because of lack of communication between the radiologists, the patients, and treating physicians. Fourth, in the era of evidence-based and personalized medicine, the report and the selection of the appropriate and cost-effective imaging method are important in the clinical management.

The book Errors in Imaging by Dr. H. Chrysikopoulos is a unique and important addition to the imaging literature. I read the book from cover to cover almost like a novel. I found many issues discussed in the book very didactic. It is amazing to rediscover the ways in which missing lesions occur. Misdiagnosis starts with a failed search not depicting the lesion and ends with a failed decision based on an erroneous evaluation of a lesion as a normal or clinically not significant finding. I am more than certain that most of us never forget the mistakes which we could have avoided. Chapter 4 suggests a structured format for the report which helps avoid missing information. It further reminds us that a report is a medicolegal document. The inclusion of *certainty* in the report, "the finding is *not clinically important* and *no further evaluation* is warranted," is particularly often used by me and I find it well received by clinicians. The process of achieving expertise in radiology is very well presented in Chap. 6. It is very interesting that I share with the author the same techniques; first, we evaluate the images with the history and clinical question waived, and then focus on them trying to confirm or to exclude the clinical suspicion. Furthermore, we first assess the normal structures and leave the abnormal ones for the end.

No matter how experienced one can be, the error is a "hell around the corner." Bad sleep during the previous night, a knock on the door from a colleague asking for a quick first opinion, phone rings, or any kind of interruption could disrupt concentration and may result in an inaccurate or erroneous report. Unfolding the reasons leading to a missed diagnosis, without any doubt, will act for the benefit of both patients and physicians contributing to continuous education and excellence in medical practice. Personal thoughts of the author and proposals for reshaping radiologic education in the end of the book are more than welcome. The selected cases are educational, the captions focusing on the teaching points are extremely helpful, and the references include almost anything published on the topic.

Dr. Chrysikopoulos's book is an important accomplishment, and this is related to his deep interest in the topic and commitment in Radiology. I congratulate him on this comprehensively written book, as he points out, "if we become aware of our mistake, we should turn this incident into an opportunity for learning." Who will benefit from the book? All radiologists: residents, fellows, consultants, and seniors will learn and further minimize the risk for misdiagnosis. I see this book as an essential acquisition for the libraries of all academic departments with teaching duties.

Apostolos Karantanas
Professor of Radiology
University of Crete
Heraklion, Greece

Chairman, Department of Medical Imaging
Heraklion University Hospital
Heraklion, Greece

Head, Hybrid Imaging
ICS - FORTH
Heraklion, Greece

Board, Greek Atomic Energy Commission
Heraklion, Greece

Ex-President ESSR
Nijmegen, The Netherlands

Acknowledgements

I am indebted to all my teachers and colleagues who sparked and supported my interests in Radiology. I would like to start with the elective course in radiology I attended as a medical student. My teachers were D.A. Aronberg, MD, S.S. Sagel, MD, and B.A. Siegel, MD at the Mallinckrodt Institute of Radiology. Their knowledge, expertise, and teaching inspired me to choose radiology as my career. During my residency at the University of California at San Diego I felt "I was standing on the shoulders of giants." The attendings that made a lasting impression on me were J.R. Amberg, MD, J.V. Forrest, MD, G. Leopold, MD, D.L. Resnick, MD, and L.B. Talner, MD. My mentor at Hygeia Hospital in Athens was J. Andreou, MD, PhD, whom I also consider a dear friend. Many years later, in Kerkyra, I met a young radiology resident, I. Papachristos, MD, with whom I held lengthy discussions about all aspects of radiology. Those discussions were the seed for this book. Throughout this project, I received advice, support, and suggestions for improving the book from numerous colleagues, friends, and relatives: J. Andreou, MD, PhD, L. Berlin, MD, I. Chrysikopoulos, MSc, MBA (my brother), S. Chrysikopoulos, MD (my father), D.A. Goussis, PhD, R. Hayek, CBF, A. Karantanas, MD, PhD, P.S.O. Kostopoulou, PhD, I. Nikolacopoulos, MSc, P. Moskowitz, MD, N. Pandis, DDS, MS, MSc, PhD, and A. Vlachos, MD. Drs. J. Andreou, L. Berlin, and A. Karantanas were very generous with their time, they read the entire manuscript, and provided valuable feedback. Mr. J. Nicolakopoulos and Dr. N. Pandis read part of the manuscript and gave me the perspective of a non-medical professional. I would like to thank members of the Springer team for a smooth collaboration, producing a textbook of high standards: A. Cerri, C Parravicini, Beauty Christobel Gunasekaran and Rajesh Gopalakrishnan. Finally, I am grateful to my wife Konstantina and my son Spyros for their unconditional love and support.

Contents

Introduction

I did my diagnostic radiology training at a major University Medical Center and I was taught by brilliant teachers. However, I did not receive any formal training about errors in radiology. As a resident, I assumed that I would mature into a competent radiologist just by gaining more *"experience."* I thought that I could easily cover any gaps, improve my skills and knowledge on my own. All I had to do is read a lot of radiology books, read a lot of journals, and "log" a lot of cases at work [1]. However, the maturation process was not as smooth as I had expected, even though I was well prepared to work without supervision. I had decided to limit my practice to CT and MRI, which were my favorite imaging modalities. My first job was in a private hospital, monitoring and reading all CT and MR scans performed in my shift. I was very lucky to receive additional training at that time. My mentor was Dr. J. Andreou, a senior radiologist, who spent considerable time with me every workday for 6 months. Together we would review all the cases I had seen and all the reports I had generated. During our sessions, I was immersed in the daily routine of a very effective consultant [2–4]. He moderated my obsession with accuracy, and he showed me that *radiology is inherently imprecise*; thus, it can be regarded as both an art and a science [5]. Fortunately, even the subjective and abstract concepts of radiology have been demystified and can be taught to a large extent [6]. My mentor emphasized two major paradigms: (a) *radiologists cannot work in a vacuum*, but our diagnostic process and our report should *support* and should *be supported* by the *clinical context* and (b) *excellence in radiology* requires *commitment* to *diligent practice*. One of his favorite quotes is quite relevant to the subject of this manuscript: "If you are *wrong* about a case *once*, you will keep *repeating* the *same mistake over and over*, unless you *question* and *examine* your *assumptions, biases,* and *mental processes*. Always *seek verification* for your diagnoses."

Thus, early on in my career I became very *conscious* of *radiology errors* and I got into the *habit* of asking my clinical colleagues for the *final diagnosis* and *feedback* [7]. Thus, I was forced to *confront* my *mistakes* and their *mechanisms*. My career took a winding path in both the private and public sector. The bulk of my practice has been CT and MRI, supplemented by a small load of plain radiographs and simple interventional procedures. This type of practice has given me the luxury of "quasi" sub-specialization. I have worked in a group setting for about 10 years, and I have worked all by myself for more than 15 years. I have had the opportunity to interpret and review initial and follow-up CT and MR studies of multiple patients with chronic diseases and various malignancies. Some of these studies were performed at other institutions, giving me the privilege to study the approach and methodology of other radiologists. I have unofficially taught trainees in radiology and other medical specialties. I have been asked to reexamine and revise reports of mine and I have been asked to consult in complex and difficult cases. Thus, over the years I have encountered all possible medical, surgical, and radiological errors and complications, and I have learned handsomely from them.

However, even to this date, I encounter challenging cases almost every day. Furthermore, every single day I realize how easy it is for a fault to intrude in my work.

Thus, 5 years ago I started a literature search for new and advanced concepts on this topic, in order to incorporate them in my practice. I was surprised to find out how much progress has been made, and this excitement motivated me to write this report.

My *purpose* was to construct a *simplified*, yet *thorough* and *concise guide* on the *nature* and *management* of *errors in imaging*. I felt that the inclusion of *personal* views would add value to this work. Specific proposals for learning and teaching are anchored in the literature and in my personal experience. My *focus* and my *interest* is on the *radiologists*. I do not discuss ancillary methods such as computer-aided detection, machine learning, or other techniques that are under investigation. System errors, substandard imaging procedures, and medicolegal implications are also beyond the scope of this manuscript [8–60].

In the concluding remarks, I argue for the need to permanently reduce errors through an *upgrade* of our *education*.

After the main text, you will find a pictorial essay of a variety of errors, blind spots, and diagnostic dilemmas that I have encountered over the years.

The list of references is lengthy, given the importance and complexity of this subject.

This manuscript was initially intended for radiology residents. However, while writing it, I felt compelled to include material that I thought would be useful for fellows and certified radiologists.

Corfu, Greece   Haris Chrysikopoulos

Abstract

Visual assessment proceeds simultaneously at two levels: a rapid overview of the entire image as a unit, and a slow deliberate scrutiny of selected parts of the image. Our visual behavior is intertwined with our cognitive labor of data analysis and data synthesis, and is supported by our experience and fund of knowledge. Our attention is easily drawn to any obvious patterns and any obvious isolated findings. At the same time we can direct our gaze and attention to specific parts of the image, at will, depending on the clinical question, the patient's history, and any obvious imaging findings. Biases and errors, such as inattentional blindness, hinder our ability to evaluate the image objectively and thus we may not "pick up" a crucial or a pertinent finding.

1.1 Overview

A briefing on the visual and cognitive processing of medical images will enhance our understanding of errors and biases. The consensus is that most errors in imaging are due to faulty perception [1–11]. Thus this topic is of extreme importance to all medical professionals. Both central and peripheral vision play an important role, as experienced observers can detect most lesions within a very short time allowance [12–20].

The initial, ultra rapid response has been called the "gestalt" or "holistic" or nonselective pathway [19, 20]. It relies on recognition of "global" patterns or templates, accumulated in one's memory during training and professional practice.

Subsequently, selected parts of the image are scrutinized at will, engaging the high resolution foveal apparatus. This slower, deliberate action or selective pathway is used to:

(a) Confirm or analyze preliminary or definite findings respectively [19, 20], and
(b) Identify subtle lesions that were not flagged in the "gestalt" phase.

At the same time, the "gestalt" absorption of information continues to operate in the background, in parallel to the selective mode.

Fixation occurs when the foveal vision captures a target, in order to initiate conscious, focused scrutiny of this finding. The fast eye movements between fixations are called saccades. Because of their rapidity, saccades do not generate useful information [12].

1.2 Research Studies: Results

Numerous studies conducted on novices and experts have unraveled their visual search behavior and have quantified their diagnostic performance [13, 19–30]. Pulmonary nodules, native

© Springer Nature Switzerland AG 2020
H. Chryssikopoulos, *Errors in Imaging*, https://doi.org/10.1007/978-3-030-21103-5_1

and artificial, have served as the favorite experimental model of investigators.

Most of these studies have yielded similar data and have reached similar conclusions:

(a) The experts identify the abnormality faster, spending fewer saccades and fewer fixations.
(b) The experts cover a smaller surface area of the image with their central (foveal) vision.
(c) The abnormality may not get reported, even if it is detected. Kundel et al. have marked three types of visual perception errors [30]:
    • Search failure: the finding remains outside the central visual field, presumably due to incomplete coverage of the image
    • Recognition failure: foveal fixation lasts less than a minimum time threshold, so that the target remains "hidden" from our attention
    • Decision error: the observer detects the lesion, but proceeds to dismiss it, thinking that it is either a normal finding or it is not significant.
(d) Perceptual and cognitive skills do not progress in tandem or at the same pace [22, 31, 32].

1.3   Research Studies vs. Real Life

Most of these studies share a common limitation: they focus on perceptual skills and ignore cognitive algorithms, creating thus an artificial set up that I call "passive search." The design of these research projects revolves around a single objective, stripped off any clinical context, such as looking for lung nodules, for the sake of detecting as many as possible. This task contrasts with the mental algorithm of experts that I call "active search." This model of experts requires integration of the imaging findings with the knowledge of disease dynamics, via analysis and synthesis [4, 33–37].

Analysis and synthesis are cognitive skills that allow us to extract vital information from the images, establish relevance to the clinical ques-

tion, and chunk them in the appropriate order. The desired result is a valid differential diagnostic list and a solid recommendation for patient management [4, 33–37].

Visual perception and visual behavior are directly influenced by knowledge and cognition, forming a virtuous feedback cycle. After multiple upgrades of this loop we achieve expertise in our domain. The expert can move easily to and fro, between observation targets, knowledge fund, data analysis, and data synthesis [36, 37].

Let's look at two examples that underscore the importance of knowing what to look for, and where to look for it:

(a) In a case of acute, fulminant otomastoiditis in a child, the expert will quickly pay close attention to the dural sinuses to determine patency or thrombosis.
(b) In a case of chronic otomastoiditis in a middle-aged individual, the expert will examine carefully the nasopharynx for an occult or obvious malignancy that obstructs the eustachian tube. If a tumor is found, the next step is to evaluate if there is extension beyond the narrow confines of the nasopharynx. Thus, the expert directs his[1] attention to the appropriate sites, utilizing his detailed knowledge of head–neck anatomy, and his knowledge of the modes and sites (local and distal) of spread of the various nasopharyngeal tumors.

So far, few investigators have tried to decipher the links between perception, knowledge, and cognitive skills [26, 27, 33, 35, 37]. Thus, we still have a lot to learn about the interrelationships of these functions. In subsequent chapters we will elaborate further on cognitive dexterities that are vital for successful imaging interpretation.

---

[1] The male gender is used generically and includes the female gender.

1.4 Inattentional Blindness

This chapter would not be complete if we did not talk about the phenomenon of inattentional blindness, which is a special case of bias/error in visual perception [38–40]. An observer fails to notice a plainly visible object or finding, because he does not anticipate its presence, and at the same time, his attention is saturated with another task or another finding. Since we cannot focus our attention on multiple tasks simultaneously, *unexpected* findings tend to remain outside our field of visual awareness. Thus we "see" only what we are looking for. I believe that this phenomenon contributes to the power of several biases. Biases act as mental and visual blinders that misdirect our attention and distort our ability to interpret objectively the imaging data in front of us. Biases are discussed in detail in Chap. 5.

References

1. Waite S, Scott J, Gale B, Fuchs T, Kolla S, Reede D. Interpretive error in radiology. AJR. 2017;208:739–49.
2. Bui-Mansfield LT. "Fool me twice": delayed diagnoses in radiology with emphasis on perpetuated errors. Video lecture. https://learning.arrs.org/course/view.php?id=518. Accessed 19 Nov 2017.
3. Rosenkrantz AB, Bansal NK. Diagnostic errors in abdominopelvic CT interpretation: characterization based on report addenda. Abdom Radiol. 2016;41:1793–9.
4. Kabadi SJ, Krishmaraj A. Strategies for improving the value of the radiology report: a retrospective analysis of errors in formally over-read studies. J Am Coll Radiol. 2017;14:459–66.
5. Bruno MA, Walker EA, Abujudeh HH. Understanding and confronting our mistakes: the epidemiology of error in radiology and strategies for error reduction. Radiographics. 2015;35:1668–76.
6. Berlin L. Radiologic errors, past, present and future. Diagnosis. 2014;1:79–84.
7. Kim YW, Mansfield LT. Fool me twice: delayed diagnoses in radiology with emphasis on perpetuated errors. AJR. 2014;202:465–70.
8. McCreadie G, Oliver TB. Eight CT lessons that we learned the hard way: an analysis of current patterns of radiological error and discrepancy with particular emphasis on CT. Clin Radiol. 2009;64:491–9.
9. Donald JJ, Barnard SA. Common patterns in 558 diagnostic radiology errors. J Med Imaging Radiat Oncol. 2012;56:173–8.
10. Funaki B, Szymski G, Rosenblum J. Significant on-call misses by radiology residents interpreting computed tomographic studies: perception versus cognition. Emerg Radiol. 1997;4:290–4.
11. Renfrew DL, Franken EA Jr, Berbaum KS, Weigelt FH, Abu-Yousef MM. Error in radiology: classification and lessons in 182 cases presented at a problem case conference. Radiology. 1992;183:145–50.
12. Kundel HL, Nodine CF. Interpreting chest radiographs without visual search. Radiology. 1975;116:527–32.
13. Kundel HL, Nodine CF, Conant EF, Weinstein SP. Holistic component of image perception in mammogram interpretation: gaze tracking study. Radiology. 2007;242:396–402.
14. Kundel HL, Nodine CF, Krupinski EA, Mello-Thoms C. Using gaze-tracking data and mixture distribution analysis to support a holistic model for the detection of cancers on mammograms. Acad Radiol. 2008;15:881–6.
15. Oestmann JW, Greene R, Bourgouin PM, Linetsky L, Llewellyn HJ. Chest "gestalt" and detectability of lung lesions. Eur J Radiol. 1993;16:154–7.
16. Oestmann JW, Greene R, Kushner DC, Bourgouin PM, Linetsky L, Llewellyn HJ. Lung lesions: correlation between viewing time and detection. Radiology. 1988;166:451–3.
17. Toms A. Shades of grey: perception and performance in radiology. The Royal College of Radiologists continued professional development library-public lectures. Date of lecture: 4 November 2015. https://videos.rcr.ac.uk/videoPlayer/?vid=384&class=video ThumbOdd. Accessed 15 Sept 2016.
18. Drew T, Evans K, Vo ML, Jacobson FL, Wolfe JM. Informatics in radiology: what can you see in a single glance and how this might guide visual search in medical images? Radiographics. 2013;33:263–74.
19. Kundel HL. Visual search and lung nodule detection on CT scans. Radiology. 2015;274:14–6.
20. Sheridan H, Reingold EM. The holistic processing account of visual expertise in medical image perception: a review. Front Psychol. 2017;8:1620. https://doi.org/10.3389/fpsyg.2017.01620.
21. Kok EM, Jarodzka H, de Bruin ABH, BinAmir HAN, Robben SGF, van Merrienboer JJG. Systematic viewing in radiology: seeing more, missing less? Adv Health Sci Educ Theory Pract. 2016;21:189–205.
22. Kelly BS, Rainford LA, Darcy SP, Kavanagh EC, Toomey RJ. The development of expertise in radiology: in chest radiograph interpretation, "expert" search pattern may predate "expert" levels of diagnostic accuracy for pneumothorax identification. Radiology. 2016;280:252–60.
23. Rubin GD, Roos JE, Tall M, et al. Characterizing search, recognition and decision in the detection of

lung nodules on CT scans: elucidation with eye track-ing. Radiology. 2015;274:276–86.

24. Drew T, Vo MLH, Olwal A, Jacobson F, Seltzer SS. Scanners and drillers: characterizing expert visual search through volumetric images. J Vis. 2013;13:1–13.

25. Wood G, Knapp KM, Rock B, Cousens C, Roobottom C, Wilson MR. Visual expertise in detecting and diagnosing skeletal fractures. Skelet Radiol. 2013;42:165–72.

26. Bertram R, Helle L, Kaakinene JK, Svedstrom E. The effect of expertise on eye movement behavior in medical image perception. PLoS One. 2013;8:e66169. https://doi.org/10.1371/journal.pone.0066169.

27. Matsumoto H, Terao Y, Yugeta A, et al. Where do neurologists look when viewing brain CT images? An eye-tracking study involving stroke cases. PLoS One. 2011;6:e28928. https://doi.org/10.1371/journal.pone.0028928.

28. Manning DJ, Barker-Mill SC, Donovan T, Crawford T. Time-dependent observer errors in pulmonary nodule detection. Br J Radiol. 2006;79:342–6.

29. Manning D, Ethell S, Donovan T, Crawford T. How do radiologists do it? The influence of experience and training on searching for chest nodules. Radiography. 2006;12:134–42.

30. Kundel HL, Nodine CF, Carmody D. Visual scanning, pattern recognition and decision-making in pulmonary nodule detection. Investig Radiol. 1987;13:175–81.

31. Norman GR, Coblentz CL, Brooks LR, Badcook CJ. Expertise in visual diagnosis: a review of the lit-erature. Acad Med. 1992;67:S78–83.

32. Brazeau-Lamontagne L, Charlin B, Gagnon R, Samson L, van der Vleuten C. Measurement of per-ception and interpretation skills during radiology training: utility of the script concordance approach. Med Teach. 2004;26:326–32.

33. Van Meeuwen LW, Jarodzka H, Brand-Gruwel S, Kirschner PA, de Bock JJPR, van Merrienboer JJG. Identification of effective visual problem solv-ing strategies in a complex visual domain. Learn Instr. 2014;32:10–21.

34. van der Gijp A, Ravesloot CJ, Jarodzka H, et al. How visual search relates to visual diagnostic performance: a narrative systematic review of eye-tracking research in radiology. Adv Health Sci Educ Theory Pract. 2017;22:765–87.

35. van der Gijp A, van der Schaaf MF, van der Schaaf IC, et al. Interpretation of radiological images: towards a framework of knowledge and skills. Adv Health Sci Educ Theory Pract. 2014;19:565–80.

36. Chrysikopoulos H. Basics of MR examinations and interpretation. In: Clinical MR imaging and physics: a tutorial. Heidelberg: Springer; 2009. p. 109–64.

37. Morita J, Miwa K, Kitasaka T, et al. Interactions of perceptual and conceptual processing: expertise in medical image diagnosis. Int J Human-Comput Stud. 2008;66:370–90.

38. Wolfe JM, Evans KK, Drew T, Aizenman A, Josephs E. How do radiologists use the human search engine? Radiat Prot Dosim. 2016;169:24–31.

39. Drew T, Vo ML, Wolfe JM. The invisible gorilla strikes again: sustained inattentional blindness in expert observers. Psychol Sci. 2013;24:1848–53.

40. Simons DJ, Chabris CF. Gorillas in our midst: sus-tained inattentional blindness for dynamic events. Perception. 1999;28:1059–74.

Abstract

Complex tasks laden with uncertainty predispose to errors and discordant opinions. Thus inter- and intra-reader disagreements reflect in part the inherent difficulty in interpreting medical images, especially if we cannot obtain confirmation of the diagnosis. So we need a working definition of errors in imaging. An error is a missed diagnosis, an inaccurate or incomplete diagnosis, the omission to specify follow-up imaging or additional studies, a suboptimal report, an unacceptable delay in delivering the report to the referring physician, or failure to communicate directly with the referring physician regarding emergencies, and other significant findings (whether urgent or not). The estimated error rate in radiology is 5–30%. Different types of errors may occur simultaneously, and some errors may be propagated for up to several years, before they get discovered. Errors potentially may have devastating consequences both for the patients and the physician who made the error, and thus safety protocols have been proposed and implemented to minimize the occurrence and the adverse impact of errors.

2.1 Errors and Discrepancies: Definition

Our clinical colleagues expect an accurate, informative, and organized report that answers their question(s) in a clear manner, within an acceptable time frame [1–4].

Decoding and translating the imaging findings into a verbal or written report is a complex task, each step of which is susceptible to a variety of pitfalls [5–12].

Thus, it is natural that different radiologists may render different interpretations for the same imaging study [7, 8]. In some cases we cannot ascertain which opinion is correct [7, 8]. In other cases, to our surprise, it turns out that the expert's opinion is incorrect [13].

Thus it is important to keep in mind the following facts:

1. Errors definitely occur, and as humans we cannot escape them [7, 8, 14, 15]. However, with the proper training and in a supportive work environment, errors can be contained to a large extent.
2. Different opinions are not always due to errors; in these instances it is more appropriate to use the terms "discrepancies" or "discordant opinions," instead of "errors" [7, 8, 16].
3. The experts cannot always serve as the "golden standard" or as the absolute "truth" [13].
4. An error does not always constitute negligence or malpractice [8, 17]. Berlin states that "negligence occurs … when the degree of error exceeds an accepted norm, [ie.] the usual and customary standards of the radiology profession" [18–21].

Table 2.1 Definition of errors in imaging

An error in imaging may be
  • A missed diagnosis
  • An inaccurate or an incomplete diagnosis
  • An omission to specify follow-up or additional studies
  • A suboptimal report (poor, vague, or inappropriate wording, not answering the clinical question, not including incidentalomas or nonpertinent, yet significant findings)
  • An unacceptable delay delivering the report or delayed communication with the referring physician regarding significant findings, whether emergent, urgent or not

So, what is an error in imaging? The answer is presented in Table 2.1.

2.2 Error and Discrepancy Rates

Multiple studies, over several decades, have documented an unexpected, high rate of errors and discrepancies. Even experienced academic radiologists, working in their area of expertise, are vulnerable to major errors [1, 7, 8, 10–13, 22–62].

One study analyzed 469 gynecologic MRIs submitted for reinterpretation at a busy oncology center [13]. These examinations had been performed and read initially at academic tertiary referral centers, community (private) hospitals, or outpatient imaging services. Histopathology or adequate imaging follow-up served as the gold standard. The second opinion of subspecialized radiologists was *not* correct in 17% of the cases, and these errors would have weighed adversely on patient management.

In another study, Abujudeh et al. asked experienced abdominal radiologists to reinterpret, in a blinded fashion, abdominal and pelvic CT scans, initially read by the same or by another radiologist. Regarding clinically significant findings and recommendations the inter- and intra-observer discrepancy rates were 26% and 32% respectively [60]. How can we reconcile such variations? Bruno reminds us that divergence in opinion "… is not in itself proof that one or another radiologist has made an interpretive error; to the contrary, it merely illustrates the degree to which high levels of uncertainty and inherent variability… limits the conclusions of imaging tests" [15].

Even plain radiographs, which provide a low level of information compared to CT, can pose significant challenges [63]. Robinson et al. recruited consultants to evaluate chest, abdominal, and skeletal radiographs in a simple, binary fashion (yes or no): are significant abnormalities present or absent? The interobserver disagreement varied from 8% to 19% [61].

Another study relied on autopsy data to quantify the association of diagnostic errors with deaths of hospitalized patients [49]. The study correlated imaging studies with 112 clinical and/or radiologic errors (which were not specified). The radiologist either initiated the diagnostic error or propagated the erroneous clinical diagnosis in 12 (11%) and 37 (33%) cases respectively. In 29 instances (26%) the radiologist was ignored, even though he provided the correct diagnosis, contrary to clinical opinion. In 24 cases (21%) the radiologist explicitly considered the correct diagnosis, but imaging failed to demonstrate the anticipated finding(s); thus these cases were attributed to limitations of the employed imaging modality.[1]

Furthermore, *different* types of *errors* can occur *simultaneously*, and some faults have a tendency to *recur* [23, 27, 51, 64, 65]. In one paper, the authors collected 656 imaging examinations (cases) that carried a total of 1269 errors [27]. In 196 cases (30% of the examinations) the errors were *propagated* in subsequent radiologic investigations. The result was a *delay* in establishing the correct diagnosis, ranging from 0 days to 12.6 years (the average delay was 251 days).[2]

---

[1]The numbers and percentages in the paper do not add up to 100%, due to typing error?

[2]I note the following limitations of this study:

1. Illustrations of recurrent/repeated mistakes were not provided,
2. No information was given about:

(a) The number of studies performed before the final diagnosis
(b) The reason(s) the patients underwent additional or follow-up imaging, and

It is difficult to determine with certainty the true error and discrepancy rates in medical imaging, despite a plethora of information in the literature. Most relevant studies lack proof of diagnosis or a gold standard, they disclose only partial data, or they are fraught with biases that lead to under- or over-estimation of the true rates [27, 49, 66]. The overall major[3] error rate, including normal and abnormal studies, is estimated at 5% [67]. However, if we exclude the normal studies, then the error rate escalates to about 30% [25]. Bruno has estimated that every single day, every radiologist commits three to four diagnostic errors [15].

2.3 Potential Impact of Errors on Patients and Imaging Professionals

The approximate annual worldwide radiologic load is 1 billion imaging studies [25]. Currently we cannot quantify the contribution of radiologists to the ultimate decisions on patient management; however, it is safe to assume that it is *significant*. Recent reports have highlighted the detrimental impact of radiological and all other medical errors on patient outcome [25, 28, 68].

Errors should not be taken lightly, regardless of their effect on the course of the patient [43–46]. The physician responsible for the error may feel *guilt* and *shame* with erosion of his[4] confidence and self-esteem. *Tension* may develop between him and referring physicians, other colleagues, administration, and other personnel. A *malpractice claim* may have *unpredictable consequences* on his *emotional* and *professional stability* [14, 69–72].

(c) How the radiologist reached the correct diagnosis? (Was it because of the use of contrast medium, difference in technique, higher quality of the study, and interval enlargement of the lesion, or was it because of another reason?)

[3]Clinically significant errors: altering patient management and outcome.

[4]The male gender is used generically and it includes the female gender.

Thus, it is in our best interest to study in depth the properties of errors. Fortunately, safety protocols have been devised that can suppress significantly and consistently the occurrence of all types of errors. *Routine implementation* of *safety algorithms* is necessary to *protect* both the *patients* and *ourselves* [11, 12, 73, 74].

References

1. Kabadi SJ, Krishmaraj A. Strategies for improving the value of the radiology report: a retrospective analysis of errors in formally over-read studies. J Am Coll Radiol. 2017;14:459–66.
2. Gunderman RB. The true purpose of a radiology report. J Am Coll Radiol. 2018;15:1450.
3. Eberhardt SC, Heilbrun ME. Radiology report value equation. Radiographics. 2018;38:1888–96.
4. Ware JB, Saurabh J, Hoang JK, Baker S, Wruble J. Effective radiology reporting. J Am Coll Radiol. 2017;14:838–9.
5. Wolfe JM, Evans KK, Drew T, Aizenman A, Josephs E. How do radiologists use the human search engine? Radiat Prot Dosim. 2016;169:24–31.
6. Newman-Toker D. A unified conceptual model for diagnostic errors: underdiagnosis, overdiagnosis, and misdiagnosis. Diagnosis. 2014;1:43–8.
7. Brady AP. Error and discrepancy in radiology: inevitable or avoidable? Insights Imaging. 2017;8:171–82.
8. Brady A, Laoide RO, McCarthy P, McDermott R. Discrepancy and error in radiology: concepts, causes and consequences. Ulster Med J. 2012;81:3–9.
9. Sabih DE, Sabih A, Sabih Q, Khan AN. Image perception and interpretation of abnormalities; can we believe our eyes? Can we do something about it? Insights Imaging. 2011;2:47–55.
10. Pinto A, Brunese L. Spectrum of diagnostic errors in radiology. World J Radiol. 2010;2:377–83.
11. Fitzgerald R. Radiological error: analysis, standard setting, targeted instruction and teamworking. Eur Radiol. 2005;15:1760–7.
12. Fitzgerald R. Error in radiology. Clin Radiol. 2001;56:938–46.
13. Lakhman Y, D'Anastasi M, Micco M, et al. Second-opinion interpretations of gynecologic oncologic MRI examinations by sub-specialized radiologists influence patient care. Eur Radiol. 2016;26:2089–98.
14. Bruno MA. Our mistakes-the human experience. Video lecture. https://learning.arrs.org/mod/url/view.php?id=400. Accessed 22 Nov 2016.
15. Bruno MA. 256 shades of gray: uncertainty and diagnostic error in radiology. Diagnosis. 2017;4:149–57.
16. Robinson PJ. Radiology's Achilles' heel: error and variation in the interpretation of the Roentgen image. Br J Radiol. 1997;70:1085–98.

17. Berlin L. Medicolegal-malpractice and ethical issues in radiology. Role of the expert witness. AJR. 2015;204:W371.
18. Berlin L. Defending the "missed" radiographic diagnosis. AJR. 2001;176:317–22.
19. Berlin L. Radiologic errors and malpractice: a blurry distinction. AJR. 2007;189:517–22.
20. Berlin L. Malpractice issues in radiology. Perceptual errors. AJR. 1996;167:587–90.
21. Berlin L, Hendrix RW. Perceptual errors and negligence. AJR. 1998;170:863–7.
22. Waite S, Scott J, Gale B, Fuchs T, Kolla S, Reede D. Interpretive error in radiology. AJR. 2017;208:739–49.
23. Bui-Mansfield LT. "Fool me twice": delayed diagnoses in radiology with emphasis on perpetuated errors. Video lecture. https://learning.arrs.org/course/view.php?id=518. Accessed 19 Nov 2017.
24. Rosenkrantz AB, Bansal NK. Diagnostic errors in abdominopelvic CT interpretation: characterization based on report addenda. Abdom Radiol. 2016;41:1793–9.
25. Bruno MA, Walker EA, Abujudeh HH. Understanding and confronting our mistakes: the epidemiology of error in radiology and strategies for error reduction. Radiographics. 2015;35:1668–76.
26. Berlin L. Radiologic errors, past, present and future. Diagnosis. 2014;1:79–84.
27. Kim YW, Mansfield LT. Fool me twice: delayed diagnoses in radiology with emphasis on perpetuated errors. AJR. 2014;202:465–70.
28. McCreadie G, Oliver TB. Eight CT lessons that we learned the hard way: an analysis of current patterns of radiological error and discrepancy with particular emphasis on CT. Clin Radiol. 2009;64:491–9.
29. Donald JJ, Barnard SA. Common patterns in 558 diagnostic radiology errors. J Med Imaging Radiat Oncol. 2012;56:173–8.
30. Funaki B, Szymski G, Rosenblum J. Significant on-call misses by radiology residents interpreting computed tomographic studies: perception versus cognition. Emerg Radiol. 1997;4:290–4.
31. Renfrew DL, Franken EA Jr, Berbaum KS, Weigelt FH, Abu-Yousef MM. Error in radiology: classification and lessons in 182 cases presented at a problem case conference. Radiology. 1992;183:145–50.
32. Wakeley CJ, Jones AM, Kabala JE, Prince D, Goddard PR. Audit of the value of double reading magnetic resonance imaging films. Br J Radiol. 1995;68:358–60.
33. Pinto A, Scuderi MG, Daniele S. Errors in radiology: definition and classification. In: Romano L, Pinto A, editors. Errors in radiology. Heidelberg: Springer; 2012. p. 1–7.
34. Bechtold RE, Chen MY, Ott DJ, Zagoria RJ, Scharling ES, Wolfman NT, Vining DJ. Interpretation of abdominal CT: analysis of errors and their causes. J Comput Assist Tomogr. 1997;21:681–5.
35. Loevner LA, Sonners AI, Schulman BJ, et al. Reinterpretation of cross-sectional images in patients with head and neck cancer in the setting of a multidisciplinary cancer center. AJNR. 2002;23:1622–6.
36. Owens EJ, Taylor NR, Howlett DC. Perceptual type error in everyday practice. Clin Radiol. 2016;71:593–601.
37. Li F, Sone S, Abe H, MacMahon H, Armato SG 3rd, Doi K. Lung cancers missed at low-dose helical CT screening in a general population: comparison of clinical, histopathologic, and imaging findings. Radiology. 2002;225:673–83.
38. Del Ciello A, Franchi P, Contegiacomo A, Cicchetti G, Bonomo L, Larici AR. Missed lung cancer: when, where and why? Diagn Interv Radiol. 2017;23:118–26.
39. Lauritzen PM, Stavem K, Andersen JG, et al. Double reading of current chest CT examinations: clinical importance of changes to radiology reports. Eur J Radiol. 2016;85:199–204.
40. Lauritzen PM, Andersen JG, Stokke MV, et al. Radiologist-initiated double reading of abdominal CT: retrospective analysis of the clinical importance of changes to radiology reports. BMJ Qual Saf. 2016;25:595–603.
41. Bisset GS III, Crowe J. Diagnostic errors in interpretation of pediatric musculoskeletal radiographs at common injury sites. Pediatr Radiol. 2014;44:552–7.
42. Driscoll DO, Halpenny D, Guiney M. Radiological error–an early assessment of departmental radiology discrepancy meetings. Ir Med J. 2012;105:172–4.
43. Gollub MJ, Panicek DM, Bach AM, Penalver A, Castellino RA. Clinical importance of reinterpretation of body CT scans obtained elsewhere in patients referred for care at a tertiary cancer center. Radiology. 1999;210:109–12.
44. Yoon LS, Haims AH, Brink JA, Rabinovici R, Forman HP. Evaluation of an emergency radiology quality assurance program at a level 1 trauma centre: abdominal and pelvic CT studies. Radiology. 2002;224:42–6.
45. Tilleman EHBM, Phoa SSKS, van Delden OM, et al. Reinterpretation of radiological imaging in patients referred to a tertiary referral centre with a suspected pancreatic or hepatobiliary malignancy: impact on treatment strategy. Eur Radiol. 2003;13:1095–9.
46. Carney E, Kempf J, DeCarvallho V, Yudd A, Nosher J. Preliminary interpretations of after-hours CT and sonography by radiology residents versus final interpretations by body imaging radiologists at a level 1 trauma center. AJR. 2003;181:367–73.
47. Queckel LG, Kessels AG, Goei R, van Engelshoven JM. Miss rate of lung cancer in the chest radiograph in clinical practice. Chest. 1999;115:720–4.
48. Siegle RL, Baram EM, Reuter SR, Clarke EA, Lancaster JL, McMahan CA. Rates of disagreement in imaging interpretation in a group of community hospitals. Acad Radiol. 1998;5:148–54.
49. Heriot GS, McKelvie P, Pitman AG. Diagnostic errors in patients dying in hospital: radiology's contribution. J Med Imaging Radiat Oncol. 2009;53:188–93.

50. Berlin L. Accuracy of diagnostic procedures: has it improved over the past five decades? AJR. 2007;188:1173–8.

51. Forrest JV, Friedman PJ. Radiologic errors in patients with lung cancer. West J Med. 1981;134:485–90.

52. White CS, Salis AL, Meyer CA. Missed lung cancer on chest radiography and computed tomography: imaging and medicolegal issues. J Thorac Imaging. 1999;14:63–8.

53. Chesebro AL, Winkler NS, Birdwell RL, Giess CS. Developing asymmetries at mammography: a multimodality approach to assessment and management. Radiographics. 2016;36:322–34.

54. Wadha A, Sullivan JR, Gonyo MB. Missed breast cancer: what can we learn? Curr Probl Diagn Radiol. 2016;45:402–19.

55. Korhonen KE, Weinstein SP, McDonald ES, Conant EF. Strategies to increase cancer detection: review of true-positive and false-negative results at digital breast tomosynthesis screening. Radiographics. 2016;36:1954–65.

56. Palazzetti V, Guidi F, Ottaviani L, Valeri G, Baldassarre S, Giusepetti GM. Analysis of mammographic diagnostic errors in breast clinics. Radiol Med. 2016;121:828–33.

57. Giess CS, Frost EP, Birdwell RL. Interpreting one-view mammographic findings: minimizing call-backs while maximizing cancer detection. Radiographics. 2014;34:928–40.

58. Gangi S, Fletcher JG, Nathan MA, et al. Time interval between abnormalities seen on CT and the clinical diagnosis of pancreatic cancer: retrospective review of CT scans obtained before diagnosis. AJR. 2004;182:897–903.

59. Garland LH. Studies on the accuracy of diagnostic procedures. Am J Roentgenol Radium Ther Nucl Med. 1959;82:25–38.

60. Abujudeh HH, Boland GW, Kaewlai R, et al. Abdominal and pelvic computed tomography (CT) interpretation: discrepancy rates among experienced radiologists. Eur Radiol. 2010;20:1952–7.

61. Robinson PJ, Wilson D, Coral A, Murphy A, Verow P. Variation between experienced observers in the interpretation of accident and emergency radiographs. Br J Radiol. 1999;72:323–30.

62. Babiarsz LS, Yousem DM. Quality control in neuroradiology: discrepancies in image interpretation among academic neuroradiologists. AJNR. 2012;33:969–80.

63. Eisenberg RL. Should "mature" radiologists be put out to pasture? Radiographics. 2016;36:937–8.

64. Lum TE, Fairbanks RJ, Pennington EC, Zwemer FL. Profiles in patient safety: misplaced femoral line guidewire and multiple failures to detect the foreign body on chest radiography. Acad Emerg Med. 2005;12:658–62.

65. Morgan B, Stephenson JA, Griffin Y. Minimising the impact of errors in the interpretation of CT images for surveillance and evaluation of therapy in cancer. Clin Radiol. 2016;71:1083–94.

66. Wu MZ, McInnes MD, Macdonald DB, Kielar AZ, Duigenan S. CT in adults: systematic review and meta-analysis of interpretation discrepancy rates. Radiology. 2014;270:717–35.

67. Graber ML. The incidence of diagnostic error in medicine. BMJ Qual Saf. 2013;22:ii21–7.

68. Makary MA, Daniel M. Medical error—the third leading cause of death in the US. BMJ. 2016;353:i2139.

69. Saber Tehrani AS, Lee HW, Mathews SC, et al. 25 year summary of US malpractice claims for diagnostic errors 1986-2010: an analysis from the National Practitioner Data Bank. BMJ Qual Saf. 2013;22:672–80.

70. Wu AW. Medical error: the second victim-the doctor who makes the mistake needs help too. BMJ. 2000;320:726–7.

71. Weiss PM. The second victim: effect of medical errors on providers. Grand rounds presentation at All Children's Hospital Johns Hopkins Medicine, recorded January 31, 2014.

72. Pratt S, Kenney L, Scott SD, Wu AW. How to develop a second victim support program: a toolkit for health care organizations. Jt Comm J Qual Patient Saf. 2012;38:235–40.

73. Gunderman RB, Nyce JM. The tyranny of accuracy in radiologic education. Radiology. 2002;222:297–300.

74. Brook OR, O'Connell AM, Thornton E, Eisenberg RL, Mendiratta-Lala M, Kruskal JB. Quality initiatives: anatomy and pathophysiology of errors occurring in clinical radiology practice. Radiographics. 2010;30:1401–10.

Abstract

The various errors can be assigned to misperception, misinterpretation, blind spots, omission, poor expression, delayed delivery of the report, or miscommunication with the referring physician. Failure to detect the abnormality is the most frequent error type. Misinterpretation of a finding leads to underdiagnosis or overdiagnosis. Blind spots are anatomic areas that do not usually flag our attention, becoming thus a convergence point for biases, perception errors, and judgment errors. Faults of omission occur (a) when we abandon our visual search before collecting all key, significant, or pertinent findings, (b) when we rush though the patient's prior imaging and prior reports, and (c) when we do not ask for assistance or verification when reading a case that challenges our comfort zone. The term "expression errors" means dictating a suboptimal report, a topic that is covered in great detail in Chap. 4. Verbal and timely communication with the referring physician is indicated for all significant findings, a topic also covered extensively in Chap. 4.

Table 3.1 Classification of errors in imaging according to the author

Types of errors in radiology
• Detection errors
• Interpretation errors
• Blind spots
• Omission errors
• Expression errors or errors formulating the report
• Errors communicating with the referring physician

are interconnected [8]. However, for the purposes of our discussion they will be treated as distinct and separate entities, presented in Table 3.1.

3.2 Detection Errors

These errors occur when we fail to perceive the abnormality. Most series report that they are the most common type of imaging error [2–4, 9–13]. In the literature we can find both qualitative and quantitative data on this class of errors; this way we can gain clarity on their nature and importance.

In a general hospital the most common unreported findings in CT and MR scans were, in descending order of frequency: enlarged lymph nodes, spine metastases, and renal carcinomas [14].

In another study, two authors analyzed 362 imaging studies (sonograms, CT, and MRI) submitted to an academic institution for a formal second opinion. Major discrepancies were noted in

3.1 Introduction

My classification of errors is shorter, compared to prior publications [1–7]. I segregate several important processes in our work, some of which

12.4% of the studies, and most of these discrepancies (64.4%) were due to perception errors [9].

Two other authors retrieved all addenda of reports of abdominopelvic CT scans performed in a university hospital over a period of approximately 7 years. The study material comprised 709 addenda that corrected 785 diagnostic errors. The most common reason (84.1% of the time) for modifying the initial report was to describe a finding that was overlooked in the initial reading [15].

Compared to plain radiographs, CT scans elicit a more complex visual response, which can also be monitored and recorded with a gaze tracking apparatus [16–19]. Such studies have shown that even experienced radiologists do not cover the entire volume of the lungs with their foveal vision in CT scans of the chest. The gaze volumes of multiple observers were quantified by two different teams [16, 17]. The results will surprise you: the average gaze volumes were 26.7% (range: 15–43%) and 69% (range 44–92%). The visual targets in one of these studies were solid, artificial, 5 mm lung nodules. They were embedded throughout the lung parenchyma, clearly separated from airways and blood vessels. Only 3 out of 13 participants recorded more than half of the nodules and the top performer detected 73% of them [16]. Another team measured the detectability of metastatic lung nodules by CT, using two different scan protocols. The nodule size varied from 1 to 18 mm (mean diameter 3.9 mm), and most of them (80%) were smaller than 5 mm. Double reading increased the sensitivity for nodule identification, for both scanning protocols: from 63% to 74% and from 64% to 79% [20].

If we turn these numbers upside down, we realize that even experienced radiologists miss a significant number of important findings.

Once a significant lesion escapes our attention, we are entirely dependent on luck or on the referring physician, to discover it within a short time frame [2]. The referring physician because of a strong conviction in his diagnosis may request a second reading from the same or from another radiologist. Alternatively, he[1] may opt for another type of imaging investigation, since our interpretation was nonproductive. If the ordering

physician questions our diagnosis, we should not let our pride get in the way; let's respect his reasoning and let's ask the question: "What if he is right?" Our ego has no business whatsoever in the care of patients [21, 22]. We should be thankful if we get another chance to intercept the lesion, possibly still early in its course. Another, less favorable scenario is that the patient deteriorates and returns for a repeat examination. This time the abnormality may show up clearly because of interval enlargement or because of dissemination [11, 23]. The worst-case scenario is that the patient suffers a major event before a correct diagnosis is made.

In any case, if we become aware of our mistake, we should turn this incident into an opportunity for learning [21, 23]. Let's retrieve the initial study and ask "Why was the lesion *not* appreciated the first time?" An honest answer should force us to commit to a safety mechanism.

I attribute many perception errors to

a. suboptimal training in errors, biases, and diagnostic algorithms,
b. incomplete visual coverage of the images or rushing through the study,
c. insufficient use of ancillary tools, such as multiplanar reconstructions (MPR) and maximum intensity projection (MIP) images.

An inexperienced reader "who does not know what to look for" and tries to "cover" an entire image with a few saccades is inviting perception, as well as other types of errors at an alarming frequency [5, 24].

3.3 Interpretation or Judgment Errors

These faults arise when we detect a finding, but we do not recognize its true nature [2, 4, 6, 25, 26]. There are two types of judgment errors:

1. A normal variant or an artifact is labeled as pathology, resulting in a false positive study (an example of overdiagnosis). In this case, there is a danger that unnecessary examinations or procedures are undertaken, possibly imposing risk to the patient.

[1]The male gender is used generically and it includes the female gender.

2. A true abnormal finding is misclassified into one of the below two outcomes:

   - It is dismissed as a normal variant or as not significant, producing the equivalent of a false negative study,
   - It is misplaced into another disease category or into another grade of clinical significance, resulting in under- or overdiagnosis. Examples include mislabeling a brochoalveolar lung carcinoma as pneumonia, or downstaging a case of disseminated ovarian carcinoma as confined within the pelvis. Overdiagnosis has not been studied adequately in radiology, usually showing up in the context of screening for malignancy [27–38]. Thus we will refer to overdiagnosis sporadically, as the situation calls for it.

3.4 Blind Spots

Blind spots are anatomic areas that we tend to overlook, unless we are primed by the request or by prior reports [11, 12, 39–46]. By extension, the term "blind spots" refers to missed lesions in these particular anatomic sites. I consider them not a pure type of error, but a mix of biases, misperception, and misjudgment. Each imaging study has its own unique signature of blind spots, which may be small in size or may be very obvious in retrospect. They may be missed in a "busy" image amidst a cluster of normal neighboring structures. For example, a lung nodule may "blend in" as a pulmonary vessel [41]. It may be difficult to discriminate lymph nodes or peritoneal implants from poorly opacified vessels or from unopacified, collapsed bowel loops [11, 42, 44]. Intracranial pathology, if symmetric, may "look normal" at first glance [8, 45, 46]. A vascular thrombus, an airway tumor, or a gastrointestinal mass may go unnoticed, if they represent incidental findings [11, 40, 41].

In my experience, the borders of tissues or organs and the interfaces between them are also "danger" areas. Focal lobulation of the surface of a kidney on a CT scan may betray an isodense carcinoma. Tracing carefully the wall of a bowel loop or the capsule of a solid abdominal organ may disclose focal discontinuity at the site of fistulization or traumatic rupture, respectively [47, 48]. Haziness of the para aortic fat in the abdomen may be an early sign of retroperitoneal fibrosis [49]. Focal nodularity or "bulging" of the interface between the mediastinum and the lung parenchyma may signal a pleural plaque or paracardiac lymphadenopathy [42]. Blurring of the cerebral grey-white junction in an epileptic patient may point to a focal cortical dysplasia [50]. Obscuration of the lentiform nucleus is a well-known sign of early ischemic cerebral infarction [51]. A thickened interface between the tracheal lumen and the great vessels of the aortic arch may be caused by a tracheal wall carcinoma [41]. I regard fat planes as very important "warning stations"; the thinner they are, the more attention they deserve [52]. For example, obliteration of the fat stripe between the pectoralis major and pectoralis minor muscles may be the only CT sign of recurrent breast carcinoma. The CT scout views may provide valuable information not included in the axial images [8, 14, 53–55]. Please keep in mind that we can render any lesion invisible by improper selection of window width and window level [45, 46].

The cranial, chest, and abdominopelvic blind spots in CT and MRI are presented in Table 3.2 [11, 12, 40–45].

Table 3.2 Blind spots in CT and MR imaging

Cranium	Chest	Abdomen–pelvis
Brainstem	Airways	Lung bases
Cerebral sulci	Lung	Pulmonary
Dural sinuses	parenchyma	arteries
Major arteries	Pleura	Stomach
Sella turcica	Lymph node	Biliary system
Suprasellar areas	stations	Pancreas
Parasellar areas	Heart	Small bowel
Cavernous sinuses	Vessels	Colon
Meckel caves	Chest wall[a]	Mesentery
Orbits	Thyroid	Kidneys
Clivus	Esophagus	Adrenal glands
Skull base	Upper	Arteries and
Nasopharynx	abdomen	veins
Parapharyngeal		Spine and
spaces		pelvic ring
		Soft tissues

[a]Bones, spinal canal, musculature, subcutaneous tissues, and breasts

3.5   Omission Errors

These mistakes usually occur: (a) when we do *not* allocate sufficient time to interpret the study, or to assess all available information about the patient, or (b) when we do *not* consult an expert or the literature for complex cases.

The result is that our interpretations and our reports turn out incomplete or erroneous.

1. *Omission to extract all the information* that is available in the imaging study [6]. Even the most humble radiologic image contains a wealth of information, and we are obligated to bring all of it to the surface [56]. How do we do that? It is very helpful to think of the question "what does the clinician need to know"? [9, 57–67]. Arriving at the answer requires several steps. First, we pick the major findings [68]. Subsequently we identify all pertinent positive and negative elements. Then we integrate all radiologic evidence with the clinical data in order to arrive at a single, specific diagnosis. If we cannot confidently achieve this result, we need to construct a short differential list, ranked in order of probability. Finally, we provide our recommendations. If the patient stands to benefit from further investigation (radiological or other type), we specify the indicated study. If it seems prudent to follow the lesion, we may opt repeating the imaging study after an appropriate time interval, and reconsider the situation at that time [6]. What follows is an example of a proper diagnostic approach to a kidney mass [69, 70]: let's assume that in an abdominal CT scan we see a kidney mass that turns out to be a malignancy. First, we determine its center of origin (renal parenchyma versus collecting system) and its growth vector. We measure its size, and we describe its borders, consistency (solid versus cystic, presence/absence of fat, calcium, necrosis, or hemorrhage), and contrast enhancement (pattern and intensity). We assess whether it breaches the renal capsule, and whether it infiltrates the pelvocalyceal system, renal sinus, peri/para renal fat, or adjacent structures. We look for preserved normal renal parenchyma, and how it behaves after intravenous contrast administration. We search for bland thrombus or tumor thrombus in the renal vein and vena cava. We look for local abnormal vascularity, i.e., is the tumor hypervascular? We search for pathologic lymph nodes and for metastatic disease, both in usual and uncommon sites. Synthesizing all of this information, we may attempt to predict tumor histology [69–71]. Finishing our report, we state which additional studies are indicated for full staging.

2. *Neglect to fully engage the patient's clinical and radiologic history.* By radiologic history, I mean prior imaging studies and/or prior imaging reports. Research has shown that proper consideration and proper utilization of the patient's clinical and radiologic profile are essential to generate a meaningful radiologic diagnosis [71–83]. Proper comparison with prior studies entails looking at the images, instead of just reading the reports. Sometimes we have to go back two or three prior studies spanning a few years or several years, in order to detect subtle changes, not apparent over a short time interval.

3. *Omission to consult an expert or resources in the literature.* We should seek assistance when confronted with a challenging or unfamiliar case [84, 85]. The need for consultation is compelling if we have not had formal subspecialty training. Fortunately, a wealth of educational material is available at our fingertips [86, 87] (www.rsna.org; www.arrs.org; https://radiopedia.org; www.ctisus.com; www.radsource.us; www.radiologyassistant.nl; www.radiologyeducation.com).

3.6   Errors Formulating the Report

With this term I mean the various errors that may occur when we commit on paper our findings, thoughts, diagnoses (or differential), and recommendations. A vague report without clear, concrete recommendations is not valuable. Thus the referring physician may have no choice but to order additional tests that are neither appropriate nor indicated. These type of errors are discussed in great detail in the next chapter, "The Radiology Report."

3.7 Errors Communicating with the Referring Physician

Delayed delivery of the report, or omission to contact directly the referring physician about emergencies or other significant findings constitute this type of errors, is also addressed in the next chapter, "The Radiology Report."

References

1. Brook OR, O'Connell AM, Thornton E, Eisenberg RL, Mendiratta-Lala M, Kruskal JB. Quality initiatives: anatomy and pathophysiology of errors occurring in clinical radiology practice. Radiographics. 2010;30:1401–10.
2. Bruno MA, Walker EA, Abujudeh HH. Understanding and confronting our mistakes: the epidemiology of error in radiology and strategies for error reduction. Radiographics. 2015;35:1668–76.
3. Kim YW, Mansfield LT. Fool me twice: delayed diagnoses in radiology with emphasis on perpetuated errors. AJR. 2014;202:465–70.
4. Renfrew DL, Franken EA Jr, Berbaum KS, Weigelt FH, Abu-Yousef MM. Error in radiology: classification and lessons in 182 cases presented at a problem case conference. Radiology. 1992;183:145–50.
5. Sabih DE, Sabih A, Sabih Q, Khan AN. Image perception and interpretation of abnormalities; can we believe our eyes? Can we do something about it? Insights Imaging. 2011;2:47–55.
6. Pinto A, Brunese L. Spectrum of diagnostic errors in radiology. World J Radiol. 2010;2:377–83.
7. Provenzale JM, Kranz PG. Understanding errors in diagnostic radiology: proposal of a classification scheme and application to emergency radiology. Emerg Radiol. 2011;18:403–8.
8. Chrysikopoulos H. Basics of MR examinations and interpretation. In: Clinical MR imaging and physics: a tutorial. Heidelberg: Springer; 2009. p. 109–64.
9. Kabadi SJ, Krishmaraj A. Strategies for improving the value of the radiology report: a retrospective analysis of errors in formally over-read studies. J Am Coll Radiol. 2017;14:459–66.
10. Berlin L. Radiologic errors, past, present and future. Diagnosis. 2014;1:79–84.
11. McCreadie G, Oliver TB. Eight CT lessons that we learned the hard way: an analysis of current patterns of radiological error and discrepancy with particular emphasis on CT. Clin Radiol. 2009;64:491–9.
12. Donald JJ, Barnard SA. Common patterns in 558 diagnostic radiology errors. J Med Imaging Radiat Oncol. 2012;56:173–8.
13. Funaki B, Szymski G, Rosenblum J. Significant on-call misses by radiology residents interpreting computed tomographic studies: perception versus cognition. Emerg Radiol. 1997;4:290–4.
14. Owens EJ, Taylor NR, Howlett DC. Perceptual type error in everyday practice. Clin Radiol. 2016;71:593–601.
15. Rosenkrantz AB, Bansal NK. Diagnostic errors in abdominopelvic CT interpretation: characterization based on report addenda. Abdom Radiol. 2016;41:1793–9.
16. Rubin GD, Roos JE, Tall M, et al. Characterizing search, recognition and decision in the detection of lung nodules on CT scans: elucidation with eye tracking. Radiology. 2015;274:276–86.
17. Drew T, Vo MLH, Olwal A, Jacobson F, Seltzer SS. Scanners and drillers: characterizing expert visual search through volumetric images. J Vis. 2013;13:1–13.
18. Bertram R, Helle L, Kaakinene JK, Svedstrom E. The effect of expertise on eye movement behavior in medical image perception. PLoS One. 2013;8:e66169. https://doi.org/10.1371/journal.pone.0066169.
19. Matsumoto H, Terao Y, Yugeta A, et al. Where do neurologists look when viewing brain CT images? An eye-tracking study involving stroke cases. PLoS One. 2011;6:e28928. https://doi.org/10.1371/journal.pone.0028928.
20. Wormans D, Ludwig K, Beyer F, Heidel W, Diederich S. Detection of pulmonary nodules at multirow-detector CT: effectiveness of double reading to improve sensitivity at standard-dose and low-dose chest CT. Eur Radiol. 2005;15:14–22.
21. Fitzgerald R. Radiological error: analysis, standard setting, targeted instruction and teamworking. Eur Radiol. 2005;15:1760–7.
22. Bruno MA. Primum non nocere: a few words on the primacy of patient safety. In: Abujudeh HH, Bruno MA, editors. Quality and safety in radiology. Oxford: Oxford University Press; 2012. p. 26–8.
23. Gunderman RB, Nyce JM. The tyranny of accuracy in radiologic education. Radiology. 2002;222:297–300.
24. Robinson PJ. Radiology's Achilles' heel: error and variation in the interpretation of the roentgen image. Br J Radiol. 1997;70:1085–98.
25. Manning DJ, Barker-Mill SC, Donovan T, Crawford T. Time-dependent observer errors in pulmonary nodule detection. Br J Radiol. 2006;79:342–6.
26. Pinto A, Scuderi MG, Daniele S. Errors in radiology: definition and classification. In: Romano L, Pinto A, editors. Errors in radiology. Heidelberg: Springer; 2012. p. 1–7.

27. Berlin L. Medicolegal-malpractice and ethical issues in radiology. Overdiagnosis, false-positive findings, and malpractice. AJR. 2014;203:W549.

28. Berlin L. Screening for early detection of breast cancer: overdiagnosis versus public education. Radiology. 2014;270:310–1.

29. Newman-Toker D. A unified conceptual model for diagnostic errors: underdiagnosis, overdiagnosis, and misdiagnosis. Diagnosis. 2014;1:43–8.

30. Garland LH. Studies on the accuracy of diagnostic procedures. Am J Roentgenol Radium Ther Nuc Med. 1959;82:25–38.

31. Zwaan L, Singh H. The challenges in defining and measuring diagnostic error. Diagnosis. 2015;2:97–103.

32. Jenniskens K, de Groot JAH, Reitsma JB, Moons KGM, Hooft L, Naaktgeboren CA. Overdiagnosis across medical disciplines: a scoping review. BMJ Open. 2017;7(12):e018448. https://doi.org/10.1136/bmjopen-2017-018448.

33. de Groot JAH, Naaktgeboren CA, Reitsma JB, Moons KGM. Methodological approaches to evaluating new highly sensitive diagnostic tests: avoiding overdiagnosis. CMAJ. 2017;189:E64–8. https://doi.org/10.1503/cmaj.150999.

34. Merritt BA, Henry TS, Cha S, et al. Tailoring radiology resident education using aggregated missed-cases data. J Am Coll Radiol. 2018;15:1013–5.

35. Wiener R, Schwartz L, Woloshin S. Time trends in pulmonary embolism in the United States: evidence of overdiagnosis. Arch Intern Med. 2011;171:831–7.

36. Hendrick RE. Obligate overdiagnosis due to mammographic screening: a direct estimate for US women. Radiology. 2018;287:391–7.

37. Monticciolo DL, Helvie MA, Hendrick RE. Current issues in the overdiagnosis and overtreatment of breast cancer. AJR. 2018;210:285–91.

38. Javitt MC. Breast cancer screening - what now, and what next? AJR. 2018;210:239–40.

39. de Groot PM, Carter BW, Abbott GF, Wu CC. Pitfalls in chest radiographic interpretation: blind spots. Sem Roentgenol. 2015;50:197–209.

40. Horton KM, Johnson PT, Fishman EK. MDCT of the abdomen: common misdiagnoses at a busy academic center. AJR. 2010;194:660–7.

41. Wu CC, Korashadi L, Abbott GF, Gilman MD. Common blind spots on chest CT: where are they all hiding? Part 1 – airways, lungs and pleura. AJR. 2013;201:W533–8.

42. Wu CC, Korashadi L, Abbott GF, Shepard JAO. Common blind spots on chest CT: where are they all hiding? Part 2, extrapulmonary structures. AJR. 2013;201:W671–7.

43. Rinaldi MF, Bartalena T, Gianneli G, et al. Incidental lung nodules on CT examinations of the abdomen: prevalence and reporting rates in the PACS era. Eur J Radiol. 2010;74:e84–8.

44. Siewert B, Sosna J, McNamara A, Raptopoulos V, Kruskal JB. Missed lesions at abdominal oncologic CT: lessons learned from quality assurance. Radiographics. 2008;28:623–38.

45. Bahrami S, Yim CM. Quality initiatives. Blind spots at brain imaging. Radiographics. 2009;29:1877–96.

46. Tchoyoson CC, Nadarajah M. System-based imaging pitfalls: brain. In: Peh WGC, editor. Pitfalls in diagnostic radiology. Heidelberg: Springer; 2015. p. 217–45.

47. Pickhardt PJ, Bhalla S, Balfe DM. Acquired gastrointestinal fistulas: classification, etiologies, and imaging evaluation. Radiology. 2002;224:9–23.

48. Kawashima A, Sandler CM, Corl FM, West OC, et al. Imaging of renal trauma: a comprehensive review. Radiographics. 2001;21:557–74.

49. Caiafa RO, Vinuesa AS, Izquierdo RS, Brufau BP, Colella JRA, Molina CN. Retroperitoneal fibrosis: role of imaging in diagnosis and follow-up. Radiographics. 2013;33:535–52.

50. Hofman PAM, Fitt GJ, Harvey AS, Kuzniecky RI, Jackson G. Bottom-of-sulcus dysplasia: imaging features. AJR. 2011;196:881–5.

51. Tomura N, Uemura K, Inugami A, Fujita H, Higano S, Shishido F. Early CT sign in cerebral infarction: obscuration of the lentiform nucleus. Radiology. 1988;168:463–7.

52. Dankbbar JW, Pameijer FA, Hendrikse J, Schmalfuss IM. Easily detected signs of perineural tumor spread in head and neck cancer. Insights Imaging. 2018;9:1089–95.

53. Berlin L. Medicolegal-malpractice and ethical issues in radiology. CT scout views and standard of care. AJR. 2014;203:W741.

54. Pinto A, Reginelli A, Pinto F, et al. Errors in imaging patients in the emergency setting. Br J Radiol. 2016;89:20150914. https://doi.org/10.1259/bjr.20150914.

55. Berlin L. Medicolegal-malpractice and ethical issues in radiology. Should CT and MRI scout images be interpreted? AJR. 2017;209:W43.

56. Eisenberg RL. Should "mature" radiologists be put out to pasture? Radiographics. 2016;36:937–8.

57. Khan R, Nael K, Erly W. Acute stroke imaging: what clinicians need to know. Am J Med. 2013;126:379–86.

58. Vancauwenberghe T, Snoeckx A, Vanbeckevoort D, Dymarkowski S, Vanhoenacker FM. Imaging of the spleen: what the clinician needs to know. Singap Med J. 2015;56:133–44.

59. Golfarb CA, Yin Y, Gilula LA, Fisher AJ, Boyer MI. Wrist fractures: what the clinician wants to know. Radiology. 2001;219:11–28.

60. Morag Y, Jacobson JA, Miller B, de Maeseneer M, Girish G, Jamadar D. MR imaging of rotator cuff injury: what the clinician needs to know. Radiographics. 2006;26:1045–65.

61. Marshall RA, Weaver ML, Sodickson A, Khurana B. Periprosthetic fractures in the emergency department: what the orthopedic surgeon wants to know. Radiographics. 2017;37:1202–17.

62. Kumbhar SS, O'Malley RB, Robinson TJ, et al. Why thyroid surgeons are frustrated with radiologists: lessons learned from pre- and postoperative US. Radiographics. 2016;36:2141–53.

63. Wieschhoff GG, Sheehan SE, Wortman JR, et al. Traumatic finger injuries: what the orthopedic surgeon wants to know. Radiographics. 2016;36:1106–28.

64. Sandstrom CK, Kennedy SA, Gross JA. Acute shoulder trauma: what the surgeon wants to know. Radiographics. 2015;35:475–92.

65. Lee SC, Jain PA, Jethwa SC, Tripathy D, Yamashita MW. Radiologists' role in breast cancer staging: providing key information for clinicians. Radiographics. 2014;34:330–42.

66. Khurana B, Sheehan SE, Sodickson A, Bono CM, Harris MB. Traumatic thoracolumbar spine injuries: what the spine surgeon wants to know. Radiographics. 2013;33:2031–46.

67. Sheehan SE, Dyer GS, Sodickson AD, Patel KI, Khurana B. Traumatic elbow injuries: what the orthopedic surgeon wants to know. Radiographics. 2013;33:869–88.

68. Zwaan L. The critical step to reduce diagnostic errors in medicine: addressing the limitations of human information processing. Diagnosis. 2014;1:139–41.

69. Allen CB, Tirman P, Jennings Clingan M, Manny J, Del Gaizo AJ, Leyendecker JR. Characterizing solid renal neoplasms with MRI in adults. Abdom Imaging. 2014;39:358–87.

70. Vendrami CL, Villavicencio CP, DeJulio TJ, et al. Differentiation of solid renal tumors with multiparametric MR imaging. Radiographics. 2017;37:2026–42.

71. Bosmans JM, Peremans L, De Schepper AM, Duyck PO, Parizel PM. How do referring clinicians want the radiologists to report? Suggestions from the COVER survey. Insights Imaging. 2011;2:577–84.

72. Berbaum KS, Franken EA, Dorfman DD, Lueben KR. Influence of clinical history on perception of abnormalities in pediatric radiographs. Acad Radiol. 1994;1:217–23.

73. White K, Berbaum K, Smith WL. The role of previous radiographs and reports in the interpretation of current radiographs. Investig Radiol. 1994;29:263–5.

74. Berlin L. Comparing new radiographs with those obtained previously. AJR. 1999;172:3–6.

75. Berlin L. Must new radiographs be compared with all previous radiographs, or only with the most recently obtained radiograph? AJR. 2000;174:611–5.

76. Hunter TB, Boyle RR. The value of reading the previous radiology report. AJR. 1988;150:697–8.

77. Aideyan UO, Berbaum K, Smith WL. Influence of prior radiologic information on the interpretation of radiographic examinations. Acad Radiol. 1995;2:205–8.

78. Leslie A, Jones AJ, Goddard PR. The influence of clinical information on the reporting of CT by radiologists. Br J Radiol. 2000;73:1052–5.

79. Gunderman RB, Phillips MD, Cohen MD. Improving clinical histories on radiology requisitions. Acad Radiol. 2001;8:299–303.

80. Berbaum KS, Franken EA. Commentary: does clinical history affect perception? Acad Radiol. 2006;13:402–3.

81. Mullins ME, Lev MH, Schellingerhout D, Koroshetz WJ, Gonzalez RG. Influence of availability of clinical history on detection of early stroke using unenhanced CT and diffusion-weighted MR imaging. AJR. 2002;179:223–8.

82. Doshi AM, Kiritsy M, Rosenkrantz AB. Strategies for avoiding recommendations for additional imaging through a comprehensive comparison with prior studies. J Am Coll Radiol. 2015;12:657–63.

83. Loy CT, Irwig L. Accuracy of diagnostic tests read with and without clinical information: a systematic review. JAMA. 2004;292:1602–9.

84. European Society of Radiology. ESR communication guidelines for radiologists. Insights Imaging. 2013;4:143–6.

85. Graber ML. Taking steps toward a safer future: measures to promote timely and accurate medical diagnosis. Am J Med. 2008;121(suppl 5):S43–6.

86. Society of Thoracic Radiology Online Educational Resources. thoracicrad.org/?portofolio=education

87. Journal of Thoracic Imaging. Residents and fellows corner. journals.lww.com/thoracicimaging/Pages/residentscorner.aspx

Abstract

I define the radiologic report as a medicolegal document that binds the reader to inform, guide, respect, and protect both the patient and the referring physician. Thus the way we construct or dictate our report should satisfy the requirements above, of course within the constraints of uncertainty of each individual case. By "information" I mean the answer to the clinical question, and the inclusion of other, significant or incidental findings. By "guidance" I mean our recommendations (if indicated) for further workup. By "respect" I mean two things: (a) providing true value to the referring physician, instead of recommending "clinical correlation," which he does anyway, and (b) not harming the patient through words or phrases that may crush his self-esteem. A clear report with specific recommendations (a) protects the patient from being subjected to inappropriate or potentially harmful tests, contrasted to a vague, incomplete report that would justify a continued, potentially misdirected search for a diagnosis, and (b) protects the referring physician from overlooking significant findings that if ignored could lead to adverse outcomes and accusations of negligence. Careful and appropriate selection of words and language are absolute requirements to avoid confusion and misunderstanding by the referring physician and the patient, when they read our report. Our level of confidence should be transparent, moderated by "common sense," and not masked by statistical hedging. The preparation and timely delivery of a worthy report are indeed acts of deep respect to the patient, the referring physician, and to ourselves. This chapter addresses all properties of a valuable report that can truly benefit the patient.

4.1 General Remarks

You will be surprised to find out how difficult it is to articulate seamlessly a meaningful radiologic report [1]. This topic has been treated in a thoughtful and meticulous manner by numerous individuals and committees [1–37]. The reader is urged to seek these sources for further information.

Some parts of this chapter have been presented earlier, but I feel that the repetition is warranted given the significance of this topic.

The radiologic report is a *medicolegal document* of great importance which reflects our knowledge, diagnostic abilities, and expression skills [1, 6, 12, 27, 30]. The way it is written and delivered determines to a great extent the strength of the rapport we build with our referring physicians [3, 4, 14, 15]. Thus we should treat our report with great respect.

The *report* should *answer the clinical question(s)* as clearly as possible, provide information about *unexpected* or *incidental*

Table 4.1 Structure of the radiology report

• Identification
• Clinical referral (or history)
• Technique
• Findings (or body of report)
• Conclusion (or impression)
• Advice (or recommendations)

findings, and *suggest further action*, when indicated [1, 2, 4, 12, 38].

Bruno et al. state "Good report writing is an independent skill that is best acquired with attention and practice .... Conscious attention must be given to ... the order in which the findings are presented, the use of simple declarative sentence structures, and a vocabulary that the readers will understand" [1].

It is recommended that we adhere to a *structured format*, such as that shown in Table 4.1 [25, 27].

We will now expand on each section of the report.

4.1.1 Identification

This component of the report includes the name and age of the patient, the name of the ordering physician or referring organization, the type and date of the examination, and whether previous imaging studies or imaging reports are available for review, comparison, or correlation.

4.1.2 Clinical Referral or Clinical History

This unit should be a summary of the clinical problem or the clinical question [11, 12, 25, 27].

4.1.3 Technique

This section is a brief description of the mechanics of the study, including technical parameters, administration of contrast medium (type, route, dosage), and radiation dose when appropriate. If there was an allergic or other type of reaction, we should describe it, record its severity, any medication(s) that were administered, the time

that the patient remained for observation in the radiology department, and any instructions given to the patient upon discharge [25, 27].

4.1.4 Findings

This is the lengthiest block of the report, devoted to the full description of the major, pertinent (positive and negative), and incidental findings [3, 5, 10, 12, 25, 27]. Predetermined templates and a structured format enhance the accuracy, thoroughness, standardization, and uniformity of our reports, and boost the satisfaction of the referring physicians [31–37].

4.1.5 Conclusion or Impression

This section is a summary of our interpretation effort. It should address explicitly the clinical question, and should either specify a precise diagnosis or provide a short differential. Other important information such as incidentalomas and adverse/allergic reactions should be restated [10–12, 27, 34, 39, 40]. The information gained from prior imaging studies or reports should be incorporated in our conclusion.

4.1.6 Advice or Recommendations

The purpose of this section is to assist the referring physician in the management of the patient. We need to consider and recommend: (a) the next step in the clarification or confirmation of a preliminary diagnosis, (b) the appropriate action in the staging or grading of known disease, or (c) a latent period for follow-up [3, 10–12, 41–53].

If additional information becomes available at a later time, or if we think of a new diagnostic possibility, we should either revise the report or write up an addendum. Any changes in our report should be immediately conveyed to the referring and treating physician [4, 5, 8, 11, 12, 54–57].

A written report should accompany every imaging examination whether or not the results were transmitted orally to the referring physician [4, 5, 54].

4.2 Incidental Findings (Incidentalomas)

We define incidentalomas as unexpected findings that are not related to the preliminary or to the working diagnosis [26, 30, 39]. Even though incidentalomas are a frequent occurrence in a variety of imaging studies, the chance of them harboring a lethal malignancy is very low, less than 1% [30, 39]. In the literature there is no consensus about the management of incidentalomas [30]. Some people are reluctant to include them in their report; there is a legitimate concern of triggering further work up that may ultimately prove an additional burden to the health care system, both in terms of costs and resources. A significant percentage of radiologists do not align with the official guidelines put forth by medical societies and committees; either because they have not read the guidelines or because they have elected to ignore them. On the other hand, an incidentaloma occasionally turns out to be either a malignancy or nonmalignant, yet significant situation. If the incidentaloma was ignored initially, then the result will certainly be harmful to the patient and probably to the initial reader as well. Berlin has a clear and strong opinion on this matter: "I believe that the moral and legal duties of radiologists are to examine carefully the radiologic images, report every finding they see, and report what the findings mean, in their professional judgment. If they believe that the incidentaloma is a benign finding, they should simply state so. Assuming that radiologists base their opinions on the ACR white papers and additional radiologic literature…" [30]. Leitman provides another strong argument in favor of reporting all incidentalomas on our reports, because of their potential value in the future [58].

4.3 Dismissing "Insignificant" Findings

This topic overlaps with the topic of incidentalomas. Some radiologists choose to ignore "insignificant" findings, claiming thus that they keep their work and their reports to a high standard [59–61].

However, there are two strong counterarguments to this line of thinking: (a) a priori it is not always possible to assign "significance" or "meaning" to any given finding [30, 58] and (b) a complete description of findings does not equate to poor thinking or a suboptimal report [62]. My stand on this is the same as for incidentalomas (please read the prior section for a refresher, if needed).

4.4 Handling Findings Unreported in Prior Imaging

Occasionally, when comparing two studies, we may realize that a finding in the reference study was not reported. How do we handle such an awkward situation? Both the patient and the referring physician have the right to know the truth. Apart from ethical dilemmas, there are practical issues of managing the patient, especially if there are any changes between the two imaging examinations [30]. Thus, the way I do it is to describe the finding in question and any interval changes (in the usual manner), regardless of relevance to the current clinical question. I make sure that the report does not allow any room for blaming the reader of the index study. For example: "The lung nodule was difficult to detect in the prior chest CT, because it was close to the bifurcation of a peripheral pulmonary artery," or "In retrospect, the mesenteric lymph node was present in the prior CT scan, but was obscured by nearby unopacified bowel loops," or "The visibility of the lesion is greater in the current study because of recent modifications in the CT protocols in our department." Small, low contrast lesions in blind spots may not provoke our attention initially, but may become evident in subsequent imaging. Thus Berlin also feels strongly about not expressing blame or judgment on the radiologist who did not record the finding [30].

4.5 Radiologic Language

We need to use specific and established terminology [10, 63–72]. Fortunately, the medical vocabulary is very rich and we can describe any abnormality in great detail. For example, the phrase "lung shadow" is vague. Instead of "shadow," we can say: ground glass nodule, dense consolidation with aerobronchograms, spiculated thick walled cavity containing air and fluid, etc.

Short declarative sentences are optimal for radiologic reporting [11, 12, 63]. For example: "A cyst is present in the right ovary" [1, 63].

The words "large" and "small" are not appropriate for findings that should be measured precisely, i.e., how large is a "large" kidney tumor? [4, 73].

Avoid abbreviations, jargon, and commonly used, but vague words that convey doubt and indecision, such as "nonspecific," "borderline," "equivocal," "suspicious," "perhaps," "indeterminate," or "not considered likely" [3, 9, 64–66, 73–76]. Low confidence modifiers also are not recommended, such as "may be consistent with" or "possibly consistent with" [9–13].

If a structure or a study is normal, then just say "normal"; do not employ words such as "unremarkable" or "negative" that denote evasion or reluctancy to call a normal study by its name [75, 77, 78].

Avoid vague quantifiers, such as "few," "several," or "multiple"; these words have a wide latitude when we translate them into numbers [79]. Give instead a specific number, or give an estimate. For example, "A total of 7 pulmonary nodules, 5 on the right and 2 on the left," "We can count 5 or 6 gallstones," "About 20 metastatic nodules scattered through the brain parenchyma."

The expressions "Clinical correlation is suggested" and "Cannot rule out" are overused; nevertheless they lack clarity, and they do not serve our purpose [4, 74, 80, 81]. Be honest "in admitting when we do not know things that are actually unknowable" [1]. Do not use the phrases "Clinical correlation is suggested" or "Cannot rule out." Instead, if the history is noncontributory, it is prudent to use the phrase "In the appropriate clinical setting these findings may represent…" [73]. This way we acknowledge our limitations and we avoid insulting our colleagues [3].

Bruno et al. suggest that we "convey our diagnostic uncertainty in straightforward prose," such as "This appearance suggests diagnosis x, … [as] the most likely possibility; … diagnosis y must

also be considered, though it is thought to be less likely because." [1]. This makes sense, since our job is to steer the referring physician towards the diagnosis that is most likely. If we say "the patient does not have x, y or z," the question remains "well, what does the patient have?" Hoang has summarized this concept in a single sentence: "Radiologists' skills are most valuable when they are used to make diagnoses, not exclude them." [81]. I allow one exception to this rule, when the referring physician asks about specific diseases (x, y, or z). If I have excluded them from my differential after thoughtful consideration, then I include in the report that "the patient does *not* have x, y, or z." Of course the conclusion of my report starts with the most likely diagnosis or with the most likely differential.

Avoid contradictory or confusing statements [81–87]. Give a solid plan of action to the referring physician. As a specific example, we will contrast two impressions of a chest imaging study of a heavy, long-time smoker, adapted from Hoang [81]:

a. "Findings most likely represent pneumonia. Cannot exclude malignancy." The last sentence gives the impression that the radiologist either does not want to or is not capable of giving a firm, definitive diagnosis.
b. "Findings most likely represent pneumonia. Given the known risk factors for malignancy, a repeat study in 6 weeks would help identify an underlying mass." This statement makes it clear that the radiologist took into account the patient's history, acknowledges the limitations of the imaging technique, and respects the referring physician.

The phrase "No change compared to prior study" as a stand-alone statement is inadequate [4, 76]. Be more specific: what has not changed? An example would be: "No change in the number, size, distribution, density and contrast enhancement of multiple lymph nodes in the mediastinum. There has been no development of hilar or axillary lymphadenopathy. Loculated or free fluid has not accumulated in the pericardial or pleural cavities. The lungs, trachea and central bronchi remain clear. The chest wall remains free of fractures, soft tissue and osseous infiltrations."

For major or significant findings, it is suggested that we indicate the image and series or scan numbers [4]. This way:

a. the referring physician can scroll through the study to find easily the relevant images and
b. if the patient returns for follow-up, we are assured that we are comparing the same lesion(s), and that we are obtaining the appropriate measurements, for the assessment of any changes.

Redundancy does not add value; on the contrary it creates the impression of hedging [3]. Ware et al. state: [Adding terms such as *identified* and *evidence of* to the negativity of a finding, as in "no evidence of aortic dissection," is redundant and should generally be avoided except in cases in which the imaging modality is clearly suboptimal for the evaluation of certain pathology…]. The phrase "interval change" is also redundant; instead, it is appropriate to specify the time interval between the studies that we are comparing [3].

4.6   Distinguishing Uncertainty from Vagueness

4.6.1   Uncertainty

At times we cannot decide if a feature of an image is real or artifactual. Other times we are not sure about the origin or about the nature of a finding. Nevertheless, we can still describe it in a proper manner, construct a coherent summary, and offer a solid recommendation. For example, a 55-year-old patient presents with a 6-month stable history of positional vertigo. The MR scan reveals a 2 mm focus of high T2 and high FLAIR signal, close to the inferior margin of the right frontal horn. The finding cannot be detected in the T1w or in the diffusion weighted sequence. There is neither perilesional edema nor contrast enhancement. The rest of the study is normal. I cannot explain the patient's symptom with this finding and I am not certain about its etiology.

However, I feel comfortable dismissing it, and thus I conclude my report by stating that "the finding is *not clinically important* and *no further evaluation* is warranted" [88, 89].

4.6.2   Vagueness

Vagueness is the opposite of clarity. A vague report obscures the value of the imaging study and may mislead the referring physician, with potential harmful consequences to the patient.[1] To highlight the difference between uncertainty and vagueness we will compare two reports of a chest radiograph that shows a spiculated 1 cm nodule (example adapted from reference 73).

a. An experienced radiologist may say: "This nodule likely represents lung cancer. A chest CT with contrast is recommended for further evaluation." The referring physician appreciates the clear, succinct report and the direct recommendation.
b. On the contrary, an inexperienced reader may say: "Diagnostic possibilities include cancer, non-calcified granuloma, artifact, metastasis, or conceivably an unusual infection. Because a tumor cannot be excluded, clinical correlation is suggested and further work-up may be of value." This time the referring physician is left helpless and confused. This report is vague, because it is just an assembly of diagnostic possibilities; it provides neither a stratification of the differential nor specific recommendations regarding the next diagnostic action.

4.7   Quantifying and Managing Uncertainty

The theme of uncertainty is inherent in our work[2] [73, 90–92]. Improper reporting of uncertainty is a variant of miscommunication. When we are not

---

[1] Please see also Sect. 4.11 on p. 10 of this chapter.
[2] Please review the related subjects of "Sensitivity versus Specificity" presented in Sect. 5.2.2.2, p. 3 of Chap. 5.

confident about our diagnosis, we use qualifiers such as "compatible with," "suggestive of," and "possibly" [73]. However, these statements are not as valuable as we may think, because there is no consensus on their exact or perceived meaning. Four studies have questioned the power and clarity of common expressions of uncertainty used by radiologists. The participants in these projects were radiologists, referring physicians, and patients. For most qualifiers there was wide variability, even among radiologists, regarding meaning and clinical significance [93–96]. The conclusion is that "Radiology reports, … do not appear to effectively convey the intended level of uncertainty to the reader" [1].

How do we deal with this potential source of confusion and misunderstanding?

Some authors have suggested limiting our responses to a few selected phrases. Langlotz proposes that there be only five possible answers to the question "Does the patient have a mass, an infarct, a pneumonia, etc.?" Our choices are: "definitely yes," "likely yes," "possibly," "likely not," and "definitely not" [73]. If our answer is "possibly" or "likely/definitely not," then we have to offer an alternative diagnosis that fulfills the "definitely/likely yes" slots.

Panicek and Hricak advocate the use of a standardized "lexicon" that assigns a specific number to the level of certainty or doubt in our diagnosis [97]. The authors allow five grades of high, medium, or low confidence in our diagnosis, expressed as a percentage (>90%, ≈75%, ≈50%, ≈25%, and <10%). However, I personally do not feel confident that I can quantify precisely the likelihood of disease, and I do not know what to do with the numbers in between the suggested cutoffs, such as 40%.

Other authors believe that we can substitute our opinion with absolute numbers, derived with statistical tools, such as the Bayes' equation [98–100]. This formula solidifies the posttest probability of disease, after the patient has undergone a diagnostic procedure (imaging or other). The final likelihood of disease depends on its pretest probability as well as the results of the procedure.

Statistical tools are very useful for application in large groups, but I strongly object to their use upon individual patients [101, 102]. What if I do not know exactly the pretest probability for a particular patient? How do I arrive at the post test probability of disease if the study is of limited diagnostic value, because the patient could not cooperate? A given patient may fall outside the "accepted" statistical boundaries. I have seen patients with documented multiple sclerosis and a completely normal brain MR scan, with their disease confined to the spinal cord. I have seen invasive breast carcinoma in very young patients, 25 years of age. Overreliance on statistics directs us away from uncommon conditions and away from uncommon presentations of common diseases, due to the prevalence and zebra effects. Consider a 69-year-old, previously healthy male patient who presents with a clinical and laboratory picture of severe adrenal insufficiency. Imaging reveals multiple, discrete, solid, high-cellularity masses: in one testis, in both adrenal glands, and in the left kidney engulfing the fat in the renal sinus, in the peri/para-renal compartments and in the left para-aortic space. Do we think of extranodal lymphoma as the most likely diagnosis? The imaging characteristics were compatible with lymphoma, and I said with a high degree of confidence "extranodal lymphoma" [103–105]. The diagnosis of lymphoma was confirmed with a core biopsy of one adrenal mass, that was 5 cm in size. To me, overemphasizing the pretest probability of extranodal lymphoma is irrelevant and misleading.

If we look at the nonmedical literature we find out that we have abused statistics as a diagnostic tool, because we have falsely equated risk with uncertainty [106–110]. In situations of risk we know exactly all parameters of the question; we know all alternatives, consequences, and probabilities. Thus we can arrive at the answer with simple calculations. On the other hand, radiology, and all other medical specialties belong to the world of uncertainty; it is not possible to gather all relevant information, and sometimes we have to act very fast, before we get access to all information we would like. Thus, we should rely heavily on knowledge, experience, heuristics, and deductive reasoning [108].

Fast and frugal trees (FFT) are a unique form of heuristics, depicted as a branching structure that stratifies the most important data of the clinical problem [111]. Each decision node is simple and easy to understand. No calculations are needed. I am not aware of any applications of FFT in medical imaging; perhaps FFT can serve as a teaching tool for expert diagnostic operations.

To conclude, I believe that the best way to command uncertainty in our reports is through careful choice of words and phrases[3] that are clear, specific, and address the clinical situation. Offering the most likely diagnosis (or differential) and providing appropriate guidance about the next step(s) of action are more important than calculating numbers or percentages.

Our findings, impression, and advice should be stated in such a way that our clinical colleagues understand easily *what we want to say* [4, 6, 11–13]. My mentor would challenge me: "Let's reverse our roles and let's pretend that you are the referring physician. Go ahead and read your own report! What's your general impression? Is it what you expected? Is it helpful? Is it organized? Is it vague or incomplete? Is it lengthy or verbose? Does it address the clinical question?" In order to drive home his point, he would add "Pick up and read a histopathology report, just the body of it, without the conclusion! Does it make any sense to you, or are you confused? Now, you get an idea how the referring physicians feel, when our reports are not tailored to them and their patients. Keep in mind that what the referring physician understands is more important than what you say" [2, 4, 112].

4.8 Errors Communicating with the Referring Physician

Many patients definitely benefit from live, direct exchange of information between the radiologist and the referring physician. If this contact is indicated, but is either *delayed* or *does not take place*, then we become responsible for *faulty or disrupted* communication [4, 6, 11, 15, 16, 56, 112].

In cases of *urgent* or *life-threatening* findings, whether expected or not, we should *immediately* contact the referring physician [4, 11, 15, 113,

114]. The time of communication and the name of the person contacted should be recorded in our report [115].

Direct communication with the referring physician should not be limited to urgent or emergent conditions. I believe that the list of indications for calling the referring physician should be expanded to include the following situations:

- When we detect significant findings, whether suspected, or not,
- When the request does not provide adequate information about the patient,
- When our impression does not match the clinical picture,
- When we think that the requested study is not optimal to address the clinical question [4, 10],
- When we modify a report or when we write up an addendum to a report,
- When we are asked to provide a formal second interpretation.

Misuse of words and phrases in reports constitutes a common cause of poor communication between radiologists and referring physicians. This topic has been covered in detail in Sects. 4.5 and 4.7 respectively.

4.9 Factors Affecting Follow Through of Our Recommendations

An important question to ask is how often the ordering physician acts upon our recommendations. Studies have shown that the noncompliance rate may reach 33% [52]. Researchers have identified three factors that increase the likelihood that follow-up imaging will be executed as per our recommendations: (a) use of strong language in our reports [116, 117], (b) giving a specific time frame for follow-up [52], and (c) direct verbal communication of the interpreting radiologist with the referring physician [118].

An example of strong wording would be "Recommend further evaluation of the brain with MRI before and after paramagnetic contrast enhancement," as opposed to a weak statement

---

[3]It is assumed that the radiologist has sufficient knowledge and experience.

"If clinically indicated, further evaluation could be performed with MRI."

A recommendation specifying the time for follow-up would be "Recommend repeat CT scan in 6 months," instead of saying "Recommend follow-up."

4.10   Personal Thoughts

I like to start the body of the report with a comment on the quality of the study. It is important to note if the study was technically suboptimal or if the patient could not cooperate [10–13, 25]. Depending on the clinical problem and the condition of the patient, I may request additional, focused imaging. I speak with the technologist, I explain my reasoning, and I provide specific instructions. Then the receptionist asks the patient to return to the department. I write up a preliminary report, stating clearly why the study is incomplete and/or suboptimal. When the patient completes the additional imaging, I either revise the report or I modify it with an addendum.

In the body of the report I routinely mention normal variants or artifacts that may mimic pathology. If the referring physician is not familiar with these situations, he may think that I missed a significant finding. For example, MR flow artifacts that project over an organ may appear as abnormal parenchymal signal or abnormal contrast enhancement. I also comment on normal anatomy that is not strictly relevant information, but may gain significance at a later date. For example, I always note an ascending, retrocecal appendix in a pelvic CT or MRI scan.

I keep the conclusion as short as possible, especially if there are multiple findings (whether pertinent, unrelated, or incidental). For example, my conclusion of an MRI scan performed after a severe pivot shift knee injury may be "Acute trauma to multiple knee structures." This way I accomplish two goals. First, the referring physician with a quick glance gets a brief summary of the situation. Second, I gently force the referring physician to read carefully the entire report.

Many physicians read only the impression, and thus may miss a significant comment in the body of the report.

4.11   The Human Face
      of the Radiology Report

At this point I feel it is appropriate to comment on another important aspect of the radiology report, it's "human face." I learnt this concept from my mentor: "Never forget that behind every report there is a real person and we are obligated to serve his wellbeing, before we sign off." We need to protect the patients from overaggressive or insecure physicians who may proceed with unnecessary tests or invasive procedures on questionable grounds, if we give them permission with a vague report [2, 119]. We also need to protect the patients from ourselves by not engaging in extreme behaviors. Some radiologists feel the need to be right and have an answer every single time, risking a misdiagnosis [90]. Other radiologists try to disguise their limitations and insecurities with ambiguous statements and frequently suggest further work up, in order to rule in or to rule out various possibilities [2, 4, 120].

Many patients read our reports and our wording may have a strong impact on their self-image. For example, I have not used the phrase "brain atrophy" in a report, or in talking to a patient (or his family) since June 1992. Instead, I grade the width of the ventricles, cisterns, and sulci and note any disproportionate enlargement of specific CSF compartments. Instead of "hippocampal and corpus callosum atrophy," I say "decreased hippocampal size and thinning of the corpus callosum."

References

1. Bruno MA, Petscavage-Thomas J, Abujudeh HH. Communicating uncertainty in the radiology report. AJR. 2017;209:1006–8.
2. Eberhardt SC, Heilbrun ME. Radiology report value equation. Radiographics. 2018;38:1888–96.
3. Ware JB, Saurabh J, Hoang JK, Baker S, Wruble J. Effective radiology reporting. J Am Coll Radiol. 2017;14:838–9.

4. Bosmans JM, Peremans L, De Schepper AM, Duyck PO, Parizel PM. How do referring clinicians want the radiologists to report? Suggestions from the COVER survey. Insights Imaging. 2011;2:577–84.

5. European Society of Radiology. ESR communication guidelines for radiologists. Insights Imaging. 2013;4:143–6.

6. European Society of Radiology. Good practice for radiological reporting. Guidelines from the European Society of Radiology (ESR). Insights Imaging. 2011;2:93–6.

7. European Society of Radiology. ESR guidelines for the communication of urgent and unexpected findings. Insights Imaging. 2012;3:1–3.

8. Langlotz C. The radiology report: a guide to thoughtful communication for radiologists and other medical professionals. North Charleston: CreateSpace; 2015.

9. Radiology reporting initiative – RSNA. www.rsna.org/Reporting_Initiative.aspx.

10. ACR Practice parameter for communication of diagnostic imaging findings. Revised 2014. www.acr.org/~/media/C5D1443C9EA4424AA12477D1AD1D927D.pdf.

11. Standards for the reporting and interpretation of imaging investigations. This document was last reviewed in 2014 by the Clinical Radiology Professional Support and Standards Board and the Clinical Radiology Faculty Board. Last update September 2015. https://www.rcr.ac.uk/publication/standards-reporting-and-interpretation-imaging-investigations. Accessed 25 Oct 2016.

12. Radiology written report guideline project. www.ranzcr.edu.au/resources/professional-documents/guidelines. Accessed 25 Oct 2016.

13. Radiology written report guidelines-short version. www.ranzcr.edu.au/resources/professional-documents/guidelines. Accessed 25 Oct 2016.

14. Pinto F, Romano S, Acampora C. Errors in radiology reporting. In: Romano L, Pinto A, editors. Errors in radiology. Heidelberg: Springer; 2012. p. 227–33.

15. Murphy DR, Singh H, Berlin L. Communication breakdowns and diagnostic errors: a radiology perspective. Diagnosis. 2014;1:253–61.

16. Hussain S. Communication of radiology results. In: Abujudeh HH, Bruno MA, editors. Quality and safety in radiology. Oxford: Oxford University Press; 2012. p. 59–67.

17. Miguel K. Teamwork and communication in radiology. In: Abujudeh HH, Bruno MA, editors. Quality and safety in radiology. Oxford: Oxford University Press; 2012. p. 68–79.

18. Pool F, Georgen S. Quality of the written radiology report: a review of the literature. J Am Coll Radiol. 2010;7:634–43.

19. Steele JL, Nyce JM, Williamson KB, Gunderman RB. Learning to report. Acad Radiol. 2002;9:817–20.

20. Kahn CE Jr, Langlotz CP, Burnside ES, Carrino JA, Channin DS, Hovsepian DM, Rubin DL. Toward best practices in radiology reporting. Radiology. 2009;252:852–6.

21. McMenamy J, Rosenkrantz AB, Jacobs J, Kim D. Use of a referring physician survey to direct and evaluate department-wide radiology quality improvement efforts. J Am Coll Radiol. 2015;12:1223–5.

22. Collard MD, Tellier J, Chowdhury AS, Lowe LH. Improvement in reporting skills of radiology residents with a structured reporting curriculum. Acad Radiol. 2014;21:126–33.

23. Gunderman RB, Ambrosius WT, Cohen M. Radiology reporting in an academic children's hospital: what referring physicians think. Pediatr Radiol. 2000;30:307–14.

24. Gunn JA, Alabre CI, Bennett SE, Kautzky M, Krakower T, Palamara K, Choy G. Structured feedback from referring physicians: a novel approach to quality improvement in radiology reporting. AJR. 2013;201:853–7.

25. Langlotz CP. Organizing the radiology report. In: The radiology report. Charleston: CreateSpace; 2015. p. 87–95.

26. Zarzour JG, Berland LL. Reporting: recommendations/guidelines. In: Donoso L, Boland GWL, editors. Quality and safety in imaging. Heidelberg: Springer; 2018. p. 85–97.

27. Ranschaert ER, Bosmans JML. Report communication standards. In: Donoso L, Boland GWL, editors. Quality and safety in imaging. Heidelberg: Springer; 2018. p. 119–43.

28. Allen B, Chatfield M, Burleson J, Thorwarth WT. Improving diagnosis in health care: perspectives from the American College of Radiology. Diagnosis. 2017;4:113–24.

29. Sureka B, Garg P. Seven C's of effective communication. AJR. 2018;210:W243.

30. Berlin L. Contemporary risk management for radiologists. Radiographics. 2018;38:1717–28.

31. Marcovici PA, Taylor GA. Journal club: structured radiology reports are more complete and more effective than unstructured reports. AJR. 2014;203:1265–71.

32. Schwartz LH, Panicek DM, Brek RA, Li Y, Hricak H. Improving communication of diagnostic radiology findings through structured reporting. Radiology. 2011;260:174–81.

33. Larson DB, Towbin AJ, Pryor RM, Donnelly LF. Improving consistency in radiology reporting through the use of department-wide standardized structured reporting. Radiology. 2013;267:240–50.

34. Langlotz CP. Toward structured reporting. In: The radiology report. Charleston: CreateSpace; 2015. p. 119–47.

35. Lather JD, Che Z, Saltzman B, Bieszczad J. Structured reporting in the academic setting: what the referring clinician wants. J Am Coll Radiol. 2018;15:772–5.

36. Tersteeg JJC, Gobardhan PD, Crolla RMPH. Improving the quality of MRI reports of preoperative patients with rectal cancer: effect of national guidelines and structured reporting. AJR. 2018;210:1240–4.

37. Alessandrino F, Pichiecchio A, Malluci G, et al. Do MRI structured reports for multiple sclerosis contain adequate information for clinical decision making? AJR. 2018;210:24–9.

38. Kabadi SJ, Krishmaraj A. Strategies for improving the value of the radiology report: a retrospective analysis of errors in formally over-read studies. J Am Coll Radiol. 2017;14:459–66.

39. Berlin L. Medicolegal-malpractice and ethical issues in radiology: the incidentaloma. AJR. 2013;200:W91.

40. Berland L, Silverman S, Gore R, et al. Managing incidental findings on abdominal CT: white paper of the ACR Incidental Findings Committee. J Am Coll Radiol. 2010;7:754–73.

41. Gore RM, Newmark GM, Thakrar KH, Mehta UK, Berlin JW. Hepatic incidentalomas. Radiol Clin N Am. 2011;49:291–322.

42. MacMahon H, Austin JHM, Gamsu G, Herold CJ, Jett JR, Naidich DP, et al. Guidelines for management of small pulmonary nodules detected on CT scans: a statement from the Fleischner society. Radiology. 2005;237:395–400.

43. Naidich DP, Bankier AA, MacMahon H, Schaefer-Prokop CM, Pistolesi M, Goo JM, et al. Recommendations for the management of subsolid pulmonary nodules detected at CT: a statement from the Fleischner society. Radiology. 2013;266:304–17.

44. Hoang JK, Langer JE, Middleton WD, et al. Managing incidental thyroid nodules detected on imaging: white paper of the ACR Incidental Thyroid Findings Committee. J Am Coll Radiol. 2015;12:143–50.

45. Berland LL. Overview of white papers of the ACR Incidental Findings Committee II on adnexal, vascular, splenic, nodal, gallbladder, and biliary findings. J Am Coll Radiol. 2013;10:672–4.

46. Pooler BD, Kim DH, Pickhardt PJ. Extracolonic findings identified in asymptomatic adults at screening CT colonography: prevalence, benefits, challenges, and opportunities. AJR. 2017;209:94–102.

47. Gore M, Pickhardt PJ, Mortele KJ, et al. Management of incidental liver lesions on CT: a white paper of the ACR Incidental Findings Committee. J Am Coll Radiol. 2017;14:1429–37.

48. Megibow AJ, Baker ME, Morgan DE, et al. Management of incidental pancreatic cysts: a white paper of the ACR Incidental Findings Committee. J Am Coll Radiol. 2017;14:911–23.

49. Herts BR, Silverman SG, Hindman NM, et al. Management of the incidental renal mass on CT: a white paper of the ACR Incidental Findings Committee. J Am Coll Radiol. 2018;15:264–73.

50. Munden RF, Carter BW, Chiles C, et al. Managing incidental findings on thoracic CT: mediastinal and cardiovascular findings. A white paper of the ACR Incidental Findings Committee. J Am Coll Radiol. 2018;15:1087–96.

51. Hoang JK, Hoffman AR, Gonzalez RG, et al. Management of incidental pituitary findings on CT, MRI, and 18F-Fluorodeoxyglucose PET: a white paper of the ACR Incidental Findings Committee. J Am Coll Radiol. 2018;15:966–72.

52. Itri JN, Raghavan K, Patel SB, et al. Developing quality measures for diagnostic radiologists: part 2. J Am Coll Radiol. 2018;15:1366–84.

53. Berlin L. Medicolegal-malpractice and ethical issues in radiology: recommending additional and follow-up radiologic examinations. AJR. 2013;201:W656.

54. Berlin L. Medicolegal-malpractice and ethical issues in radiology: ACR practice guidelines concerning addendum reports. AJR. 2013;201:W158.

55. Berlin L. Medicolegal-malpractice and ethical issues in radiology. Amended versus addended versus addendum reports. AJR. 2017;209:W109.

56. Orzel JA, Berlin L. Correction of interpretive errors. AJR. 2003;180:1477.

57. Hussain S, Allende MB, Karam AR, Hussain JS, Vijayaraghavan G. Addenda to the radiology report: what are we trying to convey? J Am Coll Radiol. 2011;8:703–5.

58. Leitman BS. Comment on the avoidance of reporting incidental findings. Letter to the editor. J Am Coll Radiol. 2018;15:7.

59. Jha S. Counterpoint: not everything significant is significant. J Am Coll Radiol. 2017;14:1554–5.

60. Heller RE III. Point: a missed lung nodule is a significant miss. J Am Coll Radiol. 2017;14:1552–3.

61. Heller RE III. Re: "A miss is still a miss". Letter to the editor. J Am Coll Radiol. 2018;15:704.

62. Posteraro RH. A miss is still a miss. J Am Coll Radiol. 2018;15:703–4.

63. Langlotz CP. Expressing an imaging observation. In: The radiology report. Charleston: CreateSpace; 2015. p. 23–30.

64. Langlotz CP. A guide to reporting style. In: The radiology report. Charleston: CreateSpace; 2015. p. 51–67.

65. Hall FM. Language of the radiology report: primer for residents and wayward radiologists. AJR. 2000;175:1239–42.

66. Coakley FV, Liberman L, Panicek DM. Style guidelines for radiology reporting: a manner of speaking. AJR. 2003;180:327–8.

67. Fardon DF, Williams AL, Dohring EJ, Murtagh FR, Gabriel Rothman SL, Sze GK. Lumbar disc nomenclature: version 2.0: recommendations of the combined task forces of the North American Spine Society, the American Society of Spine radiology and the American Society of Neuroradiology. Spine J. 2014;14:2525–45.

68. Hansell DM, Bankier AA, MacMahon H, McLoud TC, Muller NL, Remy J. Fleischner society: glossary of terms for thoracic imaging. Radiology. 2008;246:697–722.

69. Aiken AH, Rath TJ, Anzai Y, et al. ACR neck imaging reporting and data systems (NI-RADS): a white paper of the ACR NI-RADS Committee. J Am Coll Radiol. 2018;15:1097–108.

70. Corwin MT, Lee AY, Fananapazir TW, Loehfelm TW, Satkar S, Sirlin CB. Nonstandardized terminology to

describe focal liver lesions in patients at risk for hepatocellular carcinoma: implications regarding clinical communication. AJR. 2018;210:85–90.

71. Tirkes T, Shah ZK, Takahashi N, et al. Reporting standards for chronic pancreatitis by using CT, MRI, and MR cholangiopancreatography: the consortium for the study of chronic pancreatitis, diabetes, and pancreatic cancer. Radiology. 2019;290:207–15.

72. Andreotti RF, Timmerman D, Benacerraf BR, et al. Ovarian-adnexal reporting lexicon for ultrasound: a white paper of the ACR ovarian-adnexal reporting and data system committee. J Am Coll Radiol. 2018;15:1415–29.

73. Langlotz CP. Radiology reporting best practices. In: The radiology report. Charleston: CreateSpace; 2015. p. 31–50.

74. Berlin L. Medicolegal-malpractice and ethical issues in radiology. "Normal" versus "unremarkable" versus "within normal limits". AJR. 2015;204:W214.

75. Hoang JK. Keep "As Above" out of the impression. J Am Coll Radiol. 2016;13:490.

76. Hoang JK. If there is no change, just say so. J Am Coll Radiol. 2016;13:236.

77. Short RG, Befera T, Hoang JK, Tailor D. A normal thyroid by any other name: linguistic analysis of statements describing a normal thyroid gland from noncontrast chest CT reports. J Am Coll Radiol. 2018;15:1642–7.

78. Ross SL, Ascher SM, Somwaru AS, Filice R. Quantifying language before and after instituting structured CT reports. J Am Coll Radiol. 2017;14:1444–50.

79. England JR, Cheng PM, Romero M. Qualitative reporting of lesion number: do radiologists and referring physicians understand each other? J Am Coll Radiol. 2018;15:1178–81.

80. Rosenkrantz AB, Bansal NK. Diagnostic errors in abdominopelvic CT interpretation: characterization based on report addenda. Abdom Radiol. 2016;41:1793–9.

81. Hoang JK. Avoid "Cannot Exclude": make a diagnosis. J Am Coll Radiol. 2015;12:1009.

82. Hoang J. Do not hedge when there is certainty. J Am Coll Radiol. 2015;14:5.

83. Krantz PG. What's your impression? Get to the point. J Am Coll Radiol. 2017;14:451.

84. Kuzminski SJ. The devil is in the details. J Am Coll Radiol. 2017;14:148.

85. Hoang JK. Add value in radiology reports by providing a frame of reference. J Am Coll Radiol. 2017;14:585–6.

86. Feld RS. What passes on first blush may not bear scrutiny. J Am Coll Radiol. 2017;14:307.

87. Wildman-Tobriner B. Mean what you say and say what you mean. J Am Coll Radiol. 2017;14:862.

88. Hoang JK. Insignificant findings: don't leave them questioning the significance. J Am Coll Radiol. 2015;12(part A):1244.

89. Berlin L. Re: "Insignificant findings: don't leave them questioning the significance". J Am Coll Radiol. 2016;13:363.

90. Gunderman RB, Nyce JM. The tyranny of accuracy in radiologic education. Radiology. 2002;222:297–300.

91. Bruno MA. Our mistakes-the human experience. Video lecture. https://www.learning.arrs.org/mod/url/view.php?id=400. Accessed 22 Nov 2016.

92. Leitman B. Uncertainty: the problem with restricting the use of selected phrase in image reporting. J Am Coll Radiol. 2016;13:363–4.

93. Hobby JL, Tom BDM, Todd C, Bearcroft PWP, Dixon AK. Communication of doubt and certainty in radiological reports. Br J Radiol. 2000;73:999–1001.

94. Khorasani R, Bates DW, Teeger S, Rothschild JM, Adams DF, Seltzer S. Is terminology used effectively to convey diagnostic certainty in radiology reports? Acad Radiol. 2003;10:685–8.

95. Rosenkrantz AB. Differences in perceptions among radiologists, referring physicians, and patients regarding language for incidental findings reporting. AJR. 2017;208:140–3.

96. Rosenkrantz AB, Kiritsy M, Kim S. How "consistent" is "consistent"? A clinician-based assessment of the reliability of expressions used by radiologists to communicate diagnostic confidence. Clin Radiol. 2014;69:745–9.

97. Panicek DM, Hricak H. How sure are you, doctor? A standardized lexicon to describe the radiologist's level of certainty. AJR. 2016;207:2–3.

98. Johnson KM. Using Bayes' rule in diagnostic testing: a graphical explanation. Diagnosis. 2017;26:159–67.

99. Bruno MA, Hollenbeak CS. Statistical tools and methods. In: Abujudeh HH, Bruno MA, editors. Radiology noninterpretive skills: the requisites. Philadelphia: Elsevier; 2017.

100. Langlotz CP. How to think about imaging information. In: The radiology report. Charleston: CreateSpace; 2015. p. 161–87.

101. Kalanithi P. When breath becomes air. New York: Penguin Random House; 2016.

102. Harvey AM, Bordley J II, Barondness J. Differential diagnosis. 3rd ed. Philadelphia: WB Saunders Company; 1979. p. 15.

103. Leite NP, Kased N, Hanna RF, et al. Cross-sectional imaging of extranodal involvement in abdominopelvic lymphoproliferative malignancies. Radiographics. 2007;27:1613–34.

104. Johnson PT, Horton KM, Fishman EK. Adrenal mass imaging with multidetector CT: pathologic conditions, pearls and pitfalls. Radiographics. 2009;29:1333–51.

105. Davda S, Roy A, Haroon A, Sahdev A, Shahabuddin KL. All nodes lead to lymphoma – a multimodality refresher of extranodal lymphoma. ECR. 2016;2016:C-1370. https://doi.org/10.1594/ecr2016/C-1370.

106. Gigerenzer G, Edwards A. Simple tools for understanding risks: from innumeracy to insight. BMJ. 2003;327:741–4.

107. Gigerenzer G, Gaissmaier W, Kurz-Milcke E, Schwartz LM, Woloshin S. Helping doctors and patients to make sense of health statistics. Psychol Sci Public Interest. 2007;8:53–96.

108. Volz KG, Gigerenzer G. Cognitive processes in decisions under risk are not the same as in decisions under uncertainty. Front Neurosci. 2012;6:1–6.
109. Savage LJ. Foundations of statistics. New York: Wiley; 1954.
110. Binmore K. Rational decisions. Princeton: Princeton University Press; 2009.
111. Phillips ND, Neth H, Woike JK, Gaissmaier W. FFTrees: a toolbox to create, visualize, and evaluate fast-and-frugal decision trees. Judgm Decis Mak. 2017;12:344–68.
112. Wallis A, McCoubrie P. The radiology report-are we getting the message across? Clin Radiol. 2011;66:1015–22.
113. Berlin L, Murphy DR, Singh H. Breakdowns in communication of radiological findings: an ethical and medico-legal conundrum. Diagnosis. 2014;1:263–8.
114. Berlin L. Communicate all actionable findings now, not later. J Am Coll Radiol. 2014;11:924–5.
115. Berlin L. Medicolegal-malpractice and ethical issues in radiology. What is "reasonable assurance of receipt?". AJR. 2013;201:W159.
116. Harvey HB, Wu CC, Gilman MD, et al. Correlation of the strength of recommendations for additional imaging to adherence rate and diagnostic yield. J Am Coll Radiol. 2015;12:1016–22.
117. Alesawi HM, Kwee TC, Glaudemans AWJM, Yakar D. Recommendations in clinical 18F-fluoro-2-deoxy-D-glucose PET/CT reports: referring physicians' compliance and diagnostic yield. J Am Coll Radiol. 2018;15:1269–75.
118. Liao GJ, Liao JM, Lalevic D, Cook TS, Zafar HM. Time to talk: can radiologists improve follow-up of abdominal imaging findings indeterminate for malignancy by initiating verbal communication? J Am Coll Radiol. 2018;15:1627–32.
119. Berlin L. Malpractice issues in radiology. Pitfalls of the vague radiology report. AJR. 2000;174:1511–8.
120. Berlin L. Medical errors, malpractice, and defensive medicine: an ill-fated triad. Diagnosis. 2017;4:133–9.

Abstract

There are several factors that render all imaging professionals susceptible to committing errors. The emphasis of this chapter is on the cognitive limitations of individuals, specifically biases. In order to make decisions quickly we tend to simplify and speed up the intake and the processing of information. Thus we may lean heavily towards one finding or one diagnosis, even if we are misdirected and wrong. The result is that we disregard, downplay, or even reject a finding or a diagnosis, even if they are significant or correct. The two most important biases in imaging are "satisfaction of search" and "premature closing." Both of them are discussed in great detail in this chapter. Additional important biases are presented as well.

A discussion of errors would not be complete without an analysis of their causes, which I separate into extrinsic and intrinsic to the individual radiologist.

5.1 Extrinsic Sources of Errors

External factors include [1–10]:

a. A *vague or incomplete clinical history* on the request form,

b. A *non-supportive environment* due to noise, suboptimal lighting, frequent interruptions, or crowding of personnel,

c. *Very long shifts* or *excessive workload*,

d. *Not clearly defined roles* in the work place.

Further discussion of these elements is beyond the scope of this manuscript.

5.2 Internal Sources of Errors

I am particularly interested in the errors that can be traced directly to the mental faculties of the radiologist. The underlying causes are varied and quite complex, and I divide them into *mechanical* and *cognitive* groups [11]. We will address them in detail, especially the cognitive types, which frequently operate in a *stealth* mode.

5.2.1 Mechanical

The mechanical causes of errors can be attributed either:

- To our knowledge base [12–14],
- To improper preparation of our report, due to faulty dictation or superficial proof reading [15, 16].

5.2.1.1 Knowledge Base

We are required to be fluent (if not expert):

- In normal anatomy and its variants,
- In the pathophysiology and imaging manifestations of disease,
- In the intricacies of the radiologic techniques (physics, indications, limitations, and artifacts),
- In the proper and precise handling of the radiologic "language" (please see Chap. 4 for a treatise of this topic).

To this list we need to add an excellent command of radiological errors [17–19]. If our knowledge and thinking base are limited, then we are seriously handicapped and we become vulnerable to a multiplicity of errors on a frequent basis [13].

5.2.1.2 Report-Related Mechanical Faults

If we are not fully focused when reporting, *we may not say what we mean to say*. The result could be a laterality or an enumeration error.

- *Laterality errors* intrude when we inadvertently switch the side of the body that hosts the lesion, i.e., right versus left [1, 20]. If the error is propagated throughout the report, the patient is in danger of experiencing a serious complication, should he undergo an invasive procedure. If the correct side is mentioned at least once, then we can detect the discrepancy if we proof read carefully the entire report. Do not fall into the trap of looking only at the conclusion, in order to save time [15]. Obviously it is not sound practice to ask our colleagues to sign off our reports [15].
- *Enumeration errors* are similar to laterality errors. The incorrect size or the incorrect level of the finding is typed in the report (e.g., an L2 fracture erroneously stated as an L3 fracture).

All other possible errors in radiology reporting have been discussed in Chap. 4.

5.2.2 Cognitive

5.2.2.1 General Remarks

Cognitive traps are subtle, but have been elucidated in great detail [21–44]. They limit our ability to give an objective account of the imaging study, and I believe that they share common threads:

- Poor ability to examine and question our modes of thinking,
- Overconfidence or low confidence in our skills and knowledge,
- Subordination to authority or the "truth," i.e., the request form, a prior radiology report, or statistics,
- Emotional attachment to prior errors,
- Overinvestment in our self-image, instead of giving priority to the care of the patient.

In the discussion that follows, I elaborate on these themes and on related concepts.

5.2.2.2 Sensitivity Versus Specificity

We need to strike a delicate balance between sensitivity and specificity in our practice [45–47]. This decision is subjective and thus intrinsically imperfect. It is dictated by our level of knowledge, our skills, confidence, and tolerance for false positive and false negative results. We should choose our comfort zone and we should reevaluate it at regular time intervals.

Some radiologists tend to undercall, because they fear that they will lose credibility if they generate false positive studies. My personal bias is to overcall and request additional studies, when I am not sure about the *clinical significance* of a *definite lesion* or about the *existence* of a *significant lesion*. For example, let's consider a 50-year-old previously healthy patient, presenting with a solitary lung mass. Bronchoscopic biopsy reveals a primary lung carcinoma. There is no evidence of spread of disease to the abdomen, pelvis, skeleton, pleura, or intrathoracic lymph nodes. There is, however, a questionable focus of abnormal enhancement in the brain parenchyma on the initial staging CT scan of the head. In this setting I will definitely recommend further evaluation of the cranium with MRI, because I do not want to miss a brain metastasis.

On the contrary, in other cases I purposely downgrade findings, if I think that they will not add any value to the workup of the patient [48, 49].

5.2.2.3 Biases

Biases are tendencies of our cognitive functions to obey certain patterns that are not always productive. We may think of biases as filters that we use to process rapidly all the information we receive from the clinical history and the imaging examination(s). These filters provoke certain expectations, and we subsequently attempt to fulfill and verify those expectations. The various biases can keep us "locked" on a non relevant finding, a misdiagnosis, or a wrong diagnosis, forfeiting an objective interpretation. We will consider the most important and most common in our work [11, 18, 21–44, 50–53].

Satisfaction of Search Bias

This bias is defined as the failure to report at least one of multiple lesions, which coexist in a given imaging examination [18, 30–35, 42, 44]. The initial paradigm called for a single root cause, namely the "satisfaction" of the observer. In simple words, detecting a significant abnormality or an abnormality that explains the clinical diagnosis makes us "happy." Because we did a good job we let our guard down; either we terminate our search prematurely or we do not pay full attention to the rest of the study. This behavior runs the risk of overlooking additional lesions.

Multiple studies have clearly demonstrated a complex and multifactorial etiology for this phenomenon. Its unfolding depends on the relative strength of multiple elements, including [54, 55]:

a. The observer (incomplete visual search, partial recognition of the target, and decision errors),
b. The targets (size, borders, conspicuity, and similarity to each other), and
c. The features of the background that hosts the targets.

This bias is of outmost importance, so we need to keep it at the forefront of our awareness at all times. This bias is so strong that even a checklist may not protect us [56].

Premature Closure

If we arrest prematurely the formulation of a differential we may fail to include appropriate diagnoses [30, 42, 44]. Thus the correct diagnosis is not even considered as a remote possibility. This bias is also of extreme importance, not only to radiologists but to several other medical specialties as well. More details are provided in the Sect. 5.3, later in this chapter.

Aunt Minnie Bias

The Aunt Minnie trap is a special type of premature closure. When we think that we recognize a pattern, we rush to make the diagnosis that fits the pattern. Obviously if our pattern recall is faulty, or if our inventory of patterns is rudimentary, then our quick diagnosis rests on insecure grounds.

Conformity Bias or Alliterative Error

We are reluctant to challenge an established clinical or radiologic diagnosis, since we a priori accept them as the truth. Thus, even if the evidence in front of us suggests another condition, we repeat the diagnosis given to us (in the history or in a prior radiology report). Remember though that occasionally, the wrong diagnostic label is propagated for a long period of time, being replicated and strengthened with each visit to a physician or to a radiology department [42, 50, 53].

Availability Bias

The current situation can be distorted by our recent cognitive and emotional memory. For example, let's say that we recently missed a cancerous nodule on a chest radiograph. For a stretch of time, each subsequent chest radiograph will haunt us. We may recruit all of our faculties with the sole purpose of unmasking the hidden or the obvious nodule, whether the radiograph is normal or abnormal. The danger is that we overcall benign lesions and we ignore (or miss) other, significant lesions [27, 30, 44, 51].

Confirmation Bias

Sometimes we become heavily engaged in our initial impression, even if it is not correct. Our cognitive mechanisms will search for findings to support our initial hypothesis. Thus we ignore contradictory evidence that would eventually lead us to the correct diagnosis [27, 40, 41, 44].

Framing Bias

Our search and our decisions may be misdirected, if we are lured by the clinical information or the clinical question [27, 30, 44, 51]. The clinical history may act as a rigid limiting frame, rather than a malleable context. Tunnel vision and misguided anticipation are two special types of framing bias.

Tunnel Vision Bias

An unexpected finding may be completely ignored by our visual and cognitive faculties, if we focus too narrowly on confirming the history or the given clinical diagnosis. This fallacy calls that expected and unexpected findings cannot coexist [42]. This bias is related to inattentional blindness, which is presented in Chap. 1, under Sect. 1.4.

Inattentional Blindness

Inattentional blindness has been presented in Chap. 1. Briefly, it is a focal breakdown of visual perception that requires the simultaneous satisfaction of two conditions [44, 57–60]:

a. The missed finding, even though quite obvious, was *unexpected*, and
b. Our attention was funneled into another task or another finding.

Anticipation Bias

If we are alarmed by a strong or compelling history on the request form, then we feel pressured to find a lesion. If none exists, we may try to force a lesion into existence. I call this phenomenon the bias to satisfy the request.

Overload–Unload Bias

The tendency to pay less attention to the first and the last images in a cross-sectional study has been called the "extreme slice" phenomenon [53]. I will add that the same principle applies to individual organs as well, i.e., we spend relatively little time looking at the most cephalic and most caudal slices through the kidneys, etc. This type of reaction, which I call overload–unload bias, occurs in examinations that produce a large number of slices. My department has a 16 slice CT scanner. A routine, plain (without iv. contrast) abdominopelvic CT examination, including all reconstructions, exceeds 1000 images.[1] I routinely use four windows to view these CT scans: soft tissue, liver, bone, and lung. Because of information overload, we tend to disengage prematurely (unload) from one slice or one anatomic structure to proceed to another, and then we repeat the cycle until we complete the study. Thus, usually, a portion of the scan is not examined properly by our central vision, facilitating the entry of perception/detection errors.

Anchoring Bias

The first perceived finding that we deem significant becomes our pivot (our anchor) for subsequent decisions. Thus, our interpretation revolves around our anchor and we may neglect or we may underestimate the importance of other findings [30, 42, 44, 51].

Zebra Retreat

The word "zebra" in medicine refers to a rare disease or to a rare manifestation of a common disorder. The radiologist may reject his/her working diagnosis of a "zebra" because of the potential embarrassment if the "zebra" thesis is not validated [51]. Thus, the radiologist seeks shelter in a diagnosis that is statistically more robust than a "zebra."

Representativeness Bias

We feel comfortable with "classic" cases that fit all the criteria of a specific disease and we have difficulty considering or accepting atypical variants of the disease [43, 61]. However, the patients don't read our textbooks (unless they are physicians) and they are not obligated to fit the "classic" textbook description of their condition.

---

[1] 2D, 3D reconstructions and thin slice axial reconstructions from the raw data.

Overconfidence Bias

Inflation of the perception of our abilities clouds our judgment and blocks our growth [40, 41, 62]. This false sense of security leads straight to premature closure, confirmation, and anchoring biases. Furthermore, if we believe we are right, we do not seek help or additional knowledge, and we stagnate in our ignorance. This topic comes up again on Chap. 6, under Sect. 6.2.2.

Blind Spots

This topic has been presented in Chap. 3, under Sect. 3.4.

Prevalence Bias

The thoroughness and intensity of our visual search are proportional to our expectation of detecting a specific finding or a specific disease. Thus the prevalence of the disease we are investigating influences the outcome of our search [63–65]. Consider screening for breast cancer with mammography; the very nature of this task opposes the "search engine" of the mammographer [63–65].

Assumption and Disbelief Bias Regarding Foreign Bodies

The literature provides several examples of oversight of foreign bodies, even though they were in plain sight [42, 44, 66, 67]. Not all of these instances can be attributed to satisfaction of search or inattentional blindness, since they can go unnoticed on several occasions by multiple specialists. For example, a postoperative patient with a retained surgical instrument was presented in the hospital grand rounds to more than 20 physicians; however, not even one physician questioned the position of the obvious metal surgical instrument that "overlaid" the patient on his abdominal radiograph [42]. So I thought of a name for this bias, specifically "assumption and disbelief regarding foreign bodies." Let me explain: we assume that all surgical and medical operations/interventions proceed as per standard protocol. For example, no gauze or surgical instrument is left inside the patient, and any stents, tubes, central catheters, etc. are properly placed, and their good position has been verified. Sometimes we cannot believe that an injury was self-inflicted or that a serious mishap occurred during an intervention. Other times we have not seen before a particular foreign body in a particular location. Thus unconsciously we ignore the foreign body, unless: (a) we are vigilant and keep an "open mind," (b) the ordering physician raises the question of the presence of a foreign body, or (c) our attention is drawn to a lesion or a complication caused by the foreign body. An example of the latter would be a chicken bone in the midst of a mesenteric phlegmon, at the perforation site of a bowel loop. Sometimes we have to actively think of a foreign body and search deliberately for it, as the explanation of the abnormality. An example would be a palm tree thorn, broken off in the hand of a gardener who presents a couple of months later with chronic osteomyelitis and septic arthritis, yet having no immediate recollection of the implanted thorn.

Additional material about foreign bodies is presented in Chap. 7, under Sect. 7.2.3.

Please also look up related material under the Sect. 7.2.1.6 in Chap. 7.

Hindsight Bias

This bias is retrospective in nature, in contrast to the other biases described above. The hindsight bias refers to our tendency to ascribe a low degree of difficulty to a diagnosis, *after* it has been confirmed [44]. By succumbing to this bias we fall into two traps: first we dismiss the opportunity to learning from the case ("I knew it all along!") and second we hold judgment or other negative feelings toward our colleague that did not "nail" the diagnosis ("I can't believe he/she missed it!").

5.3 Interpretation Errors and Biases: Bringing It All Together

The phenomenon of "satisfaction of search" has been studied extensively at the viewing station (with native and artificial lesions) and in the laboratory [31–35, 54–56]. Simply stated, the detection of one lesion interferes with our ability to track down additional lesions, especially if there is no perceptual similarity between (among) them. For example, an obvious distal femoral fracture due to acute trauma may distract us from noticing an osteolytic focus in the proximal femur due to a metastasis. We need to be aware that this bias is a very important source of errors. For more information on this bias, please see Sect. 5.2.2.3 of this chapter.

Other biases have received limited attention in the radiology literature. On the contrary, multiple studies have unraveled the entry of biases in the daily work of other physicians, especially in primary care, internal medicine, and emergency medicine [68–75]. Thus, indirectly, we can gain valuable insight into the "mind" of radiologists.

The most frequent and significant causes of medical errors are due to the tendency of physicians to:

- Formulate preliminary diagnostic hypotheses *very early* in their encounter with patients,
- *Lock* onto these hypotheses until they exclaim their final diagnosis,
- *Experience difficulty* considering *alternative* or *additional* diagnoses, even when they get the opportunity to *reassess* all available information about the patient at a later date [40, 41, 68–70, 75].

Thus, only a *brief time window* is "open" to consider the correct diagnosis or the appropriate differential. This tight corridor of thought is reinforced with the recruitment of additional biases, in favor of the leading hypothesis, such as [68–70]:

- searching only for evidence that will confirm the leading hypothesis,
- under weighting critical cues that would steer one away from the leading, but incorrect hypothesis to a competing, but correct diagnosis,
- overweighing the status of neutral or noncritical evidence in order to dismiss the competing hypothesis, so as to remain within the confines of the initial or leading (but incorrect) hypothesis,
- settle for the statistically most common among the competing hypotheses, instead of choosing the best fit to the patient.

It is reasonable to assume that radiologists, at least early in their training, operate in a similar fashion, based on research in social and cognitive psychology [70]. This assumption carries the following conclusion, with far reaching implications: *multiple biases* hold a *strong grip* on *our diagnostic maps*, restricting our ability to "see" clearly and work in a methodical and thorough fashion.

Given the prevalence, strength, and diversity of biases, two more questions arise:

- Do we need debiasing techniques? We will deal extensively with this matter later, in Chap. 7.
- How much weight do we place on the clinical information we receive? The history provided on the request is filtered through the referring physician's biases, and it may be incomplete, vague, or inaccurate.

I favor expanding the request form to look like a mini medical report, providing information about the current complaint, past significant medical history, physical examination, relevant laboratory findings, prior imaging, and ending with a clinical impression. I feel this approach is particularly productive for patients who seek medical attention for the first time.

As an example, let's look at the request: "lung cancer-restaging and comparison with prior CT scan." In order to maximize the accuracy of the interpretation and the robustness of the report, additional information is needed, specifically what has transpired since the last CT scan. Has the patient undergone surgery, radiation, chemotherapy, embolization, or some type of tumor ablation? Is there clinical or laboratory evidence of recurrence, metastasis, or a complication of therapy? Does the patient have acute symptoms? Does the oncologist suspect an unrelated illness?

The radiologist who integrates appropriately the clinical, laboratory, and imaging data obtains a "bird's eye" view of the situation, and may be able to formulate a more accurate diagnosis (or differential), compared to the referring physician.

References

1. Busardo FP, Frati P, Santurro A, Zaami S, Fineschi V. Errors and malpractice lawsuits in radiology: what the radiologist needs to know. Radiol Med. 2015;120:779–84.
2. Berlin L. Medical errors, malpractice, and defensive medicine: an ill-fated triad. Diagnosis. 2017;4:133–9.
3. Berlin L. Liability of interpreting too many radiographs. AJR. 2000;175:17–22.
4. Berlin L. Medicolegal-malpractice and ethical issues in radiology: does interpreting too many radiologic studies increase the chance for error? AJR. 2013;201:W357.
5. Waite S, Kolla S, Jeudy J, et al. Tired in the reading room: the influence of fatigue in radiology. J Am Coll Radiol. 2017;14:191–7.
6. Krupinski EA, Berbaum KS, Caldwell RT, Schartz KM, Kim J. Long radiology workdays reduce detection and accommodation accuracy. J Am Coll Radiol. 2010;7:698–704.
7. Berlin L. Medicolegal-malpractice and ethical issues in radiology. Faster radiologic interpretation, errors, and malpractice: an unavoidable triad? AJR. 2018;210:W92–3.
8. Hanna TN, Zygmont ME, Peterson R, et al. The effects of fatigue from overnight shifts on radiology search patterns and diagnostic performance. J Am Coll Radiol. 2018;15:1709–16.
9. Hanna TN, Lamoureux C, Krupinski EA, Weber A, Johnson JO. Effect of shift, schedule, and volume on interpretive accuracy: a retrospective analysis 2.9 million radiologic examinations. Radiology. 2018;287:205–12.
10. Stec N, Arje D, Moody AR, Krupinski EA, Tyrrell PN. A systematic review of fatigue in radiology: is it a problem? AJR. 2018;210:799–806.
11. Renfrew DL, Franken EA Jr, Berbaum KS, Weigelt FH, Abu-Yousef MM. Error in radiology: classification and lessons in 182 cases presented at a problem case conference. Radiology. 1982;183:145–50.
12. European Society of Radiology (ESR). Good practice for radiological reporting. Guidelines from the European Society of Radiology (ESR). Insights Imaging. 2011;2:93–6.
13. Berlin L. Malpractice issues in radiology. Possessing ordinary knowledge. AJR. 1996;166:1027–9.
14. Halligan S. Subspecialist radiology. Clin Radiol. 2002;57:982–3.
15. Berlin L. Medicolegal-malpractice and ethical issues in radiology. Proofreading radiology reports. AJR. 2013;200:W691–2.
16. ACR Practice parameter for communication of diagnostic imaging findings. Revised 2014. www.acr.org/~/media/C5D1443C9EA4424AA12477D1AD1D927D.pdf.
17. Brady AP. Error and discrepancy in radiology: inevitable or avoidable? Insights Imaging. 2017;8:171–82.
18. Itri JN, Tappouni RR, McEachern RO, Pesch RO, Patel SH. Fundamentals of diagnostic error in imaging. Radiographics. 2018;38:1845–65.
19. Eberhardt SC, Heilbrun ME. Radiology report value equation. Radiographics. 2018;38:1888–96.
20. Sangwaiya MJ, Saini S, Blake MA, Dreyer KJ, Karla MK. Errare human est: frequency of laterality errors in radiology reports. AJR. 2009;192:W239–24.
21. Croskerry P. Clinical cognition and diagnostic error: applications of a dual process model of reasoning. Adv Health Sci Educ. 2009;14:27–35.
22. Kahneman D, Slovic P, Tversky A. Judgement under uncertainty: heuristics and biases. Cambridge: Cambridge University Press; 1982.
23. Kahneman D. Thinking fast and slow. New York: Farrar, Straus and Giroux; 2013.
24. Wallsten TS. Physician and medical student bias in evaluating diagnostic information. Med Decis Mak. 1981;1:145–64.
25. Elstein AS, Schwarz A. Clinical problem solving and diagnostic decision making: selective review of the cognitive literature. BMJ. 2002;324:729–32.
26. Gunderman RB, Sistrom C. Avoiding errors in reasoning: an introduction to logical fallacies. AJR. 2006;187:W469–71.
27. Gunderman RB. Biases in radiologic reasoning. AJR. 2009;192:561–4.
28. Koontz NA, Gunderman RB. Gestalt theory: implications for radiology education. AJR. 2008;190:1156–60.
29. Itri JN, Patel SH. Heuristics and cognitive error in medical imaging. AJR. 2018;210:1097–105.
30. Lee CS, Nagy PG, Weaver SJ, Newman-Toker DE. Cognitive and system factors contributing to diagnostic errors in radiology. AJR. 2013;201:611–7.
31. Berbaum KS, El-Khoury GY, Franken EA Jr, et al. Missed fractures resulting from satisfaction of search effect. Emerg Radiol. 1994;1:242–9.
32. Ashman CJ, Yu JS, Wolfman D. Satisfaction of search in osteoradiology. AJR. 2000;175:541–4.
33. Berbaum KS, Franken EA, Dorfman DD, Caldwell RT, Krupinski EA. Role of faulty decision making in the satisfaction of search effect in chest radiography. Acad Radiol. 2000;7(12):1098–106.
34. Samuel S, Kundel HL, Nodine CF, Toto LC. Mechanism of satisfaction of search: eye position recordings in the reading of chest radiographs. Radiology. 1995;94:895–902.
35. Berbaum KS, Schartz KM, Caldwell RT, et al. Satisfaction of search from detection of pulmonary nodules in computed tomography of the chest. Acad Radiol. 2013;20:194–201.
36. Croskerry P. The cognitive imperative: thinking about how we think. Acad Emerg Med. 2000;7:1223–31.
37. Berlin L. Malpractice issues in radiology. Outcome bias. AJR. 2004;183:557–60.

38. Berlin L. Malpractice issues in radiology. Alliterative bias. AJR. 2000;174:925–31.
39. Berlin L. Malpractice issues in radiology. Hindsight bias. AJR. 2000;175:597–601.
40. Berner ES, Graber ML. Overconfidence as a cause of diagnostic errors in medicine. Am J Med. 2008;121(5 Suppl):S2–S23.
41. Croskerry P, Norman G. Overconfidence in clinical decision making. Am J Med. 2008;121(5 Suppl):S24–9.
42. Jager G, Futterer JJ, Rutten M (2014) Cognitive errors in radiology: "thinking fast and slow". ECR 2014 poster C-0899. http://posterng.netkey.at/esr/viewing/index.php?module=viewing_poster&doi=10.1594/ecr2014/C-0899. Accessed 22 Feb 2019.
43. Norman G, Eva KW. Diagnostic error and clinical reasoning. Med Educ. 2010;44:94–100.
44. Busby LP, Courtier JL, Glastonbury CM. Bias in radiology: the how and why of misses and misinterpretations. Radiographics. 2018;38:236–47.
45. Gunderman RB, Nyce JM. The tyranny of accuracy in radiologic education. Radiology. 2002;222:297–300.
46. West RW. Radiology malpractice in the emergency room setting. Emerg Radiol. 2000;7:14–8.
47. Radiology written report guideline project. www.ranzcr.edu.au/resources/professional-documents/guidelines. Accessed 25 Oct 2016.
48. Hoang JK. Insignificant findings: don't leave them questioning the significance. J Am Coll Radiol. 2015;12.(Part A:1244.
49. Berlin L. Re: "Insignificant findings: Don't leave them questioning the significance". J Am Coll Radiol. 2016;13:363.
50. Bui-Mansfield LT. "Fool me twice": delayed diagnoses in radiology with emphasis on perpetuated errors. Video lecture. www.learning.arrs.org/course/view.php?id=518. Accessed 19 Nov 2017.
51. Bruno MA, Walker EA, Abujudeh HH. Understanding and confronting our mistakes: the epidemiology of error in radiology and strategies for error reduction. Radiographics. 2015;35:1668–76.
52. Berlin L. Radiologic errors, past, present and future. Diagnosis. 2014;1:79–84.
53. Kim YW, Mansfield LT. Fool me twice: delayed diagnoses in radiology with emphasis on perpetuated errors. AJR. 2014;202:465–70.
54. Cain MS, Mitroff SR. Memory for found targets interferes with subsequent performance in multiple in multiple-target visual search. J Exp Psychol Hum Percept Perform. 2013;39:1398–408.
55. Cain MS, Adamo SH, Mitroff SR. A taxonomy of errors in multiple-target visual search. Vis Cogn. 2013;21:899–921.
56. Berbaum KS, Krupinski EA, Schartz KM, et al. The influence of a vocalized checklist on detection of multiple abnormalities in chest radiography. Acad Radiol. 2016;23:413–20.
57. Wolfe JM, Evans KK, Drew T, Aizenman A, Josephs E. How do radiologists use the human search engine? Radiat Prot Dosim. 2016;169:24–31.
58. Drew T, Vo ML, Wolfe JM. The invisible gorilla strikes again: sustained inattentional blindness in expert observers. Psychol Sci. 2013;24:1848–53.
59. Simons DJ, Chabris CF. Gorillas in our midst: sustained inattentional blindness for dynamic events. Perception. 1999;28:1059–74.
60. Palazzetti V, Guidi F, Ottaviani L, Valeri G, Baldassarre S, Giusepetti GM. Analysis of mammographic diagnostic errors in breast clinics. Radiol Med. 2016;121:828–33.
61. Trowbridge RL. Twelve tips for teaching avoidance of diagnostic errors. Med Teach. 2008;30:496–500.
62. Kruger J, Dunning D. Unskilled and unaware of it: difficulties in recognizing one's own incompetence lead to inflated self-assessments. J Pers Soc Psychol. 1999;77:1121–34.
63. Evans KK, Birdwell RL, Wolfe JM. If you don't find it often, you often don't find it: why some cancers are missed in breast cancer screening. PLoS One. 2013;8:e64366.
64. Reed WM, Ryan JT, McEntee MF, Evanoff MG, Brennan PC. The effect of abnormality-prevalence expectation non expert observer performance and visual search. Radiology. 2011;258:938–43.
65. Wolfe JM, Horowitz TS, Van Wert MJ, Kenner NM, Place SS, Kibbi N. Low target prevalence is a stubborn source of errors in visual search tasks. J Exp Psychol Gen. 2007;136:623–8.
66. Lum TE, Fairbanks RJ, Pennington EC, Zwemer FL. Profiles in patient safety: misplaced femoral line guidewire and multiple failures to detect the foreign body on chest radiography. Acad Emerg Med. 2005;12:658–62.
67. Lee A, Lau K, Stuckey S. Case report. An endless line on the chest radiograph. BMJ Case Rep. 2014;2014:bcr2014204540.
68. Kostopoulou O. Diagnostic errors: psychological theories and research implications. In: Hurwitz B, Sheikh A, editors. Health care errors and patient safety. Hoboken: Blackwell Publishing; 2009. p. 97–111.
69. Kostopoulou O, Deveraux-Walsh C, Delaney BC. Missing celiac disease in family medicine: the importance of hypothesis generation. Med Decis Mak. 2009;29:282–90.
70. Kostopoulou O, Sirota M, Round T, Samaranayaka S, Delaney BC. The role of physician's first impressions in the diagnosis of possible cancers without alarm symptoms. Med Decis Mak. 2017;37:9–16.
71. Singh H, Giardina TD, Meyer AN, Reis MD, Thomas EJ. Types and origins of diagnostic errors in primary care settings. JAMA Intern Med. 2013;173:418–25.
72. Schiff GD, Hasan O, Kim S, et al. Diagnostic error in medicine: analysis of 583 physician-reported errors. Arch Intern Med. 2009;169:1881–7.

73. Ghandi TK, Kachalia A, Thomas EJ, et al. Missed and delayed diagnoses in the ambulatory setting: a study of closed malpractice claims. Ann Intern Med. 2006;145:488–96.

74. Okafor N, Payne VL, Chathampally Y, Miller S, Doshi P, Singh H. Using voluntary reports from physicians to learn from diagnostic errors in emergency medicine. Emerg Med J. 2016;33:245–52.

75. Graber ML, Franklin N, Gordon R. Diagnostic error in internal medicine. Arch Intern Med. 2005;165:1493–9.

Abstract

The current demands of medicine extend well beyond the diagnostic and therapeutic domains. Thus all physicians need to acquire a variety of dexterities in order to advance their practice. This chapter presents the related topics of expertise and competence. By "expertise" I mean the mastery of detection and interpretation skills". By "competence" I mean the mastery or a high level of operation of non-interpretive skills, such as team working, knowledge sharing and leadership. The focus of this chapter is expertise, what it is and how we achieve it, drawing on extensive knowledge from the fields of expertise, accelerated learning, and medical decision making.

6.1 General Remarks

In order to function as accomplished consultants, we need to attain (a) expertise in a subspecialty and (b) competency in several non-interpretive domains [1–26]. Thus, it is appropriate to introduce the topics of expertise and competency [2–26].

Gladwell popularized the notion that 10,000 hours of practice (on average) are sufficient to reach excellence [27]. This is true only in part, since *expertise is not guaranteed* after a certain *time threshold* [2–6]. A meta-analysis about general and specialist physicians reached a seemingly paradoxical conclusion [28]. We would expect that the accumulation of years of "experience" would improve the quality of health care. However, contrary to our assumptions, that study found that multiple metrics of *performance deteriorated* with *age* and with the *number of years in practice* [28].

It takes *a specific* type of *training*, *daily routine*, and *self-discipline* in order to climb from proficiency to truly extraordinary performance [6]. Furthermore, we are not doomed to professional stagnation or deterioration with advancing age. On the contrary, it is possible not only to sustain but also to continuously cultivate exceptional performance [6]. Ericsson, one of the pioneers researching this process, named it *deliberate practice* [2–6].

So, what is deliberate practice? Let's start by stating that there are *no substitutes* or *shortcuts* for hard work. Diligent practice needs to be *sustained* and *continuously refined* over *several years*, before one can achieve expert status. Of course, innate abilities are important contributors to the speed, degree, and natural ceiling of individual progress towards expertise [29, 30].

The purpose of deliberate practice is to improve the performance of the trainee, i.e., the *emphasis is* on *doing* and *thinking*, not on passive memorization or on passive consumption of information.

The features of deliberate practice are the following:

1. *Clearly defined goals* are *set* and subsequently *broken* into multiple *small milestones*, so that

© Springer Nature Switzerland AG 2020
H. Chrysikopoulos, *Errors in Imaging*, https://doi.org/10.1007/978-3-030-21103-5_6

it becomes easier for someone to progressively achieve those goals.

2. The trainee is gently asked to *push beyond his comfort zone*, so that he continuously elevates his baseline of operation.

3. *He repeats the appropriate task* over and over, *with purposeful, focused attention.*

4. *Proper feedback by the trainer* is of *paramount importance* to the success of the project. The feedback serves several functions:
   (a) To correct early on, any deviations from the desired path,
   (b) To motivate and support the efforts and labor of the trainee,
   (c) To identify any difficulties and suggest alternate approaches when a plateau persists,
   (d) To hold in place a mental framework so that the trainee can reflect on his practice and performance.

The *ultimate goal* of deliberate practice is for the trainee *to become autonomous*, and able to coach himself into greater and greater heights of performance. Indeed, there are physicians who can execute *positive* and *lasting* changes in their practice, via a self-directed process, called adaptive expertise. These individuals can leverage diagnostic challenges to acquire new knowledge, enrich their cognitive algorithms, and reflect upon their practice and habits. Furthermore, they can consciously transfer their knowledge and intellectual capacity to future problems [31].

I would like to quote a general definition of an expert physician, put forth by two medical educators: "Experts have extensive knowledge and use it effectively to address the tasks of daily practice. They know how to find additional knowledge using the resources available to them. When necessary, they are able to engage in innovative problem solving to construct new solutions to novel practice challenges. They often incorporate these new solutions into practice automatically as accrued experience, but are also able to reflect on these solutions and use the constructed knowledge to form a deeper understanding of their practice" [9].

It is worthwhile to note the following comments by Schön: "[The expert has] the ability to manage ambiguous problems, tolerate uncertainty, and make decisions with limited information" [32]. Epstein adds that "Competence… allows the practitioner to be attentive, curious, self-aware, and willing to recognize and correct errors" [33].

Let's continue with the perspective of a radiologist: "[The radiology expert has] disciplined strategy towards visual search, a wide knowledge base, the ability to use this knowledge to analyze the current situation and find recognisable patterns, a continuous upgrading of knowledge base, so that more and more cues are available for recall as new diagnostic challenges are met and finally to understand the context of the diagnostic exam, to know what to look for and why; at the same time keeping an open mind to unexpected or new findings" [34, 35].

Interpretation mastery and a solid knowledge base by themselves are no longer sufficient for professional strength. Individual authors and major organizations have argued for years that an expert achieves his full potential only when he engages successfully in non-interpretive activities, called competences or roles [15–26, 36, 37]. Examples include team working, knowledge sharing, and leadership. The core physician's competences as defined by the ACGME and CanMEDS are highlighted in Tables 6.1 and 6.2 [15, 17, 18].

In a key paper, Epstein and Hundert defined professional competence as "the habitual and judicious use of communication, knowledge, technical skills, clinical reasoning, emotions, values, and reflection in daily practice for the benefit of the individual and community being served" [21].

Table 6.1 ACGME[a] core competencies

- Patient care
- Medical knowledge
- Interpersonal and communication skills
- Professionalism
- Practice-based learning and improvement
- Systems-based practice

[a]Accreditation Council for Graduate Medical Education

Table 6.2 CanMEDS[a] roles

• Medical expert
• Communicator
• Collaborator
• Leader
• Health advocate
• Scholar
• Professional

[a]Canadian Medical Education Directives for Specialists

My own *definition* of *competence* is: *competence is the capability of the physician to satisfy his/her duties toward his/her patients and his/her colleagues with integrity, consistency, efficiency, and professionalism.*

Competence, like expertise, is achieved with diligent practice and is valued relative to the individual's professional status or level of training.

Further discussion of this topic is not relevant to the scope of this manuscript. The framework, benefits, knowledge, skills, attitudes, milestones, and assessments for each of the required competency domains have been described in detail. The interested reader is referred to the literature for further study [15–26].

6.2   How Do We Achieve Expertise in Radiology?

From now on, the term "expertise" implies expertise in detection and interpretation. No discussion of expertise would be complete without considering the topics of decision making and learning. Both of these subjects are inextricably linked to mastery.

6.2.1   Medical Decision Making (MDM)

The accepted theory of MDM invokes two cognitive modes of operation: a fast, intuitive, or system 1, and a slow, deliberate, or system 2 [38–41]. The first one relies on pattern recognition and pattern retrieval from our mental archive, thus it takes very little time. The second one employs thoughtful, effortful problem solving, and is the appropriate strategy for difficult, complex, or unknown cases.

Some cases require dynamic oscillation between the two systems. All physicians, novices, and experienced activate and operate this dual processing model of diagnostic reasoning.

Some authors believe that what separates the experts from the novices is the quality of the diagnostic hypotheses they can articulate. "In short, expertise resides in content knowledge, not in [cognitive] process" [41].

I do not agree with this conclusion and I can tell you my own experience. At the end of residency my head was full of loosely interconnected bits and chunks of information, like pieces of a giant puzzle. I had difficulty linking the relevant information and separating my thoughts into discrete modules. At that time my diagnostic reasoning was heavily dependent on recognition of rudimentary imaging patterns. My problem solving was slow, shallow, fragmented, and laden with biases. Prompted by regular feedback from my mentor and colleagues, I started reflecting upon my gaps, mistakes, and omissions. Slowly, over time, I constructed mental loops to recognize and avoid errors. The loops were refined with each pass, and gradually they enlarged to encompass blind spots, biases, and radiologic reports. For example, knowing what to look for sharpened my perception [38]. Conversely, finding what I was looking for reinforced this noble feedback cycle and confirmed its power. The validity of this form of learning has been firmly established by educators and psychologists [31, 32, 42, 43]. Numerous authors support my experience, noting both quantitative and qualitative gains in knowledge and cognitive organization, complexity, and flexibility, as one progresses to expertise [5, 13, 21, 44–47]. Multiple studies in real life situations have proven the superior performance of accomplished radiologists relative to trainees [47–58].

I do not have numbers or statistics to prove it, but it is clear to me that over the course of about 25 years, I have refined my diagnostic acumen, the accuracy of my differential lists, and the sharpness of my reports and recommendations. These improvements have compounded slowly over time, as a result of continuous reading, learning, thinking and asking.

Brown et al. have concluded that "Mastery… is a gradual accretion of knowledge, conceptual understanding, judgment and skill. These are the fruits of … the practice of new skills, and of striving, reflection, and mental rehearsal" [46, p. 18].

6.2.2 Accelerated Learning

Learning specialists have brought forward several modes of learning that are superior to the traditional methods, such as [46, 59–62]:

- Retrieval
- Elaboration
- Mixed practice over blocked practice
- Distributed and interleaved practice over massed practice
- Desirable difficulty
- Assessment and feedback

Retrieval is the recollection of new material from memory, as opposed to revisiting the original source of the material. For example, suppose we just finished reading a text. What is more beneficial for our learning? Taking a quiz or rereading the text? Retrieval practice, especially if periodic, arrests the forgetting curve, enhances retrieval networks, and facilitates data storage in long-term memory, for future use upon demand. "Cramming," i.e., rereading the same book or the same notes within a short time period, is a poor learning strategy.

Elaboration is the *active* deconstruction and reassembly of new information so that we can *explain* it to somebody else, using our *own* words (instead of passively regurgitating the material via rote memorization). Elaboration is especially strong if we link the new information to prior knowledge. An example would be an oral presentation on the MRI appearance of acute cerebral ischemic infarction, provided that: the topic is new knowledge for us, we know the pathophysiology of ischemic cerebral infarction, we know its CT appearance, we do not read off our notes, and we do not read verbatim what we display on the slides.

Another facet of the elaboration principle is to connect our home study, as much as possible, to cases that we have encountered at work.

Mixed practice consists of studying "a series of cases side by side where two factors are engineered - different presentations of the same diagnosis and similar presentations of different diagnoses. In this manner, the clinician would learn those features or aspects of the case that discriminate among different conditions." On the other hand, in *blocked* practice "one sees examples of one condition, then examples of another one, and so on" [59]. Thus, blocked practice activates the memorization but not the discrimination circuits, and is clearly inferior to mixed practice as a learning modality.

In *distributed* practice, teaching is delivered in blocks, spread out in time. Interleaving means switching from one subject or skill to another, even before the trainee has a chance to master the new material or the new skill. On the contrary, in *massed* practice all teaching is concentrated in one session. "Mass" practitioners are rewarded with steep learning at the end of the mass session, but are "punished" with steep forgetting, soon after the session is over. "Practice that's spaced out, interleaved with other learning, and varied produces better mastery, longer retention and more versatility" [46, p. 47]. [Another] "significant advantage of interleaving and variation is that they help us learn better how to assess context and discriminate between problems, selecting and applying the correct solution from a range of possibilities" [46].

Solid and meaningful learning requires *effort* when confronted with a new or a difficult task. The Diagnosis Please (DXP) cases in *Radiology* are examples of *desirable difficulty* practice [63]. I elaborate on the benefits of DXP cases in Sect. 6.2.3.2 of this chapter. In my opinion, multiple choice questions (MCQ) are a counterproductive strategy. I get to say more about MCQs in the Epilogue.

Assessment/Feedback: Many of us are poor judges of our learning, our standing, and our limitations, i.e., we do not know what we do not know [46, 64–66]. As a matter of fact, the physicians with limited experience and truncated knowledge are the ones who predictably overrate their diagnostic abilities. Even experienced physicians can be wrong occasionally, despite superb knowledge and a high degree of confidence in their diagnosis (regardless of whether the diagnosis is correct or not). Thus all of us need some form of calibration and external feedback, such as standardized tests, morbidity and mortality conferences, peer review, or informal talks with mentors and colleagues.

My conclusions for optimal home study are to:

- Approach each organ via imaging patterns; study specific diseases at a later date
- Explore all possible variations and manifestations of a single disease entity
- Cross-study the spectrum of diseases than can occur in a single anatomic compartment (e.g., study all tumors that can occur in the anterior mediastinum)
- Study clinical problems (instead of individual diseases), such as acute abdominal pain in the right lower quadrant in adults. This way you think about different diseases that produce similar symptoms and signs, and you learn how to differentiate them.
- Avoid multiple choice formats (see the Epilogue)

I am certain that the skills and knowledge gained via the above suggestions will prove very valuable in real life situations. Numerous books, pictorial essays, and review articles serve as excellent vehicles for this type of training [67–112].

6.2.3   The Author's Proposals to Radiology Residents for Accelerated Learning

Since we have accumulated precious knowledge about learning, teaching, expertise, errors, and diagnostic reasoning, I believe that we can trace the most efficient path from novice to expert status [1, 2, 5, 12, 13, 30, 31, 33, 59–62, 64, 113–127].

My suggestions are interrelated and reinforce each other. They are designed for radiology resi-

dents, to enhance knowledge and skills accrued at the viewing station. However, they should serve as guidelines, not as a rigid sequence.

6.2.3.1   Initial Steps
In my opinion the two most important actions in the first 6–9 months of residency are:

1. Establishing appropriate habits, including the deliberate practice of visual search, perception, interpretation, reporting, and asking for feedback.
2. Gaining proficiency in the diagnosis of emergencies, such as acute abdomen, trauma, and stroke [128].

Let's Expand on These

- Allocate adequate time for each study; don't rush [129, 130]. Look at the entire image including its corners. Use checklists to ensure thoroughness of visual search. Learn to spot the lesion, to separate normal from abnormal, and to recognize normal variants as such. Being able to recite a ten item differential list becomes irrelevant if we miss the lesion. After completing the search, group all relevant items together and prioritize them in order of clinical significance. Think of any pertinent positive or negative findings that are missing from your list, and if so, go back to the images and look for them [131, 132]. This feedback loop gets you in the habit of asking what the clinician needs to know. Do not attempt to formulate diagnostic candidates before exhausting the search phase. This discipline will keep you away from pseudo Aunt Minnie patterns.
- Become conscious of "radiologic language." It is premature to consider a diagnosis or a differential before describing the findings with the proper vocabulary [133–147].
- I consider these two actions, gathering and describing the findings (in a proper way), equivalent to taking a careful history and performing a thorough physical examination on a patient. You may find these steps time consuming, but they offer protection against vari-

ous errors and biases, especially satisfaction of search and premature closure.

- Formulate wide differential diagnoses, in other words keep an "open" mind, in order to avoid the bias of premature closure. Subsequently, by exclusion, narrow the differential as much as possible.
- Engage with clinical colleagues and attend their conferences to learn their "language" and what they need to know from the radiologists [148–160]. This way you can direct your search on target and construct your report with clarity and specificity.
- Use structured reports with checklists and blind spot reminders. Scrutinize the reports for their content and for errors in spelling, laterality, enumeration, or measurements.
- Ask senior radiologists and clinical colleagues for feedback. Feedback is one of the most important factors for progress.

Accelerated Learning of Imaging Signs and Patterns

I believe there is a way to build quickly our mental archive of normal and abnormal: *focus on the images* instead of the text. First study and "absorb" the figures in books, teaching files, and journal articles; then read the captions of the figures. Postpone thorough reading of the main text for a later date. The benefit of this approach is a fast and compact exposure to a variety of signs and patterns. Remember to study diseases not in isolation, but in the context of their differential, i.e., engage the principles of mixed practice [46, 59]. Please revisit the suggestions for optimal home study, in Sect. 6.2.2 of this chapter.

Think Out of the Box!

There is no reason to limit ourselves to medical resources. Some medical educators call for "different ways of knowing" [25]. For example, several years ago, Braverman, a Professor of Dermatology at Yale University, conceived a novel idea: he used works of fine art as a vehicle for teaching medical students the craft of perception and communication [161]. A recent study has confirmed the benefit of this activity on nov-

ice radiology residents [162]. Herman, a lawyer and an art historian, has expanded the scope of Braverman's work. She has devised a specialty course, the core of which is held live, in Fine Arts Museums (www.artfulperception.com). Her method has been adopted by several medical schools, both in Europe and in the USA (www.artfulperception.com/participants.php).

6.2.3.2 Intermediate Steps

- After approximately 9–12 months I think it is appropriate to study in depth *normal variants, errors, biases, pitfalls, blind spots, and "do not touch lesions."* These topics were addressed in detail in several excellent sources [131, 149, 163–286].
- After 1.5–2 years concentrate on broadening your knowledge and sharpening your judgment. I propose the following actions:
  - Select a few cases from the daily workload for detailed study via review articles, standard textbooks, teaching files, and dedicated websites. Pay considerable attention to images of the differential diagnostic possibilities [59]. Introductory textbooks on a subspecialty should be read from cover to cover during the rotation in that subspecialty. Once you have mastered the requisites, you can proceed to more detailed treatises as needed.
  - Practice the drills "*what does the clinician need to know?*," "*what can I not afford to miss?*," "*what could it be?*," and "*what else could it be?*" The first question is addressed throughout Chap. 4. The other questions are addressed in detail in Chap. 7, Sects. 7.2.1.4 and 7.2.1.5.
  - Practice thinking of *causes and complications* [129, 131, 235, 236, 244, 287–300]. For example, the detection of otomastoiditis should become a reflex for evaluating the nasopharynx. The reverse should also hold: a thickened nasopharynx should prompt a search for otomastoiditis, in addition to searching for local invasion and lymphadenopathy. For a more detailed explanation of these concepts, please Chap. 7, under the Sect. 7.2.1.6.

- Be alert for the possibility of
  - Subtle *bilateral or symmetric* abnormalities [131, 188, 301] and
  - *Absence or displacement* of structures [131, 237].
- Practice narrowing a wide differential to a few candidates, arranged in order of likelihood, keeping in mind the clinical setting and potential biases [302].
- Attend clinicopathologic conferences and visit teaching files of proven cases, both of which are powerful sources of immediate feedback.
- Allow room for *uncertainty*, which permeates our work every single day [1, 163, 177]. We may have trouble accepting uncertainty, since in our training we develop "a false expectation that *every* case has a correct answer, in light of which all other answers are more or less wrong." [303]. Furthermore, we desire to know the right answer right away. Instead, we may have to wait a long time, even years, before we get confirmation of our diagnosis [304]. Sometimes we just never find out. Thus "Doctors need to be prepared to work amid uncertainty and complexity. This calls upon their professional judgment, which is their specific expertise" [305]. Gawande, a surgeon, remarks that "We look for medicine to be an orderly field of knowledge and procedure. But it is not. It is an imperfect science, an enterprise of constantly changing knowledge, uncertain information, fallible individuals, and at the same time lives on the line" [306].
- Tackle the *Diagnosis Please (DXP) cases* in the journal *Radiology* [63]. I have found that these cases are powerful exercises on multiple cognitive levels. The first and most obvious benefit is that we have to *commit* to a single answer; *hedging* is *not* an option. We can arrive at the correct answer only if we integrate appropriately the clinical, laboratory, and imaging data. Difficult DXP cases serve to stretch our limits and to mobilize all of our resource-

fulness and creativity. These cases also test our patience, persistence, and flexibility. If our initial diagnostic attempt is not productive, we have to be willing to abandon our initial hypothesis and consider alternate routes [307]. Eventually we may go through multiple trials before we reach our limits or before we lock on to the correct diagnosis. Furthermore, we have to bear uncertainty for a few months, before the publication of the answer. The detailed discussion of the case provides valuable feedback for self-reflection.

- Volunteer to *give oral presentations* on topics of your choice during noon or afternoon conferences. Allow time for discussion, questions, answers, and feedback on the quality of your presentations. This way one achieves mini expertise on a topic, which is a strong boost to his/her self-confidence.
- *Assess your progress and weaknesses* at regular time intervals. Ask mentors and senior colleagues for guidance.
- Engage in a *research project* that will result in a *publication* [308–311]. I view research as an explicit, well-defined variant of what we do implicitly at the viewing station every day: collection, analysis, and synthesis of data in order to reach a conclusion. Furthermore, a research project is an excellent opportunity to: (a) practice collaboration, time management, communication, and self-expression, and (b) learn how to critically evaluate the medical literature. Of course, the contribution of new knowledge has a positive impact both for the individual and the greater medical community.

6.2.3.3 Final Steps (Fellowship or Last Year of Residency)

- Choose a subspecialty: true expertise can be achieved only when we narrow our practice to a particular subsection of radiology [176, 177, 312]. Dedication to a subspecialty affords repeated exposure to the same clinical problems, greater depth of knowledge, security in interpreting the relevant imaging studies, and ultimately, superb confidence and efficacy in our role as consultants.

- Work on your weak areas. Cover any gaps in required knowledge and skills with teaching files, interactive workshops, and textbooks.
- Continue the practices of prior stages.

References

1. Gunderman RB, Nyce JM. The tyranny of accuracy in radiologic education. Radiology. 2002;222:297–300.
2. Ericsson KA, editor. The road to excellence: the acquisition of expert performance in arts, sciences, sports and games. Hillsdale: Lawrence Erlbaum Associates; 1996.
3. Ericsson KA. Deliberate practice and the acquisition and maintenance of expert performance in medicine and related domains. Acad Med. 2004;79:S70–81.
4. Ericsson KA, Prietula MJ, Cokely ET. The making of an expert. Harv Bus Rev. 2007;85:114–21.
5. Ericsson KA. Acquisition and maintenance of medical expertise: a perspective from the expert-performance approach with deliberate practice. Acad Med. 2015;90:1471–86.
6. Ericsson KA, Pool R. Peak: secrets from the new science of expertise. New York: Houghton Mifflin Harcourt Publishing; 2016.
7. Mylopoulos M, Lohfeld M, Norman GR, Dhaliwal G, Eva KW. Renowned physicians' perceptions of expert diagnostic practice. Acad Med. 2012;87:1413–7.
8. Mylopoulos M, Regehr G, Ginsburg S. Exploring residents' perceptions of expertise and expert development. Acad Med. 2011;86:S46–9.
9. Mylopoulos M, Regehr G. Putting the expert together again. Med Educ. 2011;45:920–6.
10. Sargeant J, Mann K, Sinclair D, et al. Learning in practice: experiences and perceptions of high-scoring physicians. Acad Med. 2006;81:655–60.
11. Duncan JR, Beta E. Predicting system performance. In: Abujudeh HH, Bruno MA, editors. Quality and safety in radiology. New York: Oxford University Press; 2012. p. 184–95.
12. Gobet F. Understanding expertise: a multidisciplinary approach. London: Palgrave Macmillan; 2015.
13. Chi MTH, Glaser R, Farr MJ. The nature of expertise. Hillsdale: Lawrence Erlbaum Associates; 1988.
14. Accreditation Council for Graduate Medical Education (ACGME). Program requirements for graduate medical education in diagnostic radiology. Revised and effective July 1, 2016. https://cdn.ymaws.com/www.aocr.org/resource/resmgr/E2S/diagnostic_radiology_effect.pdf. Accessed 18 Jan 2018
15. The American Board of Radiology. Noninterpretive skills resource guide 2017. www.theabr.org/sites/all/themes/abr-media/pdf/Noninterpretive_Skills_Domain_Specification_and_resource_Guide.pdf. Accessed 18 Jan 2018.
16. The diagnostic radiology milestone project. 2015 July. https://www.acgme.org/Portals/0/PDFs/Milestones/DiagnosticRadiologyMilestones.pdf. Accessed 18 Jan 2018.
17. Frank JR, Snell L, Sherbino J, editors. CanMEDS 2015 physician competency framework. Ottawa: Royal College of Physicians and Surgeons of Canada; 2015.
18. CanMEDS 2015 OTR special addendum. https://Canmeds.royalcollege.ca/uploads/en/framework/CanMEDS%202015%20OTR_Special_ Addendum_EN.PDF. Accessed 18 Jan 2018.
19. Specialty training curriculum for clinical radiology. The Faculty of Clinical Radiology, The Royal College of Radiologists, 13 November 2015, London UK. https://gmc-uk.org/CR_Curriculum_2015_FINAL_approved_13_Nov_15.pdf_63900516.pdf. Accessed 18 Jan 2018.
20. Standards of practice for diagnostic and interventional radiology. Version 10.2-2017. The Royal Australian and New Zealand College of Radiologists, The Faculty of Clinical Radiology. file:///D:/My%20Files/Downloads/RANZCR%20Standards%20V10.2.pdf. Accessed 18 Jan 2018.
21. Epstein RM, Hundert EM. Defining and assessing professional competence. JAMA. 2002;287:226–35.
22. Lum A, Zaeski W. Curriculum matters! Designing curriculum for radiology resident rotations. In: Van Deven T, Hibbert KM, Chhem RK, editors. The practice of radiology education: challenges and trends. Heidelberg: Springer; 2010. p. 11–25.
23. Finley K, Probyn L. Applying CanMEDS to academic afternoons. In: VanDeven T, Hibbert KM, Chhem RK, editors. The practice of radiology education: challenges and trends. Heidelberg: Springer; 2010. p. 27–55.
24. Engel-Hills P, Chhem RK. The nature of professional expertise. In: Hibbert KM, Chhem RK, van Deven T, Wang SC, editors. Radiology education: the evaluation and assessment of clinical competence. Heidelberg: Springer; 2012. p. 3–9.
25. Hibbert KM, van Deven T, Ros S. Fundamentals of assessment and evaluation: clarifying terminology. In: Hibbert KM, Chhem RK, van Deven T, Wang SC, editors. Radiology education: the evaluation and assessment of clinical competence. Heidelberg: Springer; 2012. p. 11–9.
26. Hibbert KM, Chhem RK. Competence in the professions: expanding opportunities and emerging practices. In: Hibbert KM, Chhem RK, van Deven T, Wang SC, editors. Radiology education: the evaluation and assessment of clinical competence. Heidelberg: Springer; 2012. p. 21–8.
27. Gladwell M. Outliers: the story of success. New York: Little Brown and Company; 2008.
28. Choudhry NK, Fletcher RH, Soumerai SB. Systematic review: the relationship between clinical experience and quality of health care. Ann Intern Med. 2005;142(4):260–73.

29. Hambrick DZ, Oswald FL, Altman EM, Meinz EZ, Gobet F, Campitelli G. Deliberate practice: is that all it takes to become an expert? Intelligence. 2014;45:34–45.

30. Kulasegaram KM, Grierson LM, Norman GR. The roles of deliberate practice and innate ability in developing expertise: evidence and implications. Med Educ. 2013;47:979–89.

31. Regehr GR, Mylopoulos M. Maintaining competence in the field: learning about practice, through practice, in practice. J Contin Educ Heal Prof. 2008;28(suppl):S19–23.

32. Schon DA. The reflective practitioner. New York: Basic Books; 1983.

33. Epstein RM. Mindful practice. JAMA. 1999;282:833–9.

34. Robinson PJ. Radiology's Achilles' heel: error and variation in the interpretation of the roentgen image. Br J Radiol. 1997;70:1085–98.

35. Sabih D-E, Sabih A, Sabih Q, Khan AN. Image perception and interpretation of abnormalities; can we believe our eyes? Can we do something about it? Insights Imaging. 2011;2:47–55.

36. European Society of Radiology (ESR). ESR communication guidelines for radiologists. Insights Imaging. 2013;4:143–6.

37. Gunderman R, Chan S. Knowledge sharing in radiology. Radiology. 2003;229:314–7.

38. Bordage G. Why did I miss the diagnosis? Some cognitive explanations and educational implications. Acad Med. 1999;74(Suppl 10):S138–43.

39. Croskerry P. A universal model of diagnostic reasoning. Acad Med. 2009;84:1022–8.

40. Croskerry P. Clinical cognition and diagnostic error: applications of a dual process model of reasoning. Adv Health Sci Educ. 2009;14:27–35.

41. Monteiro SM, Norman G. Diagnostic reasoning: where we've been, where we're going. Teach Learn Med. 2013;25(suppl 1):S26–32.

42. Dewey J. How we think: a restatement of the relation of reflective thinking to the educative process. Sunnyvale: Loki's Publishing; 2017.

43. Kolb DA. Experiential learning: experience as the source of learning and development. 2nd ed. Upper Saddle River: Pearson Education; 2015.

44. Alexander PA. The development of expertise: the journey from acclimation to proficiency. Educ Res. 2003;32:10–4.

45. Alexander PA. Model of domain learning: validity for physicians. Personal communication. 2016 Nov 9.

46. Brown PC, Roediger HL III, McDaniel MA. Make it stick: the science of successful learning. Cambridge: The Belknap Press of Harvard University Press; 2014. p. 18.

47. Funaki B, Szymski G, Rosenblum J. Significant on-call misses by radiology residents interpreting computed tomographic studies: perception versus cognition. Emerg Radiol. 1997;4:290–4.

48. Itri JN, Kang HC, Krishnan S, Nathan D, Scanlon MH. Using focused missed-case conferences to reduce discrepancies in musculoskeletal studies interpreted by residents on call. AJR. 2011;197:W696–705.

49. Bruni S, Bartlett E, Yu E. Factors involved in discrepant preliminary radiology resident interpretations of neuroradiologic imaging studies: a retrospective analysis. AJR. 2012;198:1367–74.

50. Taylor SA, Halligan S, Burling D, et al. CT colonography: effects of experience and training on reader performance. Eur Radiol. 2004;14:1025–33.

51. Hillier JC, Tattersall DJ, Gleeson FV. Trainee reporting of computed tomography examinations: do they make mistakes and does it matter? Clin Radiol. 2004;59:159–62.

52. Filippi CG, Schneider B, Burbank HN, Alsofrom GF, Linnell G, Ratkovits B. Discrepancy rates of radiology resident interpretations of on-call neuroradiology MR imaging studies. Radiology. 2008;249:972–9.

53. Lal NR, Murray UM, Eldevik OP, Desmond JS. Clinical consequences of misinterpretations of neurologic CT scans by on-call radiology residents. AJNR. 2000;21:124–9.

54. Meyer RE, Nickerson JP, Burbank HP, Alsofrom GF, Linnell GJ, Filippi CG. Discrepancy rates of on-call radiology residents' interpretation of CT angiography studies of the neck and circle of Willis. AJR. 2009;193:527–32.

55. Le AH, Licurse A, Catanzano TM. Interpretation of head CT scans in the emergency department by fellows versus general staff non-neuroradiologists: a closer look at the effectiveness of a quality control program. Emerg Radiol. 2007;14:311–6.

56. Erly WK, Berger WG, Krupinski E, Seeger JF, Guisto JA. Radiology resident evaluation of head CT scan orders in the emergency department. AJNR. 2002;23:103–7.

57. Wechsler RJ, Spettell CM, Kurtz AB, et al. Effects of training and experience in interpretation of emergency body CT scans. Radiology. 1996;199:717–20.

58. Williams SM, Connelly DJ, Wadsworth S, Wilson DJ. Radiological review of accident and emergency radiographs: a 1-year audit. Clin Radiol. 2000;55:861–5.

59. Norman G, Eva KW. Diagnostic error and clinical reasoning. Med Educ. 2010;44:94–100.

60. Oakley B. A mind for numbers: how to excel at math and science (even if you flunked algebra). New York: Jeremy P. Tarcher/Penguin; 2014.

61. Thalheimer W. The decisive dozen: research background abridged. http://willthalheimer.typepad.com/files/decisive-dozen-research-v1.2.pdf. Accessed 8 Nov 2016.

62. Kohn A. Brain science: overcoming the forgetting curve. 2014 Apr 10. https://www.learningsolutions-mag.com/articles/1400/brain-science-the-forgetting-curve. Accessed 18 Nov 2016.

63. Diagnosis Please. DXP. http://dxp.rsna.org.

64. Berner ES, Graber ML. Overconfidence as a cause of diagnostic errors in medicine. Am J Med. 2008;121(5 Suppl):S2–S23.

65. Croskerry P, Norman G. Overconfidence in clinical decision making. Am J Med. 2008;121(5 Suppl):S24–9.
66. Friedman CP, Gatti GG, Franz TM, et al. Do physicians know when their diagnoses are correct? Implications for decision support and error reduction. J Gen Intern Med. 2005;20:334–9.
67. Wittenberg J, Harisinghami MK, Jhaveri K, Varghese J, Mueller PR. Algorithmic approach to CT diagnosis of the abnormal bowel wall. Radiographics. 2002;22:1093–109.
68. Villanova JC, Barcelo J, Smirniotopoulos JG, Perez-Andres R, et al. Hemangioma from head to toe: MR imaging with pathologic correlation. Radiographics. 2004;24:367–85.
69. Nasseri F, Eftekhari F. Clinical and radiologic review of the normal and abnormal thymus: pearls and pitfalls. Radiographics. 2010;30:413–28.
70. Nishino M, Ashiku SK, Kocher OK, Thurer RL, Boiselle PM, Hatabu H. The thymus: a comprehensive review. Radiographics. 2006;26:335–48.
71. Juanpere S, Canete N, Ortuno P, Martinez S, Sanchez G, Bernado L. A diagnostic approach to the mediastinal masses. Insights Imaging. 2013;4:29–52.
72. Tomiyama N, Honda O, Tsubamoto M, et al. Anterior mediastinal tumors: diagnostic accuracy of CT and MRI. Eur J Radiol. 2009;69:280–8.
73. Yeung MY, Gasser B, Gangi A, et al. Imaging of cystic masses of the mediastinum. Radiographics. 2002;22:S79–93.
74. Brancatelli G, Vilgrain V, Federle MP, et al. Budd-Chiari syndrome; spectrum of imaging findings. AJR. 2007;188:W188–76.
75. Blachar A, Federle MP, Brancatelli G. Hepatic capsular retraction: spectrum of benign and malignant etiologies. Abdom Imaging. 2002;27:690–9.
76. Rumboldt Z, Castillo M, Huang B, Rossi A, editors. Brain imaging with MRI and CT: an image pattern approach. New York: Cambridge University Press; 2012.
77. Yock DH Jr. Magnetic resonance imaging of CNS disease: a teaching file. 2nd ed. St. Louis: Mosby; 2002.
78. Reed JC. Chest radiology: plain film patterns and differential diagnoses, expert consult, online and print. 6th ed. Philadelphia: Elsevier Mosby; 2011.
79. Levine SM, Lambiase RE, Petchprapa CN. Cortical lesions of the tibia: characteristic appearances at conventional radiography. Radiographics. 2003;23:157–77.
80. Resnick D. Tumors and tumor-like lesions of bone: routine radiographic abnormalities. In: Resnick D, Petterson H, editors. Skeletal radiology, NICER series on diagnostic imaging. London: Merit Communications; 1992. p. 278–90.
81. Mittal PK, Little B, Harri PA, et al. Role of imaging in the evaluation of male infertility. Radiographics. 2017;37:837–54.
82. Raptis CA, Sridhar S, Thompson RW, Fowler KJ, Bhalla S. Imaging of the patient with thoracic outlet syndrome. Radiographics. 2016;36:984–1000.
83. Ditkofsky N, Singh A. Challenges in magnetic resonance imaging for suspected acute appendicitis in pregnant patients. Curr Probl Diagn Radiol. 2015;44:297–302.
84. Chang PT, Schooler GR, Lee EY. Diagnostic errors of right lower quadrant pain in children: beyond appendicitis. Abdom Imaging. 2015;40:2071–90.
85. Casciani E, De Vincentiis C, Mazzei MA, et al. Errors in imaging the pregnant patient with acute abdomen. Abdom Imaging. 2015;40:2112–26.
86. Hegazi TM, Belair JA, McCarthy EJ, Roedl JB, Morrison WB. Sports injuries around the hip: what the radiologist should know. Radiographics. 2016;36:1717–45.
87. Liszewski MC, Lee EY. Neonatal lung disorders: pattern recognition approach to diagnosis. AJR. 2018;210:964–75.
88. Rha SE, Byun JY, Jung SE, et al. Atypical CT and MRI manifestations of mature ovarian cystic teratomas. AJR. 2004;183:743–50.
89. Choi HHI, Manning MA, Mehrotra AK, Wagner S, Jha RC. Primary hepatic neoplasms of vascular origin: key imaging features and differential diagnoses with radiology-pathology correlation. AJR. 2017;209:W350–9.
90. Orru E, Calloni SF, Tekes A, Huisman TAGM, Soares BP. The child with macrocephaly: differential diagnosis and neuroimaging findings. AJR. 2018;210:848–59.
91. Wu JS, Hochman MG. Soft-tissue tumors and tumorlike lesions: a systematic approach. Radiology. 2009;253:297–316.
92. Paulson EK, Thompson WM. Review of small-bowel obstruction: the diagnosis and when to worry. Radiology. 2015;275:332–42.
93. Costa AF, Thipphavong S, Arnason T, Stueck AE, Clarke SE. Fat-containing liver lesions on imaging: detection and differential diagnosis. AJR. 2018;210:68–77.
94. Travinh E, Lanzman B, Provenzale J, Wintermark M. Imaging evaluation of the adult presenting with new-onset seizure. AJR. 2019;212:15–25.
95. Patnana M, Menias CO, Pickhardt PJ, et al. Liver calcifications and calcified liver masses: pattern recognition approach on CT. AJR. 2018;211:76–86.
96. Jha RC, Khera SS, Kalaria AD. Portal vein thrombosis: imaging the spectrum of disease with an emphasis on MRI features. AJR. 2018;211:14–24.
97. Trofimova A, Vey BL, Mullins ME, Wolf DS, Kadom N. Imaging of children with nontraumatic headaches. AJR. 2018;210:8–17.
98. Swenson DW, Ayyala RS, Sams C, Lee EY. Practical imaging strategies for acute appendicitis in children. AJR. 2018;211:901–9.
99. Semionov A, Kosiuk J, Ajlan AA, Discepola F. Thoracic diseases with musculoskeletal manifestations and vice versa: a review. AJR. 2018;211:1000–9.
100. Tavare AN, Robinson P, Altoos R, et al. Postoperative imaging of sarcomas. AJR. 2018;211:506–18.

101. Tirkes T. Chronic pancreatitis: what the clinician wants to know from MR imaging. Magn Reson Imaging Clin N Am. 2018;26:451–61.

102. Burk KS, Knipp D, Sahani DV. Cystic pancreatic tumors. Magn Reson Imaging Clin N Am. 2018;26:405–20.

103. Kranz PG, Malinzak MD, Amrhein TJ. Approach to imaging in patients with spontaneous intracranial hemorrhage. Neuroimaging Clin N Am. 2018;28:353–74.

104. Stanton CL, Fatterpekar GM. Imaging interpretation of temporal bone studies in a patient with tinnitus. Magn Reson Imaging Clin N Am. 2016;26:207–25.

105. Learned KO, Nasseri F, Mohan S. Imaging of the postoperative orbit. Neuroimaging Clin N Am. 2015;25:457–76.

106. Siegelman ES, Chauhan A. MR characterization of focal liver lesions. Magn Reson Imaging Clin N Am. 2014;22:295–313.

107. Zampolin R, Edfarb A, Miller T. Imaging of lumbar spine fusion. Neuroimaging Clin N Am. 2014;24:269–86.

108. Maroldi R, Ravanelli M, Farina D, et al. Post-treatment evaluation of paranasal sinuses after treatment of sinonasal neoplasms. Neuroimaging Clin N Am. 2015;25:667–85.

109. Willson MC, Ross JS. Postoperative spine complications. Neuroimaging Clin N Am. 2014;24:305–26.

110. Caserta MP, Sakala M, Shen P, Gorden L, Wile G. Presurgical planning for hepatobiliary malignancies. Magn Reson Imaging Clin N Am. 2014;22:447–65.

111. Bittane RM, de Moura AB, Lien RJ. The postoperative spine: what the spine surgeon needs to know. Neuroimaging Clin N Am. 2014;24:295–303.

112. Singh A, Bhalla AS, Jana M. Bronchiectasis revisited: imaging-based pattern approach to diagnosis. Curr Probl Diagn Radiol. 2019;48:53–60.

113. Dweck C. The new psychology of success. New York: Ballantine Books; 2006.

114. Carey B. How we learn: the surprising truth about when, where, and why it happens. New York: Penguin Random House; 2015.

115. Norman G. Medical education: past, present and future. Perspect Med Educ. 2012;1:6–14.

116. Norman G. Building on experience – the development of clinical reasoning. NEJM. 2006;355:2251–2.

117. Miglioretti DL, Gard CC, Carney PA, et al. When radiologists perform best: the learning curve in screening mammogram interpretation. Radiology. 2009;253:632–40.

118. Pusic M, Pecaric M, Boutis K. How much practice is enough? Using learning curves to assess the deliberate practice of radiograph interpretation. Acad Med. 2011;86:731–6.

119. Wolf FM, Miller JG, Bozynski ME, et al. Effects of experience and case difficulty on the interpretation of pediatric radiographs. Acad Med. 1994;69(suppl 10):S31–3.

120. Nodine CF, Kundel HL, Mello-Thomas C, et al. How experience and training influence mammography expertise. Acad Radiol. 1999;6:575–85.

121. Sarkany DS, Shenoy-Bhangle AS, Catanzano TM, Fineberg TA, Eisenberg RL, Slanetz PJ. Running a radiology residency program: strategies for success. Radiographics. 2018;38:1729–43.

122. Alves T, Kalume-Brigido M, Yablon C, Bhargava P, Fessell D. The 9 habits of highly effective radiologists. Curr Probl Diagn Radiol. 2018;47:203–5.

123. Fayad LM. The champion's creed: shared value of athletes and academicians. Curr Probl Diagn Radiol. 2017;46:393–4.

124. Papa J. Learning sciences principles that can inform the construction of new approaches to diagnostic training. Diagnosis. 2014;1:125–9.

125. Greene R. Mastery. New York: Penguin Books; 2012.

126. Hambrick DZ, Campitelli G, Macnamara BN, editors. The science of expertise: behavioral, neural, and genetic approaches to complex skill (Frontiers of cognitive psychology) Routledge. New York: Taylor & Francis Group; 2018.

127. Clark RC. Building expertise: cognitive methods for training and performance improvement. 3rd ed. San Francisco: Pfeiffer, Wiley; 2008.

128. Ganguli S, Camacho M, Yam CS, Pedrosa I. Preparing first-year radiology residents and assessing their readiness for on-call responsibilities. AJR. 2009;192:539–44.

129. Trowbridge RL. Twelve tips for teaching avoidance of diagnostic errors. Med Teach. 2008;30:496–500.

130. Groopman J. The eye of the beholder. In: How doctors think. Boston: Houghton Mifflin Company; 2007. p. 177–202.

131. Chrysikopoulos H. Basics of MR examinations and interpretation. In: Clinical MR imaging and physics: a tutorial. Heidelberg: Springer; 2009. p. 109–64.

132. Zwaan L. The critical step to reduce diagnostic errors in medicine: addressing the limitations of human information processing. Diagnosis. 2014;1:139–41.

133. European Society of Radiology (ESR). Good practice for radiological reporting. Guidelines from the European Society of Radiology (ESR). Insights Imaging. 2011;2:93–6.

134. Langlotz CP. Expressing an imaging observation. In: The radiology report. Charleston: CreateSpace; 2015. p. 23–30.

135. Hall FM. Language of the radiology report: primer for residents and wayward radiologists. AJR. 2000;175:1239–42.

136. Fardon DF, Williams AL, Dohring EJ, Murtagh FR, Gabriel Rothman SL, Sze GK. Lumbar disc nomenclature: version 2.0: recommendations of the combined task forces of the North American Spine Society, the American Society of Spine radiology and the American Society of Neuroradiology. Spine J. 2014;14:2525–45.

137. Hansell DM, Bankier AA, MacMahon H, McLoud TC, Muller NL, Remy J. Fleischner society: glossary of terms for thoracic imaging. Radiology. 2008;246:697–722.

138. Aiken AH, Rath TJ, Anzai Y, et al. ACR neck imaging reporting and data systems (NI-RADS): a white paper of the ACR NI-RADS committee. J Am Coll Radiol. 2018;15:1097–108.

139. Corwin MT, Lee AY, Fananapazir TW, Loehfelm TW, Satkar S, Sirlin CB. Nonstandardized terminology to describe focal liver lesions in patients at risk for hepatocellular carcinoma: implications regarding clinical communication. AJR. 2018;210:85–90.

140. Tirkes T, Shah ZK, Takahashi N, et al. Reporting standards for chronic pancreatitis by using CT, MRI, and MR cholangiopancreatography: the consortium for the study of chronic pancreatitis, diabetes, and pancreatic cancer. Radiology. 2019;290:207–15.

141. Andreotti RF, Timmerman D, Benacerraf BR, et al. Ovarian-adnexal reporting lexicon for ultrasound: a white paper of the ACR ovarian-adnexal reporting and data system committee. J Am Coll Radiol. 2018;15:1415–29.

142. Hoang JK. If there is no change, just say so. J Am Coll Radiol. 2016;13:236.

143. Short RG, Befera T, Hoang JK, Tailor D. A normal thyroid by any other name: linguistic analysis of statements describing a normal thyroid gland from noncontrast chest CT reports. J Am Coll Radiol. 2018;15:1642–7.

144. Hoang JK. Avoid "cannot exclude": make a diagnosis. J Am Coll Radiol. 2015;12:1009.

145. Hoang J. Do not hedge when there is certainty. J Am Coll Radiol. 2015;14:5.

146. Krantz PG. What's your impression? Get to the point. J Am Coll Radiol. 2017;14:451.

147. Kuzminski SJ. The devil is in the details. J Am Coll Radiol. 2017;14:148.

148. Vaid S, Vaid N, Rawat S, Ahuja AT. An imaging checklist for pre-FESS CT: framing a surgically relevant report. Clin Radiol. 2011;66:459–70.

149. Kabadi SJ, Krishmaraj A. Strategies for improving the value of the radiology report: a retrospective analysis of errors in formally over-read studies. J Am Coll Radiol. 2017;14:459–66.

150. Khan R, Nael K, Erly W. Acute stroke imaging: what clinicians need to know. Am J Med. 2013;126:379–86.

151. Vancauwenberghe T, Snoeckx A, Vanbeckevoort D, Dymarkowski S, Vanhoenacker FM. Imaging of the spleen: what the clinician needs to know. Singap Med J. 2015;56:133–44.

152. Golfarb CA, Yin Y, Gilula LA, Fisher AJ, Boyer MI. Wrist fractures: what the clinician wants to know. Radiology. 2001;219:11–28.

153. Morag Y, Jacobson JA, Miller B, De Maeseneer M, Girish G, Jamadar D. MR imaging of rotator cuff injury: what the clinician needs to know. Radiographics. 2006;26:1045–65.

154. Marshall RA, Weaver ML, Sodickson A, Khurana B. Periprosthetic fractures in the emergency department: what the orthopedic surgeon wants to know. Radiographics. 2017;37:1202–17.

155. Kumbhar SS, O'Malley RB, Robinson TJ, et al. Why thyroid surgeons are frustrated with radiologists: lessons learned from pre- and postoperative US. Radiographics. 2016;36:2141–53.

156. Wieschhoff GG, Sheehan SE, Wortman JR, et al. Traumatic finger injuries: what the orthopedic surgeon wants to know. Radiographics. 2016;36:1106–28.

157. Sandstrom CK, Kennedy SA, Gross JA. Acute shoulder trauma: what the surgeon wants to know. Radiographics. 2015;35:475–92.

158. Lee SC, Jain PA, Jethwa SC, Tripathy D, Yamashita MW. Radiologists' role in breast cancer staging: providing key information for clinicians. Radiographics. 2014;34:330–42.

159. Khurana B, Sheehan SE, Sodickson A, Bono CM, Harris MB. Traumatic thoracolumbar spine injuries: what the spine surgeon wants to know. Radiographics. 2013;33:2031–46.

160. Sheehan SE, Dyer GS, Sodickson AD, Patel KI, Khurana B. Traumatic elbow injuries: what the orthopedic surgeon wants to know. Radiographics. 2013;33:869–88.

161. Dolev JC, Friedlaender LK, Braverman IM. Use of fine art to enhance diagnostic skills. JAMA. 2001;286:1020–1.

162. Goodman TR, Kelleher M. Improving novice radiology trainees' perception using fine art. J Am Coll Radiol. 2017;14:1337–40.

163. Eberhardt SC, Heilbrun ME. Radiology report value equation. Radiographics. 2018;38:1888–96.

164. Waite S, Scott J, Gale B, Fuchs T, Kolla S, Reede D. Interpretive error in radiology. AJR. 2017;208:739–49.

165. Bui-Mansfield LT. "Fool me twice": delayed diagnoses in radiology with emphasis on perpetuated errors. Video lecture. https://learning.arrs.org/course/view.php?id=518. Accessed 19 Nov 2017.

166. Rosenkrantz AB, Bansal NK. Diagnostic errors in abdominopelvic CT interpretation: characterization based on report addenda. Abdom Radiol. 2016;41:1793–9.

167. Bruno MA, Walker EA, Abujudeh HH. Understanding and confronting our mistakes: the epidemiology of error in radiology and strategies for error reduction. Radiographics. 2015;35:1668–76.

168. Berlin L. Radiologic errors, past, present and future. Diagnosis. 2014;1:79–84.

169. Kim YW, Mansfield LT. Fool me twice: delayed diagnoses in radiology with emphasis on perpetuated errors. AJR. 2014;202:465–70.

170. McCreadie G, Oliver TB. Eight CT lessons that we learned the hard way: an analysis of current patterns of radiological error and discrepancy with particular emphasis on CT. Clin Radiol. 2009;64:491–9.

171. Donald JJ, Barnard SA. Common patterns in 558 diagnostic radiology errors. J Med Imaging Radiat Oncol. 2012;56:173–8.

172. Brady AP. Error and discrepancy in radiology: inevitable or avoidable? Insights Imaging. 2017;8:171–82.

173. Brady A, Laoide RO, McCarthy P, McDermott R. Discrepancy and error in radiology: concepts, causes and consequences. Ulster Med J. 2012;81:3–9.

174. Sabih DE, Sabih A, Sabih Q, Khan AN. Image perception and interpretation of abnormalities; can we believe our eyes? Can we do something about it? Insights Imaging. 2011;2:47–55.

175. Pinto A, Brunese L. Spectrum of diagnostic errors in radiology. World J Radiol. 2010;2:377–83.

176. Fitzgerald R. Radiological error: analysis, standard setting, targeted instruction and teamworking. Eur Radiol. 2005;15:1760–7.

177. Fitzgerald R. Error in radiology. Clin Radiol. 2001;56:938–46.

178. Owens EJ, Taylor NR, Howlett DC. Perceptual type error in everyday practice. Clin Radiol. 2016;71:593–601.

179. Li F, Sone S, Abe H, MacMahon H, Armato SG 3rd, Doi K. Lung cancers missed at low-dose helical CT screening in a general population: comparison of clinical, histopathologic, and imaging findings. Radiology. 2002;225:673–83.

180. Del Ciello A, Franchi P, Contegiacomo A, Cicchetti G, Bonomo L, Larici AR. Missed lung cancer: when, where and why? Diagn Interv Radiol. 2017;23:118–26.

181. de Groot PM, Carter BW, Abbott GF, Wu CC. Pitfalls in chest radiographic interpretation: blind spots. Semin Roentgenol. 2015;50:197–209.

182. Horton KM, Johnson PT, Fishman EK. MDCT of the abdomen: common misdiagnoses at a busy academic center. AJR. 2010;194:660–7.

183. Wu CC, Korashadi L, Abbott GF, Gilman MD. Common blind spots on chest CT: where are they all hiding? Part 1 – airways, lungs and pleura. AJR. 2013;201:W533–8.

184. Wu CC, Korashadi L, Abbott GF, Shepard JAO. Common blind spots on chest CT: where are they all hiding? Part 2, extrapulmonary structures. AJR. 2013;201:W671–7.

185. Rinaldi MF, Bartalena T, Gianneli G, et al. Incidental lung nodules on CT examinations of the abdomen: prevalence and reporting rates in the PACS era. Eur J Radiol. 2010;74:e84–8.

186. Siewert B, Sosna J, McNamara A, Raptopoulos V, Kruskal JB. Missed lesions at abdominal oncologic CT: lessons learned from quality assurance. Radiographics. 2008;28:623–38.

187. Bahrami S, Yim CM. Quality initiatives. Blind spots at brain imaging. Radiographics. 2009;29:1877–96.

188. Tchoyoson CC, Nadarajah M. System-based imaging pitfalls: Brain. In: Peh WGC, editor. Pitfalls in diagnostic radiology. Heidelberg: Springer; 2015. p. 217–45.

189. Keats TE, Anderson MW. Atlas of normal variants that may simulate disease. 9th ed. Philadelphia: Elsevier Saunders; 2013.

190. Bancroft LW, Bridges M, editors. MRI. Normal variants and pitfalls. Philadelphia: Wolters Kluwer, Lippincott Williams and Wilkins; 2012.

191. Robbins J, Kusmirek J, Barroilhet L, Anderson B, Bradley K, Sadowski E. Pitfalls in imaging of cervical cancer. Semin Roentgenol. 2016;51:17–31.

192. Katabathina VS, Flaherty E, Prasad SR. Cross-sectional imaging of renal masses; imaging technique-related potential pitfalls and solutions. Semin Roentgenol. 2016;51:32–9.

193. Katabathina VS, Shiao J, Flaherty E, Prasad SR. Cross-sectional imaging of renal masses; imaging interpretation-related potential pitfalls and possible solutions. Semin Roentgenol. 2016;51:40–8.

194. Belfield J, Kennish S. Pitfalls in stone imaging. Semin Roentgenol. 2016;51:49–59.

195. Taner AT, Schieda N, Siegelman ES. Pitfalls in adrenal imaging. Semin Roentgenol. 2015;50:260–72.

196. Fournier LS, Bennani S, Bats AS, et al. Pitfalls in imaging of advanced ovarian cancer. Semin Roentgenol. 2015;50:284–93.

197. Tappouni R, Sakala MD, Hosseinzadeh K. Mimics of hepatic neoplasms. Semin Roentgenol. 2015;50:305–19.

198. Kaza R, Al-Hawary M, Sokhandon F, Shirkhoda A, Francis IR. Pitfalls in pancreatic imaging. Semin Roentgenol. 2015;50:320–7.

199. Anis M, Caroline D. Pitfalls in imaging after gastrointestinal surgery. Semin Roentgenol. 2015;50:328–34.

200. Godoy MCB, Truong MT, Cartr BW, Viswanathan C, de Groot P, Ko JP. Pitfalls in pulmonary nodule characterization. Semin Roentgenol. 2015;50:164–74.

201. Betancourt-Cuellar SL, Carter BW, Palacio D, Erasmus JJ. Pitfalls and limitations in non-small cell lung cancer staging. Semin Roentgenol. 2015;50:175–82.

202. Viswanathan C, Carter BW, Shroff G, Godoy MCB, Marom EM, Truong MT. Pitfalls in oncologic imaging: complications of chemotherapy and radiotherapy in the chest. Semin Roentgenol. 2015;50:183–91.

203. Godoy MCB, Marom EM, Carter BW, Sorensen J, Truong MT, Abbott GF. Computed tomography imaging of lung infection in the oncologic setting: typical features and potential pitfalls. Semin Roentgenol. 2015;50:192–6.

204. Carter BW, Betancourt SL, Viswanathan C, Mawlawi O, Marom EM, Truong MT. Potential pitfalls in interpretation of positron emission tomography/computed tomography findings in the thorax. Semin Roentgenol. 2015;50:210–6.

205. Palacio D, Benveniste MF, Betancourt-Cuellar SL, Gladish GW. Multidetector computed tomography pulmonary angiography pitfalls in the evaluation of pulmonary embolism with emphasis in technique. Semin Roentgenol. 2015;50:217–25.

206. Manlove W, Raptis CA, Bhalla S. Pitfalls in computed tomography of the aorta. Semin Roentgenol. 2015;50:229–34.
207. Shroff GS, Viswanathan C, Godoy MCB, Marom EM, Sabloff BS, Truong MT. Pitfalls in oncologic imaging: pericardial recesses mimicking adenopathy. Semin Roentgenol. 2015;50:235–40.
208. Carter BW, de Groot P, Godoy MCB, Marom EM, Wu CC. Imaging of the mediastinum: vascular lesions as potential pitfall. Semin Roentgenol. 2015;50:241–50.
209. Lichtenberger JP III, Carter BW, Abbott GF. Pitfalls in imaging of the chest wall. Semin Roentgenol. 2015;50:251–7.
210. Peh WCG, editor. Pitfalls in diagnostic radiology. Berlin: Springer; 2015.
211. Peh WCG, editor. Pitfalls in musculoskeletal radiology. Berlin: Springer; 2017.
212. Hansell DM. Pitfalls in the HRCT diagnosis of fibrosing lung disease. Society of Thoracic Radiology 2014 online course. https://ebixadam. s3.amazonaws.com/Oakstone%20Media/988/988-05/05.mp4. Accessed 18 Oct 2017.
213. Romano L, Pinto A, editors. Errors in radiology. Milan: Springer; 2012.
214. Lackner KJ, Krug KB. Avoiding errors in radiology. Case-based analysis of causes and preventive strategies. Stuttgart: Thieme; 2011.
215. Coackley FV, editor. Pearls and pitfalls in abdominal imaging: pseudotumors, variants and other difficult diagnoses. New York: Cambridge University Press; 2010.
216. Moulding FJ, Roach SC, Carrington BM. Unusual sites of lymph node metastases and pitfalls in their detection. Clin Radiol. 2004;59:558–72.
217. Gangi S, Fletcher JG, Nathan MA, et al. Time interval between abnormalities seen on CT and the clinical diagnosis of pancreatic cancer: retrospective review of CT scans obtained before diagnosis. AJR. 2004;182:897–903.
218. Takhtani D. CT neuroangiography: a glance at the common pitfalls and their prevention. AJR. 2005;185:772–83.
219. Gaur S, Dialani V, Slanetz PJ, Eisenberg RL. Architectural distortion of the breast. AJR. 2013;201:W662–70.
220. Leung JWT, Sickles EA. Developing asymmetry identified on mammography: correlation with imaging outcome and pathologic findings. AJR. 2007;188:667–75.
221. Bahl M, Baker JA, Kinsey EN, Ghate SV. Architectural distortion on mammography: correlation with pathologic outcomes and predictors of malignancy. AJR. 2015;205:1339–45.
222. Tabar L, Tot T, Dean PB. Breast cancer- the art and science of early detection with mammography: perception, interpretation and histopathologic correlation. Stuttgart: Thieme; 2004.
223. Kalli S, Lanfranchi M, Alexander A, Mkim S, Freer PE. Spectrum of extramammary malignant neoplasm in the breast with radiologic-pathologic correlation. Curr Probl Diagn Radiol. 2016;45:392–401.
224. Gupta P, Potti TA, Wuertzer SD, Palchoke DA. Spectrum of fat-containing soft-tissue masses at MR imaging: the common, the uncommon, the characteristic and the sometimes confusing. Radiographics. 2016;36:753–66.
225. Lee SH, Seo JB, Kang JW, Chae EJ, Park SH, Lim TH. Incidental cardiac and pericardial abnormalities on chest CT. J Thorac Imaging. 2008;23:216–26.
226. Anderson S. Acute abdominal CT pitfalls. Video presentation. https://learning.arrs.org/mod/page/view.php?id=7336. Accessed 22 Oct 2016.
227. Nicola R. Abdominal ultrasound pitfalls. Video presentation. https://learning.arrs.org/mod/page/view.php?id=7337. Accessed 22 Oct 2016.
228. Menashe SJ, Iyer RS, Parisi MT, Otto RK, Stanescu AL. Pediatric chest radiographs: common and less common errors. AJR. 2016;207:903–11.
229. Helms CA. Fundamental of skeletal radiology. 4th ed. Philadelphia: Elsevier; 2014.
230. Torabi M, Hosseinzadeh K, Federle MP. CT of non-neoplastic hepatic vascular and perfusion disorders. Radiographics. 2008;28:1967–82.
231. Blachar A, Federle MP, Brancatelli G, Peterson MS, Oliver JH III, Li W. Radiologic performance in the diagnosis of internal hernia by using specific CT findings with emphasis on transmesenteric hernia. Radiology. 2001;221:422–8.
232. Kamaya A, Federle MP, Desser TS. Imaging manifestations of abdominal fat necrosis and its mimics. Radiographics. 2011;31:2021–34.
233. Blachar A, Federle MP, Ferris JV, et al. Radiologists's performance in the diagnosis of liver tumors with central scars by using specific CT criteria. Radiology. 2002;223:532–9.
234. Blachar A, Barnes S, Adam SZ, et al. Radiologists's performance in the diagnosis of acute intestinal ischemia, using MDCT and specific CT findings, using a variety of CT protocols. Emerg Radiol. 2011;18:385–94.
235. Furlan A, Fakhran S, Federle MP. Spontaneous abdominal hemorrhage: causes, CT findings and clinical implications. AJR. 2009;193:1077–87.
236. Blachar A, Federle MP, Pealer KM, Abu Abeid S, Graif M. Radiographic manifestations of normal postoperative anatomy and gastrointestinal complications of bariatric surgery, with emphasis on CT imaging findings. Semin Ultrasound CT MR. 2004;25:239–51.
237. Potchen EJ. Measuring observer performance in chest radiology: some experiences. J Am Coll Radiol. 2006;3:423–32.
238. Patlas MN, Dreizin D, Menias CO, et al. Abdominal and pelvic trauma: misses and misinterpretations at multidetector CT. Radiographics. 2017;37:703–4.
239. Lakhani A, Khan SR, Bharwani N, Stewart V, Rockall AG, Khan S, Barwick TD. FDG PET/CT pitfalls in gynecologic and genitourinary oncologic imaging. Radiographics. 2017;37:577–94.

240. Shroff GS, Carter BW, Viswanathan C, et al. Challenges in interpretation of staging PET/CT in thoracic malignancies. Curr Probl Diagn Radiol. 2017;46:330–41.

241. Marko J, Wojfman DJ, Aubin AL, Sesterhenn IA. Testicular seminoma and its mimicks: from the radiologic pathologic archives. Radiographics. 2017;37:1085–98.

242. Senar AC, Dinu LE, Artigas JM, Larrosa R, Navarro Y, Angulo E. Foreign bodies on lateral neck radiographs in adults: imaging findings and common pitfalls. Radiographics. 2017;37:323–45.

243. Nagpal P, Maller V, Garg G, et al. Upper extremity runoff: pearls and pitfalls in computed tomography angiography and magnetic resonance angiography. Curr Probl Diagn Radiol. 2017;46:115–29.

244. Villavicencio CP, Adam SZ, Nikoliadis P, Yaghmai V, Miller FH. Imaging of the urachus: anomalies, complications, and mimics. Radiographics. 2016;36:2049–63.

245. Hayeri MR, Ziai P, Shehata ML, Teytelboym OM, Huang BK. Soft-tissue infections and their imaging mimics: from cellulitis to necrotizing fasciitis. Radiographics. 2016;36:1888–910.

246. Bolog NV, Andreisek G. Reporting knee meniscal tears: technical aspects, typical pitfalls and how to avoid them. Insights Imaging. 2016;7:385–98.

247. Dannheim K, Bhargava P. A rare finding of brown fat in bone marrow as a mimick for metastatic disease. Am J Hematol. 2016;91:545–6.

248. Kitzing YX, Prado A, Varol C, Karczmar GS, Maclean F, Oto A. Benign conditions that mimick prostate carcinoma: MR imaging features with histopathologic correlation. Radiographics. 2016;36:162–75.

249. Albano D, La Grutta L, Grassedonio E, et al. Pitfalls in whole body MRI with diffusion weighted imaging performed on patients with lymphoma: what radiologists should know. Magn Reson Imaging. 2016;34:922–31.

250. Flavell RR, Naeger DM, Aparici CM, Hawkins RA, Pampaloni MH, Behr SC. Malignancies with low fluoro-deoxyglucose uptake at PET/CT: pitfalls and prognostic importance. Radiographics. 2016;36:293–4.

251. Bachler P, Baladron MJ, Menias C, et al. Multimodality imaging of liver infections: differential diagnosis and potential pitfalls. Radiographics. 2016;36:1001–23.

252. Vernuccio F, Borhani AA, Dioguardi Burgio M, Midiri M, Furlan A, Brancatelli G. Common and uncommon pitfalls in pancreatic imaging: it is not always cancer. Abdom Radiol. 2015;41:283–94.

253. Ropp A, Waite S, Reede D, Patel J. Did I miss that: subtle and commonly missed findings on chest radiographs. Curr Probl Diagn Radiol. 2015;44:277–89.

254. Roumanis PS, Bhargava P, Aubin GK, et al. Atypical magnetic resonance imaging findings in hepatocellular carcinoma. Curr Probl Diagn Radiol. 2015;44:237–45.

255. Scaglione M, Iaselli F, Sica G, Feragalli B, Refky N. Errors in imaging of traumatic injuries. Abdom Imaging. 2015;40:2091–8.

256. Darras K, Andrews GT, McLoughlin PD, Khorrami-Arani N, Roston A, Forster BB. Pearls for interpreting computed tomography of the cervical spine in trauma. Radiol Clin N Am. 2015;53:657–74.

257. Tyson S, Hatem SF. Easily missed fractures of the upper extremity. Radiol Clin N Am. 2015;53:717–36.

258. Yu JS. Easily missed fractures in the lower extremity. Radiol Clin N Am. 2015;53:737–55.

259. Gyftopoulos S, Chitkara M, Bencardino JT. Misses and errors in upper extremity trauma radiographs. AJR. 2014;203:477–91.

260. Hong GS, Lee CW, Kim MH, Kim C. Appendiceal location analysis and review of the misdiagnosis rate of appendicitis associated with deep pelvic cecum on multidetector computed tomography. Clin Imaging. 2016;40:714–9.

261. Kim S, Lim HK, Lee JY, Lee J, Kim MJ, Lee AS. Ascending retrocecal appendicitis: clinical and computed tomographic findings. J Comput Assist Tomogr. 2006;30:772–6.

262. Fardanesch M, White C. Missed lung cancer on chest radiography and computed tomography. Semin Ultrasound CT MR. 2012;33:280–7.

263. Mandato Y, Reginelli A, Galasso R, Iacobellis F, Berritto D, Cappabianca S. Errors in the radiological evaluation of the alimentary tract: part I. Semin Ultrasound CT MR. 2012;33:300–7.

264. Reginelli A, Mandato Y, Solazzo A, Berritto D, Iacobellis F, Grassi R. Errors in the radiological evaluation of the alimentary tract: part II. Semin Ultrasound CT MR. 2012;33:308–17.

265. Sica G, Guida F, Bocchini G, et al. Errors in imaging assessment of polytrauma patients. Semin Ultrasound CT MR. 2012;33:337–46.

266. Wei CJ, Tsai WC, Tiu CM, Wu HT, Chiou HJ, Chang CY. Systematic analysis of missed extremity fractures in emergency radiology. Acta Radiol. 2006;47:710–7.

267. Dominguez S, Liu P, Roberts C, Mandell M, Richman PB. Prevalence of traumatic hip and pelvic fractures in patients with suspected hip fracture and negative initial standard radiographs-a study of emergency department patients. Acad Emerg Med. 2005;12:366–70.

268. Hernandez JA, Swischuk LE, Yngve DA, Carmichael KD. The angled buckle fracture in pediatrics: a frequently missed fracture. Emerg Radiol. 2003;10:71–5.

269. Prokesch RW, Chow LC, Beaulieu CF, Bammer R, Jeffrey RB Jr. Isoattenuating pancreatic adenocarcinoma at multi-detector row CT: secondary signs. Radiology. 2002;224:764–8.

270. El-Sherief AH, Wu CC, Schoenhagen P, et al. Basics of cardiopulmonary bypass: normal and abnormal postoperative CT appearances. Radiographics. 2013;33:63–72.

271. Chakarun CJ, Forrester DM, Gottsengen CJ, Patel DB, White EA, Matuck GR Jr. Giant cell tumor of bone: review, mimics, and new developments in treatment. Radiographics. 2013;33:197–211.

272. Elsayes KM, Menias CO, Morshid AI, et al. Spectrum of pitfalls, pseudolesions, and misdiagnoses in noncirrhotic liver. AJR. 2018;211:97–108.

273. Elsayes KM, Chernyak V, Morshid AI, et al. Spectrum of pitfalls, pseudolesions, and potential misdiagnoses in cirrhosis. AJR. 2018;211:87–96.

274. Banaste N, Caurier B, Bratan F, Bergerot JF, Thomson V, Millet I. Whole-body CT in patients with multiple traumas: factors leading to missed injury. Radiology. 2018;289:374–83.

275. Weirich JM, Bannas P, Regier M, et al. Low-dose CT for evaluation of suspected urolithiasis: diagnostic yield for assessment of alternative diagnoses. AJR. 2018;210:557–63.

276. Fu CJ, Chen HW, Chen LH, et al. Extraspinal malignancies found incidentally on lumbar spine MRI: prevalence and etiologies. J Radiol Sci. 2013;38:85–91.

277. Glastonbury CM, Salzman KL. Pitfalls in the staging of nasopharyngeal carcinoma. Neuroimaging Clin N Am. 2013;23:9–25.

278. Aiken AH. Pitfalls in the staging of cancer of oral cavity cancer. Neuroimaging Clin N Am. 2013;23:27–45.

279. Corey A. Pitfalls in the staging of cancer of the oropharyngeal squamous cell carcinoma. Neuroimaging Clin N Am. 2013;23:47–66.

280. Chen AY, Hudgins PA. Pitfalls in the staging squamous cell carcinoma of the hypopharynx. Neuroimaging Clin N Am. 2013;23:67–79.

281. Baugnon KL, Beitler JJ. Pitfalls in the staging of the laryngeal squamous cell carcinoma. Neuroimaging Clin N Am. 2013;23:81–105.

282. Friedman ER, Saindane AM. Pitfalls in the staging of the major salivary gland neoplasms. Neuroimaging Clin N Am. 2013;23:107–22.

283. Saindane AM. Pitfalls in the staging of cancer of the thyroid. Neuroimaging Clin N Am. 2013;23:123–45.

284. Saindane AM. Pitfalls in the staging of lymph node metastasis. Neuroimaging Clin N Am. 2013;23:147–66.

285. Wildman-Tobriner B, Allen BC, Maxfield CM. Common resident errors when interpreting computed tomography of the abdomen and pelvis: a review of types, pitfalls, and strategies for improvement. Curr Probl Diagn Radiol. 2019;48:4–9.

286. Kruskal JB, Anderson SW, Soto JA, editors. Pitfalls in clinical imaging: categorical course syllabus 2012. Reston: ARRS; 2012.

287. Tsai R, Raptis D, Raptis C, Mellnick VM. Complications after gynecologic and obstetric procedures: a pictorial review. Curr Probl Diagn Radiol. 2018;47:189–99.

288. Velayudhan V, Chaudhry ZA, Smoker WRK, Shinder R, Reede DL. Imaging of intracranial and orbital complications of sinusitis and atypical sinus infection: what the radiologist needs to know. Curr Probl Diagn Radiol. 2017;46:441–51.

289. Panizza PSB, Viana PCC, Horvat N, et al. Inflammatory bowel disease: current role of imaging in diagnosis and detection of complications: gastrointestinal imaging. Radiographics. 2017;37:701–2.

290. Venkatanarasimha N, Damodharan K, Gogna A, et al. Diagnosis and management of complications from percutaneous biliary tract interventions. Radiographics. 2017;37:665–80.

291. Desai KR, Pandhi ME, Seedial SM, et al. Retrievable IVC filters: comprehensive review of device-related complications and advanced retrieval techniques. Radiographics. 2017;37:1236–45.

292. Plowman RS, Javidan-Nejad C, Raptis CA, et al. Imaging of pregnancy-related vascular complications. Radiographics. 2017;37:1270–89.

293. Talbot BS, Gange CP Jr, Chaturvedi A, Klionsky N, Hobbs SK, Chaturvedi A. Traumatic rib injury: patterns, imaging pitfalls, complications, and treatment. Radiographics. 2017;37:628–51.

294. Dillman JR, Trout AT, Smith EA, Towbin AJ. Hereditary renal cystic disorders. Radiographics. 2017;37:924–46.

295. Nikola R, Shaqdan KW, Aran S, Singh AK, Abujudeh HH. Detecting aortic graft complications: a spectrum of computed tomography findings. Curr Probl Diagn Radiol. 2016;45:330–9.

296. McGettigan MJ, Menias CO, Gao ZJ, Mellnick VM, Hara AK. Imaging of drug induced complications in the gastrointestinal system. Radiographics. 2016;36:71–87.

297. Del Campo L, Leon NG, Palacios DC, Lagana C, Tagarro D. Abdominal complications following hematopoetic stem cell transplantation. Radiographics. 2014;34:396–412.

298. Nixon JN, Biyam DR, Stanescu L, Phillips GS, Finn LS, Paris MT. Imaging of pediatric renal transplants and their complications: a pictorial review. Radiographics. 2013;33:1227–51.

299. Low G, Crockett AM, Leung K, et al. Imaging of vascular complications and their consequences following transplantation in the abdomen. Radiographics. 2013;33:633–52.

300. Weinstein S, Osei-Bonsu S, Aslam R, Yee J. Multidetector CT of the postoperative colon: review of normal appearances and common complications. Radiographics. 2013;33:515–32.

301. Koontz NA, Gunderman RB. Gestalt theory: implications for radiology education. AJR. 2008;190:1156–60.

302. Jain B. The key role of differential diagnosis in diagnosis. Diagnosis. 2017;4:239–40.

303. Gunderman RB. Education and the art of uncertainty. Radiology. 2005;237:801–2.

304. Low G, Dharmana H, Saravana-Barwan S, Girgis S. Diagnosis please case 235: hepatic adenomatosis due to inflammatory adenomas. Radiology. 2016;281:639–45.

305. Fish D, de Cossart L. Thinking outside the (tick) box: rescuing professionalism and professional judgment. Med Educ. 2006;40:403–4.

306. Gawande A. Complications: a surgeon's notes on an imperfect science. London: Profile books; 2001.

307. Centor R. Stumbling towards a diagnosis. Diagnosis (Berl). 2014;1:63–4.

308. Karlik SJ. Building a teaching module in clinical inquiry for radiology residents. In: Van Deven T, Hibbert KM, Chhem R, editors. The practice of radiology education: challenges and trends. Heidelberg: Springer; 2010. p. 57–69.

309. Schmidt MH. Fostering research in a Canadian radiology training program: a residency research direc-tor's perspective. In: Van Deven T, Hibbert KM, Chhem R, editors. The practice of radiology education: challenges and trends. Heidelberg: Springer; 2010. p. 207–12.

310. Pfeifer CM, Heitkamp DE. Point: losing the zero-sum game: it's time to eliminate required research in radiology residency. J Am Coll Radiol. 2018;15:658–60.

311. Anderson S. Counterpoint: research by radiology residents is meaningful and important. J Am Coll Radiol. 2018;15:661–2.

312. Halligan S. Subspecialist radiology. Clin Radiol. 2002;57:982–3.

Abstract

This chapter addresses ways to block errors and biases, with the emphasis placed on the individual imaging professional, not on the system. I present a maze of checklists, questions, and filters to stop errors and biases "on their tracks." This chapter is the most "dense" in terms of knowledge and information and displays a fresh way of thinking about errors and biases. Following the proposed algorithms is cumbersome and time consuming at first, but continuous practice leads to a safer navigation through the diagnostic dilemmas of everyday practice. So keep your eyes on the "prize": improved outcomes for the patients, an overall decrease in the cost of health care, and a healthy sense of pride for us.

7.1 General Remarks

Any problem solving starts with an awareness that a problem exists. Once it is identified, we can proceed with its description and analysis. Then we can work on possible solutions.

Fortunately, awareness and knowledge about errors, quality, and safety are very high, thanks to the pioneering and elegant work of several institutions and bold individuals [1–53]. Several strategies have been devised to constrain and suppress imaging errors, each serving a specific function.

It takes multiple, interdigitating layers of safety to build a strong protection against errors, given their variability and complexity. The success of this project requires coordinated teamwork and each one of us fulfilling his share.

We will address separately the roles of the:

- Individual imaging professional,
- Administration and heads of nonteaching radiology services,
- Administration and department heads of teaching institutions and major radiology/ healthcare organizations.

7.2 Error Reducing Strategies for Individual Radiologists

Most errors on a personal level are due to misperception, misjudgment, and miscommunication [31, 32]. My opinion is that the most significant underlying mechanisms are limited knowledge, cognitive biases, and insufficient allocation of time to read the study.

These elements have been discussed in Chaps. 3, 4, and 5. We have not yet talked about debiasing (or metacognitive) methods. I have purposely delayed this discussion, until the reader had gained a solid understanding of biases and errors. Debiasing techniques are taxing, since they demand intensive mental effort and self-discipline. With persistent practice, eventually they become second nature.

7.2.1 Diagnostic Algorithms and Methods for Neutralizing Biases

The literature is rich in theoretical frameworks on debiasing and decision making, but I could not extract a complete practical strategy [24, 54–73]. So far, multiple and varied investigations have not found effective tools to counteract cognitive errors [69]. These studies have enrolled nurses, medical students, trainees, and expert physicians from several specialties, including radiology. A meta-analysis of 42 such published papers reached the conclusion that "the evaluations typically involved trainees in artificial settings, making it difficult to extrapolate the results to actual practice" [71]. I would add that we have to take into consideration the evolution in diagnostic reasoning that takes place with progressive and advanced training [68, 74–76]. Thus, I doubt that conclusions about performance of students and junior residents can be extrapolated to senior trainees and certified radiologists.

As a matter of fact, in my personal experience, I have found that *consistent* use of *debiasing* strategies is *extremely useful* for both the *suppression* and the *timely correction* of *errors*. To override biases, I have modified my routine over the years to include the following filters, presented in Table 7.1.

7.2.1.1 Bypassing the Request, the Patient's History, and Prior Imaging Reports [63, 67, 70]

As a resident I worked on thousands of teaching files without a priori knowledge of the clinical

Table 7.1 Debiasing filters

- Bypassing the request, the patient's history and prior imaging reports
- Bypassing statistical limitations
- Satisfaction of searching the entire image and the entire study
- What can I not afford to miss?
- What could it be? Or what else could it be?
- Looking behind the scenes for causes and complications
- Timing factors
- Pause and reboot

history [66]. This way, without any bias, I patiently trained myself to look for subtle clues of disease. I still practice this habit to this date. About one-third of the cases that come through my desk are examined twice: once before and once after I read the request. The first time I "squeeze" the images for any information and I formulate my impression. The second time I may concentrate on a particular area or I may review the entire study "from scratch," depending on the clinical context. I may or may not change my initial interpretation. I certainly do not consider that my first impression is always right. My intention is to remain flexible to change direction, if indicated by the clinical picture.

7.2.1.2 Bypassing Statistical Limitations

By statistical biases I mean overreliance on incidence, prevalence, pre- and post-test probabilities of disease, instead of careful assessment and appropriate weighting of the imaging finding(s). For a more thorough discussion of this topic, please see Chap. 4, Sect. 4.7.

There are three statistical rules that I follow:

(a) Common things are common. However a particular patient may fall outside the statistical boundaries that we accept as highly probable vs. unlikely for our presumptive diagnosis.

(b) Unusual expressions of a common disorder are more common than typical manifestation of a rare disease [76, 77].

(c) An individual patient may be afflicted by two or more conditions at the same time! Thus we have to consider this unusual scenario if we cannot fit all pieces of the puzzle in a single diagnosis.

7.2.1.3 Satisfaction of Searching the Entire Image and the Entire Study

In order to avoid the trap of satisfaction of search, I do two things:

(a) I use checklists to ensure that I look at the entire image, both in its center and along its periphery. In cross-sectional imaging, I follow each organ or structure through its entirety, slice by slice, keeping in it within my central field of view [78–80]. Then I review each slice moving my central field of view from right to left or from center to periphery (or vice versa) in order to integrate my "puzzle" of visual information.

(b) I neglect the obvious lesion until I have completed visual investigation of the rest of the study. Let me give you two examples.

- Suppose I start reading an abdominal CT scan, to further evaluate a 5 cm solid liver nodule detected by sonography. I place the liver at the end of my search procedure, so that I am not distracted by the obvious finding.

- Suppose alternatively that in the cranial slices of a chest CT study I detect a spiculated 2 cm mass in the apex of the right lung. At that time, I reverse course, I temporarily neglect the lung apices, and I start my search at the bottom slice, working my way up (in a caudo-cranial direction). This way I don't forget to evaluate carefully the parts of the upper abdomen that are included in the scan (e.g., liver, adrenal glands, upper lumbar spine, etc.).

7.2.1.4 "What Can I Not Afford to Miss?"

I have mentioned this crucial question several times so far [63, 81, 82]. The answer to this question is: I cannot afford to miss emergencies, or conditions that may progress rapidly, or that may cause irreversible harm, if detected at a later date. Some obvious examples are tumors, thrombi, hemorrhage, airway obstruction, gastrointestinal perforation, brain aneurysms, other vascular malformations, etc.

Let me give you two examples from my daily practice.

(a) In chest CT scans of oncology patients I pay particular attention to the pulmonary arteries for thromboembolic disease, to the trachea and central bronchi for an intraluminal mass, and to the spine for pathologic fractures or an intracanalicular mass that may cause thecal sac compression.

(b) In abdominopelvic scans before I start my dictation, regardless of the history on the request, I look again at the pancreas, the gastrointestinal tract, and the internal genital organs for subtle tumors.

7.2.1.5 What Else Could It Be? Or What Could It Be?

Perhaps we have come up with a diagnosis and we are confident that we are correct. It is still a useful habit to ask "What else could it be?" [6, 71]. Perhaps we have not seen a particular lesion or pattern before, and the question becomes "What could it be?" Searching for the right answer may require complex thinking. In order to secure all possible routes to the appropriate diagnosis (or differential) I have devised an elaborate algorithm, presented in Table 7.2.

(a) Anatomic localization

To address the question "What could it be?" I always start by determining the precise anatomic origin of the abnormality [76, 83–86]. If I am not certain about it, then I need to expand my differential; I have to consider as potential sources of origin (a) all structures that reside in the specific compartment that hosts the lesion, and (b) the structures in all neighboring spaces. For example, a dorsally exophytic or pedunculated gastric mass may be mistaken for a pancreatic process [87]. A localized malignant peritoneal mesothelioma

Table 7.2 Algorithm to answer the questions "What could it be?" or "What else could it be?"

- Anatomic localization
- Uncommon manifestation of a common disease
- Uncommon localization of a common disease
- Neoplasia (tumor)
- Tumor-like conditions and tumor mimics
- Syndromes and congenital associations
- Lymphoma, tuberculosis, sarcoidosis, and Castleman's disease (special situation—SpSi #1)
- Hemangiomas and their benign variants, excluding lymphatic and arterial/venous malformations (SpSi #2)
- Amyloidosis and inflammatory pseudotumor (SpSi #3)

in the region of the splenic flexure may be indistinguishable from a colonic adenocarcinoma, a gastrointestinal stromal tumor, or an extraperitoneal sarcoma [88].

It may be difficult to ascertain the origin of large tumors, either benign or malignant, if they have established wide contact with neighboring structures. This question is especially important in the abdominal and pelvic cavities, where masses may attain a considerable size before they become symptomatic. Various imaging signs are powerful in suggesting the anatomic origin of a tumor [83–86, 89–94]. We will now present such signs that are applicable in oncologic CT and MRI cases of the abdomen and pelvis.

- Crescent sign
  A tumor may forcefully compress an organ, without infiltrating it. The externally compressed organ becomes deformed and assumes a crescent shape [83, 85, 86].
- Beak sign
  The beak is a triangular or curved tongue of tissue that belongs to the organ of origin of a neoplasm with an exophytic component. The edge of the organ is stretched into a beak as the tumor expands beyond the confines of the organ [85, 86]. A "pseudo beak" sign has also been described, due to partial volume effects, in cases of external compression [85].
- "Embedded organ sign"
  A mass, if pliable and if restricted by anatomic boundaries, may grow circumferentially and "drape" itself (partly or entirely) around the organ or viscus of origin. Thus the organ or viscus appears "embedded" within the tumor, or it appears to invaginate within the tumor [85].
- Pedicle or Stalk sign
  A neoplasm may achieve most of its growth outside the organ or viscus of origin. The connection between the two may be a wide bridge or a narrow stalk, which if identified betrays the organ or viscus of origin [85].
- Bridging vessel sign
  The bridging vessels are useful in pointing out the presence of a bridge or stalk that

connects the tumor to the organ or viscus of origin [85].
- The prominent feeding artery and prominent draining vein sign
  If we can trace the afferent and efferent vessels of the tumor to branches of major abdominopelvic arteries and veins, then we can state with confidence the origin of the mass [85, 89, 90].
- Renal displacement and renal rotation sign
  If a retroperitoneal tumor causes both displacement and rotation of the kidney, then it most likely arises outside the kidney [91].
(b) "Could it be an uncommon manifestation of a common disease?"
  If the lesion is not homogeneous, we can mentally "dissect" it into its components. Perhaps we get a breakthrough if we examine each part of the lesion separately. A simple example is a cystic meningioma [76, 95]. If we subtract the cyst(s), then it becomes easier to deal with the solid component and state with confidence that it represents a meningioma; assembling all information, we can then reach the conclusion that the mass is a cystic variant of the "classic" meningioma.
(c) "Could it be an uncommon localization of a common disease?"
  Suppose we see a lesion of mixed composition in an adrenal gland: soft tissue elements are mixed with macroscopic fat and calcifications. What would we think if we saw such a mass in an ovary or in the mediastinum? [96]. So the question we can ask ourselves is: "Have I seen something like that in another anatomic location?"
(d) "Could it be a tumor?" We tend to associate certain imaging patterns with benign conditions. For example, let's consider a previously healthy patient with fever, productive cough, and an air bronchogram in his chest radiograph. Our initial diagnosis would be pneumonia. However, bronchoalveolar cell carcinoma may masquerade as pneumonia [97]. Lymphangioleiomyomatosis is often misclassified under the heading of cystic diseases of the lungs, but actually it is a nonmalignant neoplasm (http://surgpathcriteria.stanford.edu/lung/lymphangioleiomyomatosis/index.html)

Table 7.3 Categories of tumor-like diseases and tumor mimics

- Focal entrapment of fluid or blood
- Deposition of noncellular material
- Growth of abnormal, non-neoplastic cells
- Abnormal proliferation of normal cells
- Mixture of inflammatory, granulomatous, fibrotic, and necrotic reactions
- Degeneration
- Congenital

[98, 99]. It is rare, occurring almost exclusively in young women of reproductive age, and it may belong to the tuberous sclerosis complex. Abnormal, inhomogeneous cells, probably of smooth muscle origin, spread in a disorderly manner (as sheets or nodules) along the walls of bronchioles, lymphatics, and peripheral pulmonary vessels. The result is stenosis and obstruction of the affected channels leading to pulmonary cysts, air trapping, reticular lung opacities, chylous pleural effusions, and pneumothorax. Distended lymphatics and enlarged nodes due to downstream lymphatic obstruction can also occur in the abdomen and pelvis. Lymphangioleiomyomatosis is not to be confused with pulmonary lymphangiomatosis; pulmonary lymhangiomatosis is mentioned below, in the section "could it be a tumor-like condition or a tumor mimic?"

I have placed lymphoma in a special category that includes tuberculosis, sarcoidosis, and Castleman disease, presented later in this chapter (in the sequence indicated in Table 7.20).

(e) "Could it be a tumor-like condition or a tumor mimic?"

I have divided tumor-like processes and tumor mimics into seven categories, based on their pathogenesis, as shown in Table 7.3.

Focal Entrapment of Fluid or Blood
The prototype example is a pleural pseudotumor, which is a focal accumulation of pleural fluid between two leaves of a lung fissure [84]. If it achieves a biconvex shape, it may raise alarm for a lung mass. Usually, measurements of CT densities reveal the true nature of these pseudotumors. If they become infected, we may see thick walls and septations with contrast enhancement, peri-

focal reaction, and elevation of CT density above that of water.

Another example of this type of pseudotumor is a chronic intra- or extra-osseous hematoma, which can cause bizarre remodeling of bone [100, 101].

Deposition of Noncellular Material in a Focal, Multifocal, or Multiorgan Fashion
The prototype example is amyloidosis, characterized by glycoprotein precipitation in the extracellular space. There is a primary and a secondary variety of amyloidosis, with a wide spectrum of manifestations [102, 103].

Growth of Abnormal, Non-neoplastic Cells
We will employ Erdheim Chester disease as an example; it is characterized by the accumulation of lipid-laden foamy histiocytes. It can present either as a purely skeletal disorder or as multisystem disease. These deposits show intense contrast enhancement in cranial, orbital, and spinal bone marrow MR scans [104]. A peculiar phenomenon is the weak contrast enhancement of thoracic and abdominal disease, both on CT and MRI [105].

Some cortical malformations of the brain represent another example of this category of tumor mimics. I have placed these malformations under the heading "Congenital," in this section.

Abnormal Proliferation of Normal Cells
Pulmonary lymphangiomatosis is characterized by proliferation, dilatation, and abnormal interconnection of lymphatic channels [84, 106]. Most commonly it involves the lungs, mediastinum, and pleura in a diffuse fashion. These abnormal lymph vessels can coalesce into discrete unilocular cysts that do not enhance with intravenous contrast [107]. This entity is not to be confused with lymphangioleiomyomatosis, described previously, in this Chapter, in Sect. 7.2.1.5, under the heading "Could it be a tumor?"

Mixture of Inflammatory, Granulomatous, Fibrotic, and Necrotic Reactions
With this term I mean localized aggregation of acute and chronic inflammatory cells, myofibroblastic spindle cells, granulomatous reaction, fibrosis, and necrotic debris. The combination

and the proportion of the above inflammatory elements vary from case to case.

The contrast enhancement may be intense and inhomogeneous. There may be edema and/or reactive changes in the surrounding or invaded tissues.

Examples include:

1. Inflammatory pseudotumor: it can develop in a variety of anatomic locations, as single or multiple foci, and it can closely resemble a malignancy [108].
2. Fungal infections: they can occur in local and disseminated forms, both in the immune-compromised and immune-competent hosts. They can run either a rapid or an indolent course. They can have an aggressive-infiltrative appearance, and they can spread to contiguous structures without respect for fascial or other types of barriers [109–111].
3. Tumefactive demyelinating plaques: they may resemble a glioma on routine CT and MR imaging [112].

Degeneration

By degenerative changes I mean the residues and sequela of wear and tear, prior trauma, prior inflammation/infection, and prior toxic insults or metabolic derangements. Examples include Schmorl's nodes in the spine, rounded atelectasis in the lungs, and focal fatty infiltration of the liver and pancreas.

Schmorl's nodes can be primary or secondary, and this distinction is of paramount importance [113–116]. The primary variety is attributed to wear and tear. In the acute phase, it is accompanied by an intense inflammatory reaction that can spread throughout the vertebral body, and may spill over into adjacent end plates. It may produce intense, localized pain and may mimic neoplastic replacement of the bone marrow. Secondary Schmorl's nodes are the result of bone weakening due to sepsis or due to malignant infiltration of the spongiosa [116].

Rounded atelectasis is complete, focal loss of aeration of lung parenchyma that becomes deformed in an unusual, spiral fashion. It is thought that the causative factor is inflammation or irritation of the pleura that becomes thickened, scarred, and triggers infolding of the adjacent lung parenchyma. It may be unifocal or multifocal, and unilateral or bilateral. Rounded atelectasis has a characteristic shape; nonetheless it may be confused with a lung mass [117].

Parenchymal islets of fat accumulation in the liver and pancreas appear hypodense on CT, and can resemble neoplastic foci. We can establish the correct diagnosis without a doubt performing MRI, with a simple in-opposed phase gradient echo sequence [118].

Congenital Conditions

For the purposes of this section I limit the term "Congenital conditions" to

1. Congenital or developmental cysts
2. Ectopic tissue
3. Malformed tissue

Low lying organs such as a pelvic kidney or a wandering spleen are not included in this category.

- A variety of congenital/developmental cysts can reside in the CNS, neck, chest abdomen, and pelvis. They can cause diagnostic difficulties (a) when they contain proteinaceous fluid or viscous material, instead of watery fluid and (b) when complicated by superinfection or malignant degeneration. Care needs to be exercised not to confuse these cysts with neoplasms that have undergone necrosis or cystic degeneration [119, 120].
- Ectopic tissue presents as a space occupying lesion; either it is anatomically separated from the native orthotopic organ, or it remains embedded within the organ of origin. Examples include heterotopic or accessory spleen, accessory pancreas, and focal heterotopia of cerebral gray matter. Congenitally misplaced splenic tissue usually lands within the pancreatic tail, and may mimic a neuroendocrine neoplasm [118, 121]. Accessory pancreatic tissue can be found at a distance or in close proximity to the main gland, usually in the wall of the

gastrointestinal tract [122]. Ectopic pancreatic nodules may trigger intussusception of the intestine, as well as any of the diseases of the native gland (eg. pancreatitis, etc). Subependymal or subcortical islets of heterotopic gray matter result from focal interruption of the normal neuronal migration [123–125].

- Focal cortical brain malformations constitute a spectrum of disorders affecting the cerebral cortex and the subjacent white matter. Microscopically there is variable disruption of the normal laminar arrangement, accompanied by gliosis, astrocytosis, and the presence of large, bizzare, distorted neurons. Ectopic neurons reside in the subcortical white matter. This group of disorders may be confused with astrocytomas in CT and routine MR imaging [124–127].

I have placed hemangioma and its benign variants, excluding lymphatic and arterial/venous malformations, in a separate category, called special situation (SpSi) #2, to be discussed shortly, on the following page.

(f) Syndromes and Congenital Associations. These diseases are characterized by a cluster or spectrum of findings/abnormalities in organs or tissues, either close to each other or far removed from another. Neurofibromatosis is an example of a syndrome [128]. Renal dysplasia or aplasia is an example of a congenital disorder with a high chance of additional malformations or malfunctions [129, 130]. Please cross reference this type of diseases with Sect. 7.2.1.8 of this chapter. I have selected three special groups of neoplastic and non-neoplastic diseases that I call special situations (SpSi) or "chameleons," because they are capable of presenting with a wide clinical and imaging spectrum. Thus they frequently enter the differential list for a variety of tumors and tumor mimics. These three groups are discussed below, as (g), (h), and (i).

(g) Lymphoma, tuberculosis, sarcoidosis, and Castleman disease—SpSi #1.

These entities share the peculiarity that they can break all the rules, since they have a multiplicity of common and uncommon manifesta-

tions. The initial targets of lymphoma, tuberculosis, and sarcoidosis may be extranodal, extrapulmonary, and extrathoracic respectively. Thus, at times they can present a formidable diagnostic challenge [131–134]. Castleman disease is a unifocal or multicentric, non-neoplastic lympho-proliferative disorder. It can present as a systemic disease and can mimic a variety of neoplasms in the neck, thorax, abdomen, and pelvis. Furthermore, it is associated with paraneoplastic syndromes, hematologic dyscrasias and malignancies, human immunodeficiency virus, and lymphocytic interstitial pneumonitis, increasing the difficulty of correct diagnosis by noninvasive means.

(h) Hemangiomas and their benign variants, excluding lymphatic and arterial/venous malformations—SpSi #2.

These entities can occur throughout the body as single or multiple processes, with simultaneous visceral and osseous involvement. At times they can assume an aggressive appearance, mimicking primary or metastatic malignancy [76, 135–137].

(i) Amyloidosis and inflammatory pseudotumor—SpSi #3.

Amyloidosis and inflammatory pseudotumor have already been presented in this chapter, under the headings "Deposition of noncellular material" and "Mixture of inflammatory, granulomatous, fibrotic, and necrotic reactions" respectively (please refer to Table 7.3).

7.2.1.6 Looking Behind the Scenes for Causes and Complications

- Some imaging findings beg the question: "what is the underlying cause?" [76]. For example consider a child with hip pain without trauma or fever. MRI reveals extensive bone marrow edema in the femur and a hip joint effusion. In this case, one of our diagnostic considerations is a femoral osteoid osteoma [138, 139].

- Some imaging findings, in a patient with a known disease, beg another question: "Has the underlying disease changed due to its natural history or due to prior treatment?" [76]. Let us consider a patient with Paget's disease in the pelvic ring and new onset of pain. A CT scan shows a new area of osteolysis with cortical disruption in the Pagetic bone. One of our considerations should be malignant degeneration into a sarcoma [140, 141].

- Other imaging findings point to an immediate or a delayed complication of prior medical/surgical intervention or treatment. Examples include radiation pneumonitis and radiation fibrosis of the lungs.

7.2.1.7 Time Factors

Diseases with real or potential harm to the patient are usually a dynamic process [142, 143]; the evolution may be slow or rapid and it may accelerate in the later stages of the disease. Thus if the imaging findings do not support the clinical diagnosis, we should consider immediate reimaging after contrast administration or reimaging after an appropriate time interval. "Fogging" of a cerebral or cerebellar ischemic infarct constitutes such an example. "Fogging" is a transitory pseudonormalization of the infarcted/ischemic brain parenchyma, becoming "invisible" (a) on CT and MR in the subacute phase, and (b) on CT immediately after endovascular treatment [144–149].

7.2.1.8 Pause and Reboot

Sometimes I encounter studies with multiple findings that do not tie neatly with each other or with the clinical history. After considering several possibilities I may not be able to come up with a satisfactory answer. If the patient does not require immediate attention, I pause and proceed to the next case. I come back to the problem case at a later time, when I feel ready to tackle it again. My thinking is that *perhaps I missed a finding, I did not consider the correct diagnosis, the patient harbors a syndrome, the patient suffers from a congenital syndrome with associated disorders, or perhaps the patient hosts two unrelated conditions.*

7.2.2 Special Considerations for Oncology Patients

Oncology patients face complex, unique, and evolving challenges, requiring great care in reading their imaging studies. Thus I decided to devote an entire section on the potential CT and MR pitfalls in this group of patients. Some of these concepts have been presented elsewhere in this book, but they are worth repeating in this section.

7.2.2.1 General Remarks

The following items need to be at the front of our checklist:

A. What can I not afford to miss [42, 81, 150].
   We need to be vigilant in:
   (a) Staging the tumor correctly,
   (b) Detecting emergencies such as spinal cord compression, airway obstruction, vascular occlusion or thrombosis,
   (c) Preserving the quality of life of these patients.
B. Multiple CT "windows" and multiplanar reconstructions (MPRs)
   Use multiple CT "windows" and MPRs to "capture" subtle lesions [42, 81, 151–155]. MPRs are suggested as ancillary tools for the detection of (a) pulmonary emboli and (b) spinal fractures, due to metastases, osteopenia, or minor trauma [156–158].
C. Thin maximum intensity projection images (MIPs)
   Create a stack of thin MIPs in order to "isolate" lung nodules from lung vessels [81, 159]
D. Coexistence of two unrelated conditions
   Consider the possibility that a new finding is not related to the patient's known neoplasm, i.e., the patient may harbor two different conditions simultaneously [42, 81, 160, 161]
E. Complications of treatment or malignancy
   Think of potential complications of treatment and of potential complications of the underlying malignancy as explanations for new or deteriorating imaging findings [81]
F. Additional tips that I have found very useful
   1. Coronal MPRs are excellent for evaluating certain blind spots, such as the paravertebral gutters, the subphrenic spaces, and the root of the mesentery.
   2. Coronal MPRs also provide a global overview of the gastrointestinal tract and a

good second look at the pancreaticoduo-denal interface.

3. Sagittal MPRs are advantageous for assessing the presacral and precoccygeal spaces, and the pouch of Douglas.
4. I consider that the evaluation of hollow viscera and hollow structures (such as the gallbladder, GI tract and urinary bladder) is complete only after viewing them in three orthogonal axes [151].
5. Occasionally I find ascites in the pelvis and lower paracolic gutters, without obvious peritoneal implants. In such cases I revisit the subdiaphragmatic spaces, relying heavily on coronal reconstructions. The search is for subtle, plaque-like implants on the peritoneum or on the surface of the liver and spleen.

7.2.2.2 Posttreatment Considerations

Novel approaches to cancer therapy include immune modulation and blockade of tumor neovascularity. These may result in unusual patterns of tumor response, and in unusual complications [81, 162–179]. Knowledge of these mechanisms is essential for: (a) the correct interpretation of confusing or seemingly contradictory appearances and (b) timely warning that a finding may represent a complication of treatment.

A. Tumor Response
  1. Pseudo-progression

     We may encounter the paradox of a stable or increasing tumor size, or the appearance of new metastases, despite a definite improvement in the general condition and the laboratory markers of the patient. This apparent contradiction has been termed pseudo-progression of disease.

     An increase in tumor size may be due to inflammation or intratumoral edema, precipitated by radiation therapy, neoadjuvant chemotherapy, or immunotherapy. This phenomenon has been observed in both solid and nonsolid organs, such as the brain and lungs.

Necrosis of the tumor is not necessarily accompanied by a reduction in size. "Sterile" remnants after initial shrinking may remain stable in size for long periods of time [180].

Tumor necrosis as a response to therapy produces obvious alterations in its CT density and MR signal patterns, as well as an obvious attenuation or even cessation of contrast uptake by the tumor.

Acute hemorrhage within or around the tumor may also occur as a response to treatment. The overall size of the tumor will increase (including the hemorrhagic component), but we will note an obvious increase in CT density and T1 signal intensity.

(a) Pseudoprogression of liver malignancy on CT.

   Some malignant tumors may be nearly isodense to liver on CT, both before and after intravenous contrast administration. Thus, these lesions may evade detection in the initial scan. Successful therapy may devitalize the tumors, in which case they will become easily visible because of their low density, poor vascularization, and low or negligible perfusion in the posttreatment scan. Thus we may be fooled that we are dealing with new lesions.

(b) Pseudoprogression of liver malignancy in the setting of steatosis.

   Previously CT isoattenuating malignant lesions will stand out as hyperdense nodules, if the surrounding liver parenchyma accumulates fat. Thus we may think that there has been interval development of new lesions.

(c) Thymic rebound hyperplasia.

   Rebound thymic hyperplasia may occur post chemotherapy or radiation therapy, and can mimic mediastinal recurrence or lymphadenopathy [181].

(d) Osseous "flare."

Osseous "flare" is another example of pseudoprogression, in the setting of skeletal metastatic disease. The explanation is that a favorable response to therapy allows the accumulation of bony matrix in osteolytic lesions. Thus, previously occult, lytic metastases appear as sclerotic foci in a follow-up CT scan, mimicking new, osteoblastic deposits.

2. Pseudo-pseudo progression.

Pseudo-pseudo progression is a term coined by Morgan et al. to describe the false impression of disease progression, when there is a significant delay between imaging and treatment [81]. In this situation the pretreatment scans may not be an accurate representation of the disease status at the onset of treatment (as they may underestimate the size and the number of neoplastic foci). Thus the first posttreatment scan will not provide a valid comparison, possibly leading us to the incorrect conclusion that the treatment was not effective.

3. Pseudoimprovement of neoplastic disease of the liver assessed by CT.

Most primary and metastatic liver tumors appear hypodense relative to normal hepatic parenchyma on CT. Thus there may be poor differentiation of tumor from hepatic parenchyma against a background of fatty infiltration. So, if there is accumulation of fat in the liver after treatment, we may get the false impression of resolution or improvement in follow-up CT scans.

B. Complications of Therapy

I will only mention the most common adverse reactions associated with the newer anticancer agents [165, 168, 174–179]:

Chest

(a) Sarcoid-like insult to the lung parenchyma and lymph nodes in the hila and mediastinum
(b) Interstitial pneumonitis
(c) Pleural effusions

Gastrointestinal Tract Wall

(a) Pneumatosis
(b) Perforation
(c) Delayed dehiscence of anastomoses

Vascular System

Minor and major thrombotic and hemorrhagic incidents in both small and large vascular territories.

C. Pseudocirrhosis of the Liver

Pseudocirrhosis is a term to describe a gross nodular distortion of the contour and the architecture of the liver that resembles cirrhosis [182, 183]. The pathophysiology and histopathology are different from the typical cirrhosis, e.g., due to alcohol abuse or viral hepatitis. Pseudocirrhosis occurs in some patients who harbor metastatic disease to the liver, most commonly from primary breast carcinoma. There are three mechanisms of pseudocirrhosis.

(a) A rapid reduction in the number and the size of liver metastases can result in nodularity of the liver contour and parenchyma, due to scarring and capsular retraction.
(b) Toxic insult to the liver from chemotherapy may devolve to nodular regenerative hyperplasia.
(c) Diffuse proliferation of metastatic disease can incite an extensive desmoplastic reaction around the cancerous nodules.

7.2.2.3 Conclusion

In conclusion, when we read comparison CT or MR scans of oncology patients we need to take into account any changes in both the neoplastic foci and the host organ. Specifically, we look for any alterations in size, contour, CT density, MR signal intensity, (in)homogeneity, strength, and pattern of contrast enhancement. Of course we need to take into account the clinical course of the patient and the specifics of the therapeutic regimen.

7.2.2.4 Screening for Cancer

Any screening process for malignancy is a low prevalence task, with the inherent disadvantage of a relatively high number of false negative studies. For a reminder for this phenomenon, please see the "Prevalence Bias" in Chap. 5, Sect. 5.2.2.3 [184–186]. This phenomenon begs the question: how can we increase the yield of screening? Is it possible to "trick" the readers into greater accuracy by artificially elevating the prevalence rate of abnormal examinations? [186].

Proper manipulation of the flow of images may prime the brain to detect subtle cancers.

7.2.3   Special Considerations for Medical Devices/Instruments and Foreign Bodies

The term "medical devices and instruments" includes anything we use in order to carry out a medical, surgical, or interventional procedure, whether it is a placement of a nasogastric tube, a laparoscopic cholecystectomy, or an endoscopic placement of a biliary stent to alleviate a malignant stricture. By foreign body I mean any type of foreign material, metal or nonmetal, that is implanted, ingested, impacted, or left behind in the patient, either by accident, on purpose or inadvertently. Examples include cardiac pacemakers, rods, and screws for spinal stabilization, a gauze forgotten in the patient's abdomen after a colectomy, a thorn in a gardener's hand, a gallstone or a bezoar impacted in the small bowel, etc. [184–196]. Medical devices/instruments and foreign bodies can migrate, kink, fracture, get left behind, get occluded (by clot, sludge, or tumor overgrowth), cause a reaction or abscess, perforate soft tissues or vessels, and obstruct the intestinal tract [90, 92, 184, 193–195, 197–203]. Thus we need to become familiar with the various medical devices, and every single time we see them, we need to check their position, continuity, integrity, and think of possible complications. Immediate or delayed deterioration of a patient following a procedure should alert us to the possibility of an iatrogenic mishap, or misplacement/failure of a medical device. We should also be alert for the presence of a foreign body, even if there is no relevant history.

7.3   Error Management in Nonteaching Radiologic Centers and Departments

7.3.1   Quality Control

Quality assurance committees and discrepancy meetings are absolute prerequisites for error man-

agement [204–222]. Quality control can be implemented in two ways. The first is via random sampling for double reading, while maintaining statistical validity [209–215]. In cases of obvious discrepancies or suspected errors, a final opinion can be reached either by consensus or by a third party, such as a senior expert radiologist [211–213]. Objective benchmarks have been established in order to assess the performance of radiology departments and individual radiologists, including trainees. This knowledge has important implications in guiding and counseling individuals, as well as devising a curriculum for trainees [210, 211, 214, 215]. Any radiologist can determine where he stands relative to his peers. Another method of learning is to focus on cases, instead of individual radiologists, for the benefit of the entire section or department. Group discussions with wide participation revolve around the analysis and prevention of errors and pitfalls [218–224]. The cases can be collected in a nonrandom way, from the daily work load, case conferences, and official second readings.

7.3.2   Error Discussion

It is advised that we engage in feedback and open discussion as a team, in a blame-free, non-punitive manner [32, 208, 218, 220–232]. This way radiologists do not feel stigmatized and they become open to suggestions for improvement.

Even major organizations advocate a shame-free, open discussion of errors and adverse incidents for the benefit of the patients and the entire medical community, such as the Royal College of Radiologists and the Agency for Healthcare Research and Quality (https://www.rcr.ac.uk/clinical-radiology/being-consultant/read/read-newsletters) [231]. Both of them provide a platform for electronic publishing of errors and incidents for educational purposes only.

7.3.3   Safeguarding the Patient's Identity in Examinations, Reports, and Files

Occasionally a patient is subjected to the wrong imaging examination, a report is dictated or filed under another patient's name, or a copy of the examination goes in another patient's file [233]. An automated, fail proof filter should ensure that these mistakes are eliminated.

7.3.4 Allocation of Resources

7.3.4.1 Subspecialists

Some imaging studies carry a high risk for errors or place a high burden on the radiologists and thus should be read only by subspecialists [82]. Two authors measured the additional time cost of reading abdominopelvic CT scans in two patient populations: non-oncologic patients complaining of abdominal pain versus oncologic patients. For the latter group the interpretation time was 40% greater [234].

All imaging studies can be stratified according to complexity and risk for error [82, 235]. Staff radiologists can also be "graded" according to their diagnostic capabilities. Thus each imaging study can be matched to the appropriate person. Underperforming radiologists should be prohibited from interpreting high demand studies until they successfully complete additional, focused training [235].

7.3.4.2 Double Reading

It has been shown that double reading increases diagnostic accuracy [1, 232, 236–242].

In some countries, double reading of screening mammograms is considered the standard of care. One radiology group employs "partial" double reading of all high-risk studies. The interpreting radiologist is alerted automatically about the dangers of the study. A second radiologist is recruited to answer in real time whether predetermined pathology is present or absent [82]. Thus, the second reader answers the question "what can I not afford to miss."

A procedure should be in place to resolve any conflicts in opinion between the two readers, in a timely and non-biased manner [232, 238, 243].

Unfortunately, many departments in small communities cannot support double reading or on-site subspecialists, due to financial constraints and manpower shortage.

7.3.4.3 Official Second Interpretation

Some patients after their initial evaluation and initial imaging get referred to tertiary medical centers, where an official second interpretation may be rendered by a subspecialist radiologist [17, 89, 236, 244–250]. Several researchers have compared the first and second readouts, but have not exposed four factors in favor of the second reader, including: (a) direct communication with the requesting physician, (b) a simplified task to answer very specific targeted questions, (c) possible access to additional data in the form or imaging or laboratory tests, performed after the initial readout, and (d) possible participation in a multidisciplinary board discussing the patient in question.

Thus, the results of this research should not surprise anybody, reflecting the importance of subspecialization and team collaboration: the second report resulted in a change in patient management in a significant percentage of cases.

7.3.4.4 Arresting Propagation of Errors

In order to avoid repetition or propagation of the same error a team of radiologists adheres stritly to the following rule: no radiologist reports more than two consecutive surveillance scans in a given patient [81].

7.3.4.5 Teleradiology

Teleradiology is a solution to the shortage of subspecialists, albeit not a perfect one [32, 251]. In small communities, interpersonal relationships are very important. In my experience both the patients and the referring physicians feel more comfortable consulting a radiologist that they have met and have known for some time [251]. Many patients prefer to discuss the results of their imaging studies with a radiologist they trust, even before revisiting their referring physician. Thus teleradiologists are considered outsiders and are viewed with skepticism in small communities. Local, on-site radiologists in small departments have one more advantage over teleradiologists: flexibility in expediting urgent or emergent situations. In my department for some CT scans the total turnaround time is less than 15 min (from the time the patient arrives at the front desk to the time that the referring physician is called with the results of the study).

Concluding, I cannot offer a solid solution to the problem of nonspecialist services in small communities.

7.3.4.6 Safeguarding the Radiology Report

A mechanism should ensure that each dictated report is assigned to the correct patient. The appropriate, structured templates could be automatically provided to the radiologist, according to the clinical history and the type of imaging study. Each template could incorporate warnings or reminders to look for blind spots and specific findings that should not be missed [82, 235, 252]. The reports should be scanned by laterality and enumeration tracking software [252]. The dictation software could keep the report "locked" until the radiologist has double checked the patient's name, measurements, and key words or phrases (for example, right/left, the size of a mass, or the level of an intervertebral disk hernia). Only then, the radiologist can sign off the report and send it to the archives, the patient's file, the referring physician, and, if indicated, to the entire team caring for the patient.

7.4 The Role of Teaching Institutions

The principles described above for individual radiologists and nonteaching centers apply to teaching institutions as well.

Academic or university organizations should carry additional duties that include [253–260]:

- Addressing, assessing, implementing, improving, and devising error management strategies,
- Examining, revising, and upgrading the training curriculum and the standards of our practice whenever necessary,
- Holding clinical-radiologic conferences on a regular schedule, with the aim of inspiring physicians from different specialties to work

together as a team. These interdisciplinary meetings should address explicitly the needs of each department, in order to foster a successful collaboration. A team of physicians is stronger than the sum of its parts [31, 32, 261].

I firmly believe that proper training is the best strategy to reduce errors and minimize their impact. Education on errors and their management should be an important and active part of any medical curriculum [262–264]!

References

1. Robinson PJ. Radiology's Achilles' heel: error and variation in the interpretation of the Roentgen image. Br J Radiol. 1997;70:1085–98.
2. Gunderman RB, Nyce JM. The tyranny of accuracy in radiologic education. Radiology. 2002;222:297–300.
3. Itri JN, Tappouni RR, McEachern RO, Pesch RO, Patel SH. fundamentals of diagnostic error in imaging. Radiographics. 2018;38:1845–65.
4. Schiff GD. Minimizing diagnostic error: the importance of follow-up and feedback. Am J Med. 2008;121(5 suppl):S38–42.
5. Brook OR, O'Connell AM, Thornton E, Eisenberg RL, Mendiratta-Lala M, Kruskal JB. Quality initiatives: anatomy and pathophysiology of errors occurring in clinical radiology practice. Radiographics. 2010;30:1401–10.
6. Graber ML. Taking steps toward a safer future: measures to promote timely and accurate Medical diagnosis. Am J Med. 2008;121(suppl 5):S43–6.
7. Kelly AM. Basic definitions. In: Abujudeh HH, Bruno MA, editors. Quality and safety in radiology. Oxford: Oxford University Press; 2012.
8. Roddie ME. Approach to characterizing radiological errors. In: Peh WCG, editor. Pitfalls in diagnostic radiology. Heidelberg: Springer; 2015.
9. Berlin L. Radiologic errors and malpractice: a blurry distinction. AJR. 2007;189:517–22.
10. Berlin L. Medicolegal-malpractice and ethical issues in radiology. Overdiagnosis, false-positive findings, and malpractice. AJR. 2014;203:W549.
11. Berlin L. Malpractice issues in radiology. Perceptual errors. AJR. 1996;167:587–90.
12. Berlin L, Hendrix RW. Perceptual errors and negligence. AJR. 1998;170:863–7.
13. Berlin L. Errors of omission. AJR. 2005;185:1416–21.
14. Waite S, Scott J, Gale B, Fuchs T, Kolla S, Reede D. Interpretive error in radiology. AJR. 2017;208:739–49.
15. Bui-Mansfield LT. "Fool me twice": delayed diagnoses in radiology with emphasis on perpetuated errors.

Video Lecture. www.learning.arrs.org/course/view.php?id=518. Accessed 19 Nov 2017.

16. Rosenkrantz AB, Bansal NK. Diagnostic errors in abdominopelvic CT interpretation: characterization based on report addenda. Abdom Radiol (NY). 2016;41:1793–9.

17. Kabadi SJ, Krishmaraj A. Strategies for improving the value of the radiology report: a retrospective analysis of errors in formally over-read studies. J Am Coll Radiol. 2017;14:459–66.

18. Bruno MA, Walker EA, Abujudeh HH. Understanding and confronting our mistakes: the epidemiology of error in radiology and strategies for error reduction. Radiographics. 2015;35:1668–76.

19. Berlin L. Radiologic errors, past, present and future. Diagnosis (Berl). 2014;1:79–84.

20. Kim YW, Mansfield LT. Fool me twice: delayed diagnoses in radiology with emphasis on perpetuated errors. AJR. 2014;202:465–70.

21. McCreadie G, Oliver TB. Eight CT lessons that we learned the hard way: an analysis of current patterns of radiological error and discrepancy with particular emphasis on CT. Clin Radiol. 2009;64:491–9.

22. Donald JJ, Barnard SA. Common patterns in 558 diagnostic radiology errors. J Med Imaging Radiat Oncol. 2012;56:173–8.

23. Renfrew DL, Franken EA Jr, Berbaum KS, Weigelt FH, Abu-Yousef MM. Error in radiology: classification and lessons in 182 cases presented at a problem case conference. Radiology. 1982;183:145–50.

24. Eberhardt SC, Heilbrun ME. Radiology report value equation. Radiographics. 2018;38:1888–96.

25. Ware JB, Saurabh J, Hoang JK, Baker S, Wruble J. Effective radiology reporting. J Am Coll Radiol. 2017;14:838–9.

26. Newman-Toker D. A unified conceptual model for diagnostic errors: underdiagnosis, overdiagnosis, and misdiagnosis. Diagnosis (Berl). 2014;1:43–8.

27. Brady AP. Error and discrepancy in radiology: inevitable or avoidable? Insights Imaging. 2017;8:171–82.

28. Brady A, Laoide RO, McCarthy P, McDermott R. Discrepancy and error in radiology: concepts, causes and consequences. Ulster Med J. 2012;81:3–9.

29. Sabih DE, Sabih A, Sabih Q, Khan AN. Image perception and interpretation of abnormalities; can we believe our eyes? Can we do something about it? Insights Imaging. 2011;2:47–55.

30. Pinto A, Brunese L. Spectrum of diagnostic errors in radiology. World J Radiol. 2010;2:377–83.

31. Fitzgerald R. Radiological error: analysis, standard setting, targeted instruction and teamworking. Eur Radiol. 2005;15:1760–7.

32. Fitzgerald R. Error in Radiology. Clin Radiol. 2001;56:938–46.

33. Bruno MA. Our mistakes-the human experience. Video Lecture. www.learning.arrs.org/mod/url/view.php?id=400. Accessed 22 Nov 2016.

34. Bruno MA. 256 shades of gray: uncertainty and diagnostic error in radiology. Diagnosis (Berl). 2017;4:149–57.

35. Garland LH. Studies on the accuracy of diagnostic procedures. Am J Roentgenol Radium Ther Nuc Med. 1959;82:25–38.

36. Abujudeh HH, Boland GW, Kaewlai R, et al. Abdominal and pelvic computed tomography (CT) interpretation: discrepancy rates among experienced radiologists. Eur Radiol. 2010;20:1952–7.

37. Robinson PJ, Wilson D, Coral A, Murphy A, Verow P. Variation between experienced observers in the interpretation of accident and emergency radiographs. Br J Radiol. 1999;72:323–30.

38. Babiarsz LS, Yousem DM. Quality control in neuroradiology: discrepancies in image interpretation among academic neuroradiologists. Am J Neuroradiol. 2012;33:969–80.

39. Wakeley CJ, Jones AM, Kabala JE, Prince D, Goddard PR. Audit of the value of double reading magnetic resonance imaging films. Br J Radiol. 1995;68:358–60.

40. Pinto A, Scuderi MG, Daniele S. Errors in radiology: definition and classification. In: Romano L, Pinto A, editors. Errors in radiology. Heidelberg: Springer; 2012.

41. Bechtold RE, Chen MY, Ott DJ, Zagoria RJ, Scharling ES, Wolfman NT, Vining DJ. Interpretation of abdominal CT: analysis of errors and their causes. J Comput Assist Tomogr. 1997;21:681–5.

42. Owens EJ, Taylor NR, Howlett DC. Perceptual type error in everyday practice. Clin Radiol. 2016;71:593–601.

43. Li F, Sone S, Abe H, MacMahon H, Armato SG 3rd, Doi K. Lung cancers missed at low-dose helical CT screening in a general population: comparison of clinical, histopathologic, and imaging findings. Radiology. 2002;225:673–83.

44. Del Ciello A, Franchi P, Contegiacomo A, Cicchetti G, Bonomo L, Larici AR. Missed lung cancer: when, where and why? Diagn Interv Radiol. 2017;23:118–26.

45. Palazzetti V, Guidi F, Ottaviani L, Valeri G, Baldassarre S, Giusepetti GM. Analysis of mammographic diagnostic errors in breast clinics. Radiol Med. 2016;121:828–33.

46. Wu MZ, McInnes MD, Macdonald DB, Kielar AZ, Duigenan S. CT in adults: systematic review and meta-analysis of interpretation discrepancy rates. Radiology. 2014;270:717–35.

47. Kohn LT, Corrigan JM, Donaldson MS. Executive summary in: to err is human: building a safer health system. Washington: National Academy Press; 2000. p. 1–16.

48. Vincent C, Neale G, Woloshynowych M. Adverse events in British hospitals: preliminary retrospective record review. BMJ. 2001;322:517–9.

49. Wachter RM. Why diagnostic errors don't get any respect-and what can be done about them. Health Aff. 2010;29:1605–10.

50. Halsted MJ. Hearing the alarms: defining medical errors. J Am Coll Radiol. 2005;2:299–300.
51. Sanders L. Sick thinking. In: Every patient tells a story. New York: Broadway Books; 2010. p. 193–215.
52. Groopman J. Introduction. In: How doctors think. Boston: Houghton Mifflin Company; 2008. p. 1–26.
53. Graber ML. The incidence of diagnostic error in medicine. BMJ Qual Saf. 2013;22:ii21–7.
54. Raskin MM. Survival strategies for radiology: some practical tips on how to reduce the risk of being sued and losing. J Am Coll Radiol. 2006;3:689–93.
55. Croskerry P. Clinical cognition and diagnostic error: applications of a dual process model of reasoning. Adv Health Sci Edu. 2009;14:27–35.
56. Kahneman D, Slovic P, Tversky A. Judgement under uncertainty: heuristics and biases. Cambridge: Cambridge University Press; 1982.
57. Kahneman D. Thinking fast and slow. New York: Farrar, Straus and Giroux; 2013.
58. Wallsten TS. Physician and medical student bias in evaluating diagnostic information. Med Decis Making. 1981;1:145–64.
59. Itri JN, Patel SH. Heuristics and cognitive error in medical imaging. Am J Roentgenol. 2018;210:1097–105.
60. Lee CS, Nagy PG, Weaver SJ, Newman-Toker DE. Cognitive and system factors contributing to diagnostic errors in radiology. AJR. 2013;201:611–7.
61. Berner ES, Graber ML. Overconfidence as a cause of diagnostic errors in medicine. Am J Med. 2008;121(5 Suppl):S2–S23.
62. Croskerry P, Norman G. Overconfidence in clinical decision making. Am J Med. 2008;121(5 Suppl):S24–9.
63. Trowbridge RL. Twelve tips for teaching avoidance of diagnostic errors. Med Teach. 2008;30:496–500.
64. Croskerry P, Singhal G, Mamede S, et al. Cognitive debiasing 1: origins of bias and theory of debiasing. BMJ Qual Saf. 2013;22(Suppl 2):ii58–64.
65. Croskerry P, Singhal G, Mamede S, et al. Cognitive debiasing 2: impediments to and strategies for change. BMJ Qual Saf. 2013;22(Suppl 2):ii65–72.
66. Henriksen K, Brady J. The pursuit of better diagnostic performance: a human factors perspective. BMJ Qual Saf. 2013;22:ii1–5.
67. Rencic J. Twelve tips for teaching expertise in clinical reasoning. Med Teach. 2011;33:887–92.
68. Delaney C, Golding C. Teaching clinical reasoning by making thinking visible: an action research project with allied health clinical educators. BMC Med Educ. 2014;14:20–9.
69. Norman GR, Monteiro SD, Sherbino J, Ilgen JS, Schmidt HG, Mamede S. The causes of errors in clinical reasoning: cognitive biases, knowledge deficits, and dual process thinking. Acad Med. 2016. https://doi.org/10.1097/ACM.0000000000001421.
70. Trowbridge RL, Dhaliwal G, Cosby KS. Educational agenda for diagnostic error reduction. BMJ Qual Saf. 2013;22:ii28–32.
71. Graber ML, Kissam S, Payne VL, et al. Cognitive interventions to reduce diagnostic error: a narrative review. BMJ Qual Saf. 2012;21:535–57.
72. Lee CS, Kadom N, Nagy P. Reducing errors from cognitive biases through quality improvement projects. J Am Coll Radiol. 2017;14:852–3.
73. Singhal G. Perspectives from a pediatrician about diagnostic errors. Diagnosis (Berlin). 2014;1:69–74.
74. Elstein AS, Schwarz A. Clinical problem solving and diagnostic decision making: selective review of the cognitive literature. BMJ. 2002;324:729–32.
75. Epstein RM, Hundert EM. Defining and assessing professional competence. JAMA. 2002;287:226–35.
76. Chrysikopoulos H. Basics of MR examinations and interpretation. In: Clinical MR imaging and physics: a tutorial. Heidelberg: Springer; 2009. p. 109–64.
77. Cahan A. Diagnosis is driven by probabilistic reasoning: counter-point. Diagnosis (Berlin). 2016;3:99–101.
78. Rubin GD, Roos JE, Tall M, et al. Characterizing search, recognition and decision in the detection of lung nodules on CT scans: elucidation with eye tracking. Radiology. 2015;274:276–86.
79. Drew T, Vo MLH, Olwal A, Jacobson F, Seltzer SS. Scanners and drillers: characterizing expert visual search through volumetric images. J Vis. 2013;13:1–13.
80. Groopman J. The eye of the beholder. In: How doctors think. Boston: Houghton Mifflin Company; 2007. p. 177–202.
81. Morgan B, Stephenson JA, Griffin Y. Minimising the impact of errors in the interpretation of CT images for surveillance and evaluation of therapy in cancer. Clin Radiol. 2016;71:1083–94.
82. Radisphere. Concurrence review. www.radiosphereradiology.com/standards/diagnostic-accuracy/concurrence-review/. Accessed 24 Oct 2016.
83. Nishino M, Hayakawa K, Minami M, Yamamoto A, Ueda H, Takasu K. Primary retroperitoneal neoplasms: CT and MR imaging findings with anatomic and pathologic diagnostic clues. Radiographics. 2003;23:45–57.
84. Walker C, Takasugi JE, Chung JA, et al. Tumorlike conditions of the pleura. Radiographics. 2012;32:971–85.
85. Kim SW, Kim HC, Yang DM, Won KY. Gastrointestinal stromal tumors (GISTs) with a thousand faces: atypical manifestations and causes of misdiagnosis on imaging. Clin Radiol. 2016;71:3130–42.
86. Shaaban AM, Revzani M, Tubay M, Elsayes KM, Woodward PJ, Menias CO. Fat-containing retroperitoneal lesions: imaging characteristics, localization, and differential diagnosis. Radiographics. 2016;36:710–34.
87. Sandrasegaran K, Rajesh A, Rydberg J, Rushing DA, Akisik FM, Henley JD. Pictorial essay. Gastrointestinal stromal tumors: clinical, radiologic and pathologic features. AJR. 2005;184:803–11.

88. Levy A, Arnaiz J, Shaw JC, Sobin LH. From the archives of AFIP. Primary peritoneal tumors: imaging features with pathologic correlation. Radiograhics. 2008;28:583–607.

89. Lakhman Y, D'Anastasi M, Micco M, et al. Second-opinion interpretations of gynecologic oncologic MRI examinations by sub-specialized radiologists influence patient care. Eur Radiol. 2016;26:2089–98.

90. Asayama Y, Yosimitsu K, Aibe H, et al. MDCT of the gonadal veins in females with large pelvic masses: value in differentiating ovarian versus uterine origin. AJR. 2006;186:440–8.

91. Wu YH, Song B, Xu J, et al. Retroperitoneal neoplasms within the perirenal space in infants and children: differentiation of renal and non-renal origin in enhanced images. Eur J Radiol. 2010;75:279–86.

92. George AE, Russell EJ, Kricheff II. White matter buckling: CT sign of extraaxial mass. AJR. 1980;135:1031–6.

93. Russel EJ, Naidich TP. The enhancing septal/alveal wedge: a septal sign of intraaxial mass. Neuroradiology. 1982;23:33–40.

94. Muranda P, Purohit BS, Thota V, Rashad A, Tan TY. Pictorial review of the imaging anatomy and common pathology of the parotid space. Poster ECR 2014/C-2384. 2014. https://posterng.net-key.at/esr/viewing/index.php?module=viewing_poster&doi=10.1594/ecr2014/C-1092. Accessed 12 Dec 2017.

95. Wasenko JJ, Hocchauser L, Stopa LG, Winfield JA. Cystic meningiomas: MR characteristics and surgical correlations. Am J Neuroradiol. 1994;15:1959–65.

96. Bhatia V, Sharma S, Sood S, Mardi K, Venkat B. Diagnosis please: case 231: retroperitoneal adrenal teratoma presenting a trichoptysis. Radiology. 2016;280:317–21.

97. Patsios D, Roberts HC, Paul NS, et al. Pictorial review of the many faces of bronchioloalveolar cell carcinoma. Br J Radiol. 2007;80:1015–23.

98. Abbott GF, Rosado-de-Christenson ML, Frazier AA, Franks TJ, Pugattch RD, Galvin JR. Lymphangioleiomyomatosis: radiologic- pathologic correlation. Radiographics. 2005;25:803–28.

99. Avila NA, Dwyer AJ, Moss J. Imaging features of lymphangioleiomyomatosis: diagnostic pitfalls. AJR. 2011;196:982–6.

100. Taljanovic MS, Hoover K. System-based imaging pitfalls: musculoskeletal system. In: Peh WCG, editor. Pitfalls in diagnostic radiology. Berlin: Springer; 2015. p. 145–83.

101. Park JS, Ryu KN. Pictorial essay. Hemophilic pseudotumor involving the musculoskeletal system: spectrum of radiologic findings. AJR. 2004;183:55–61.

102. Howard S, Jagganathan J, Krajewski K, et al. Multimodality imaging in amyloidosis. Cancer Imaging. 2012;12:109–17.

103. Georgiades CS, Neyman E, Barish MA, Fishman EK. Amyloidosis: review and CT manifestations. Radiographics. 2004;24:405–16.

104. Sedrak P, Ketonen L, Hou P, et al. Erdheim-Chester disease of the central nervous system: new manifestations of a rare disease. Am J Neuroradiol. 2011;32:2126–31.

105. Antunes C, Graca B, Donato P. Thoracic, abdominal and musculoskeletal involvement in Erdheim-Chester disease: CT, MR and PET imaging findings. Insights Imaging. 2014;5:473–82.

106. Raman SP, Pipavath SNJ, Raghu G, Schmidt RA, Godwin JD. Imaging of thoracic lymphatic diseases. AJR. 2009;193:1504–13.

107. Yang DH, Goo HW. Generalized lymphangiomatosis: radiologic findings in three pediatric patients. Korean J Radiol. 2006;7:287–91.

108. Patnana M, Sevrukov AB, Elsayes KM, Viswanathan C, Lubner M, Menias CO. Inflammatory pseudotumor: the great mimicker. AJR. 2012;198:W217–27.

109. Heo SH, Shin SS, Kim JW, et al. Imaging of actinomycosis in various organs: a comprehensive review. Radiographics. 2014;34:19–33.

110. Morland D, Hassler S. Diagnosis please. Case 219: pelvic actinomycosis mimicking malignant tumor. Radiology. 2015;276:304–8.

111. Middlebrooks EH, Frost CJ, De Jesus RO, Massini TC, Schmafuss IM, Mancuso AA. Acute invasive fungal rhinosinusitis: a comprehensive update of CT findings and design of an effective diagnostic imaging model. Am J Neuroradiol. 2015;36:1529–35.

112. Given CA, Stevens BS, Lee C. The MRI appearance of tumefactive demyelinating lesions. AJR. 2004;182:195–9.

113. Wu HT, Morrison WB, Schweitzer ME. Edematous Scmorl's nodes on thoracolumbar MR imaging: characteristic patterns and changes over time. Skeletal Radiol. 2006;35:212–9.

114. Hauger O, Cotten A, Chateil JF, Borg O, Moinard M, Diard F. Giant cystic Schmorl's nodes. Imaging findings in six patients. AJR. 2001;176:969–72.

115. Nogueira-Barbosa MH, Crema MD, da Silva Herrero CFP, Pasqualini W, Defino HLA. The several faces of Schmorl's node: pictorial essay. Coluna. 2015;14:320–3.

116. Rodacki MA, Castro CE, Castro DS. Diffuse vertebral body edema due to calcified intraspongious disk herniation. Neuroradiology. 2005;47:316–21.

117. Sobocinska M, Sobocinski B, Jarmzemska A, Searfin B. Rounded atelectasis of the lung: a pictorial review. Pol J Radiol. 2014;79:203–9.

118. Vernuccio F, Borhani AA, Dioguardi Burgio M, Midiri M, Furlan A, Brancatelli G. Common and uncommon pitfalls in pancreatic imaging: it is not always cancer. Abdom Radiol. 2015;41:283–94.

119. Dahan H, Arrive L, Wendum D, le Pointe D, Djouri H, Tubiana JM. Retrorectal developmental cysts in adults: clinical and radiologic-histopathologic review, differential diagnosis, and treatment. Radiographics. 2001;21:575–84.

120. Yang DM, Jung DH, Kim H, et al. Retroperitoneal cystic masses: CT, clinical, and pathologic find-

ings and literature review. Radiographics. 2004;24:1353–65.

121. Yildiz AE, Ariyurek MO, Karcaaltincaba M. Splenic anomalies of shape, size, and location: pictorial essay. Sci World J. 2013. https://doi.org/10.1155/2013/321810. Accessed 13 Dec 2017.

122. Revzani M, Menias C, Sandrasegaran K, Olpin JD, Elsayes KM, Shaaban AM. Heterotopic pancreas: histopathologic features, imaging findings, and complications. Radiographics. 2017;37:484–99.

123. Donkol RH, Mogdazy KM, Abolenin A. Assessment of gray matter heterotopia by magnetic resonance imaging. World J Radiol. 2012;4:90–6.

124. Abdel Razek AA, Kandell AY, Elsorogy LG, Elmongy A, Basett AA. Disorders of cortical formation: MR imaging features. Am J Neuroradiol. 2009;30:4–11.

125. Barkovich AJ, Guerrini R, Kuzniecky RI, Jackson GD, Dobyns WB. A developmental and genetic classification for malformations of cortical development: update 2012. Brain. 2012;135:1348–69.

126. Hofman PAM, Fitt GJ, Harvey AS, Kuzniecky RI, Jackson G. Bottom-of-sulcus dysplasia: imaging features. AJR. 2011;196:881–5.

127. Colombo N, Tassi L, Galli C, et al. Focal cortical dysplasias: MR imaging, histopathology, and clinical correlations in surgically treated patients with epilepsy. Am J Neuroradiol. 2003;24:724–33.

128. Fortman BJ, Kuszyk BS, Urban BA, Fishman EK. Neurofibromatosis type 1: a diagnostic mimicker at CT. Radiographics. 2001;21:601–12.

129. Westland R, Schreuder MF, Ket JC, van Wijk JA. Unilateral renal agenesis: a systematic review on associated anomalies and renal injury. Nephrol Dial Transplant. 2013;28:1844–55.

130. Hall-Craggs MA, Kirkham A, Creighton SM. Renal and urologic abnormalities occurring with Mullerian anomalies. J Pediatr Urol. 2013;9:27–32.

131. Ha CS, Medeiros LJ, Charnsangavej C, Crump M, Gospodarowitz MK. Plenary session-oncodiagnosis panel: 2004. Lymphoma Radiographics. 2006;26:607–20.

132. Burrill J, Williams CJ, Bain G, Conder G, Hine AL, Misra RR. Tuberculosis: a radiologic review. Radiographics. 2007;27:1255–127.

133. Koyama M, Ueda H, Togashi K, Umeoka S, Kataoka M, Nagai S. Radiologic manifestations of sarcoidosis in various organs. Radiographics. 2004;24:87–104.

134. Bonekamp D, Horton KM, Hruban RH, Fishman EK. Castleman disease: the great mimic. Radiographics. 2011;31:1793–807.

135. Vilanova JC, Barcelo J, Smirniotopoulos JG, et al. Hemangioma from head to toe: MR imaging with pathologic correlation. Radiographics. 2004;24:367–85.

136. Friedman DP. Symptomatic vertebral hemangiomas: MR findings. AJR. 1996;167:359–64.

137. Chrysikopoulos H, Roussakis A, Tsakraklides V, Vassilouthis J. Sclerotic skeletal hemangiomatosis presenting with spinal cord compression-CT and MRI findings. Br J Radiol. 1996;69:965–7.

138. Chai JW, Hong SH, Choi JY, et al. Radiologic diagnosis of osteoid osteoma: from simple to challenging findings. Radiographics. 2010;30:737–49.

139. Klontzas ME, Zibis AH, Karantanas AH. Osteoid osteoma of the femoral neck: use of the half-moon sign in MRI diagnosis. AJR. 2015;205:353–7.

140. Theodorou DJ, Theodorou SJ, Kakitsubata Y. Imaging of Paget disease of bone and its musculoskeletal complications: review. AJR. 2011;196:S64–75.

141. Smith SE, Murphey MD, Motamedi K, Mulligan ME, Resnick CS, Gannon FH. Radiologic spectrum of Paget disease of bone and its complications with pathologic correlation. Radiographics. 2002;22:1191–216.

142. Zwaan L, Singh H. The challenges in defining and measuring diagnostic error. Diagnosi. 2015;2:97–103.

143. Heyhoe J, Lawton R, Armitage G, Conner M, Ashurst NH. Understanding diagnostic error: looking beyond diagnostic accuracy. Diagnosi. 2015;2:205–9.

144. De Cocker LJ, Lovblad KO, Hendrikse J. MRI of cerebellar infarction. Eur Neurol. 2017;77:137–46.

145. Yannes M, Frabizzio JV, Shah QA. Reversal of CT hypodensity after acute ischemic stroke. J Vasc Interv Neurol. 2013;6:10–4.

146. Choi P, Srinkath V, Phan T. "Fogging" resulting in normal MRI 3 weeks after ischemic stroke. BMJ Case Rep. 2011;2011:bcr042011410.

147. O'Brien P, Sellar RJ, Wardlaw JM. Fogging on T2-weighted MR after acute ischemic stroke: how often might this occur and what are the implications? Neuroradiology. 2004;46:635–41.

148. Uchino A, Sawada YA, Imaizumi T, Mineta T, Kudo S. Report of fogging effect on fast FLAIR magnetic resonance images of cerebral infarctions. Neuroradiology. 2004;46:40–3.

149. Dekeyzer S, Reich A, Othman AE, Wiesmann M, Nikoubashman O. Infarct fogging on immediate postinterventional CT-a not infrequent occurrence. Neuroradiology. 2017;59:853–9.

150. Wu J, Goyal L, Nipp R, Wo J, Qadan M, Uppot RN. The tipping point: critical changes in the management of malignant tumors of the gastrointestinal tract. Curr Probl Diagn Radiol. 2019;48:61–74.

151. Johnson PT, Badger D, Horton KM, Fishman EK. Mitigating misdiagnosis in radiology: educational CT CME case conference for peer review and interpretive improvement. J Am Coll Radiol. 2016;13:1244–6.

152. Johnson PT, Horton KM, Fishman EK. How not to miss or mischaracterize a renal cell carcinoma: protocols, pearls and pitfalls. AJR. 2010;194:W307–15.

153. Espinosa LA, Kelly AM, Hawley C, et al. Clinical utility of multiplanar reformation in pulmonary CT angiography. AJR. 2010;194:70–5.

154. Bae KT, Mody GN, Balfe DM, et al. CT depiction of pulmonary emboli: display window settings. Radiology. 2005;236:677–84.
155. Sahi K, Jackson S, Wiebe E, et al. The value of "liver windows" settings in the detection of small renal cell carcinomas on unenhanced computed tomography. Can Assoc Radiol J. 2014;65:71–6.
156. Mitchell RM, Jewell P, Javaid MK, McKean D, Ostlere SJ. Reporting of vertebral fragility fractures: can radiologists help reduce the number of hip fractures? Arch Osteoporos. 2017;12:71. https://doi.org/10.1007/s11657-017-0363-y.
157. Obaid H, Husamaldin Z, Bhatt R. Underdiagnosis of vertebral collapse on routine multidetector computed tomography scan of the abdomen. Acta Radiol. 2008;49:795–800.
158. Lenchick L, Rogers LF, Delmas PD, Gennant HK. Diagnosis of osteoporotic vertebral fractures: importance of recognition and description by radiologists. AJR. 2004;183:949–58.
159. Kawel N, Seifert B, Luetlof M, Boehm T. Effect of slab thickness on the CT detection of pulmonary nodules: use of sliding thin-slab maximum intensity projection and volume rendering. AJR. 2009;192:1324–9.
160. Liu ZY, Sun JJ, He KW, Zhuo PY, Yu ZY. Primary or metastatic hepatic carcinoma? A breast cancer patient after adjuvant chemotherapy and radiotherapy postoperatively with intrahepatic cholangiocarcinoma and review of the literature. World J Surg Oncol. 2016;14:183–6.
161. Akanabe S, Ohira M, Kobayashi T, et al. Intrahepatic cholangiocarcinoma coinciding with a liver metastasis from a rectal carcinoma: case report. Surg Case Rep. 2016;2:94–7.
162. Nishino M, Hatabu H, Hodi FS. Imaging of cancer immunotherapy: current approaches and future directions. Radiology. 2019;290:9–22.
163. Milliron B, Mittal PK, Canacho JC, Datir A, Moreno CC. Gastrointestinal stromal tumors: imaging features before and after treatment. Curr Probl Diagn Radiol. 2017;46:17–25.
164. Kwak JJ, Tirumani SH, Van den Abbele AD, Koo PJ, Jacene HA. Cancer immunotherapy: imaging assessment of novel treatment response patterns and immune related adverse events. Radiographics. 2015;35:424–37.
165. Wang LL, Leach JL, Breneman JC, McPherson CM, Gaskill-Shipley MF. Critical role of imaging in the neurosurgical and radiotherapeutic management of brain tumors. Radiographics. 2014;34:702–21.
166. Tirumani SH, Kim KW, Nishino M, et al. Update on the role of imaging of metastatic colorectal cancer. Radiographics. 2014;34:1908–28.
167. Shinagare AB, Jagannathan JP, Krajewsji KM, Ramaiya NH. Liver metastases in the era of molecular targeted therapy: new faces of treatment response. AJR. 2013;201:W15–28.
168. Brufau BP, Cerqueda CS, Villalba LB, Izquierdo RS, Gonzalez BM, Molina CN. Metastatic renal cell carcinoma: radiologic findings and assessment of response to targeted antiangiogenic therapy by using multidetector CT. Radiographics. 2013;33:1691–716.
169. Tirkes T, Hollar MA, Tann M, Kohli MD, Akisik F, Sandrasegaran K. Response criteria in oncologic imaging: review of traditional and new criteria. Radiographics. 2013;33:1323–41.
170. Clark T, Maximin S, Meier J, Pokharel S, Bhargava P. Hepatocellular carcinoma: review of epidemiology, screening, imaging diagnosis, response assessment, and treatment. Curr Probl Diagn Radiol. 2015;44:479–86.
171. Cruite I, Osan S, Dighe M. An update on criteria for assessing tumor response to treatment. Curr Probl Diagn Radiol. 2013;42:209–19.
172. Anzidei M, Napoli A, Zaccagna F, et al. Liver metastases from colorectal cancer treated with conventional and antiangiogenetic chemotherapy: evaluation with liver computed tomography perfusion and magnetic resonance diffusion-weighted imaging. JCAT. 2011;35:690–6.
173. Choi H, Charnsangavej C, Faria SC, et al. Correlation of computed tomography and positron emission tomography in patients with metastatic gastrointestinal stromal tumor treated at a single institution with imatinibmesylate: proposal of new computed tomography response criteria. J Clin Oncol. 2007;25:1753–9.
174. Nishino M, Hatabu H, Sholl LM, Ramaiya NH. Thoracic complications of precision cancer therapies: a practical guide for radiologists in the new era of cancer care. Radiographics. 2017;37:1371–87.
175. Viswanathan C, Truong MT, Sabegiel TL, et al. Abdominal and pelvic complications of nonoperative oncologic therapy. Radiographics. 2014;34:941–61.
176. Katabathina VS, Restrepo CS, Betancour Cuellar SL, Riascos RF, Menias CO. Imaging of oncologic emergencies: what every radiologist should know. Radiolographics. 2013;33:1533–53.
177. Abramson RG, Abramson VG, Chan E, et al. Complications of targeted drug therapies for solid malignancies: manifestations and mechanisms. AJR. 2013;200:475–83.
178. Walker CM, Saldana DA, Gladish GW, et al. Cardiac complications of oncologic therapy. Radiographics. 2013;33:1801–15.
179. Ulaner GA, Lyall A. Identifying and distinguishing treatment effects and complications from malignancy at FDG PET/CT. Radiographics. 2013;33:1817–34.
180. Di Cesare E, Cerone G, Enrici RM, Tombolini V, Anselmo P, Masciocchi C. MRI characterization of residual mediastinal masses in Hodgkin's disease: long term follow-up. Magn Reson Imaging. 2004;22:31–8.
181. Gawande RS, Khurana A, Messig S, et al. Differentiation of normal thymus from anterior mediastinal lymphoma and lymphoma recurrence at pediatric PET/CT. Radiology. 2012;262:623–2.

182. Adike A, Karlin N, Menias C, Carey EJ. Pseudocirrhosis: a case series and literature review. Case Rep Gastroenetrol. 2016;10:381–91.

183. Lee SL, Chang ED, Na SJ, et al. Pseudocirrhosis of breast cancer metastases to the liver treated by chemotherapy. Cancer Res Treat. 2014;46:98–103.

184. Evans KK, Birdwell RL, Wolfe JM. If you don't find it often, you often don't find it: why some cancers are missed in breast cancer screening. PLoS One. 2013;8:e64366.

185. Reed WM, Ryan JT, McEntee MF, Evanoff MG, Brennan PC. The effect of abnormality-prevalence expectation non expert observer performance and visual search. Radiology. 2011;258:938–43.

186. Wolfe JM, Horowitz TS, Van Wert MJ, Kenner NM, Place SS, Kibbi N. Low target prevalence is a stubborn source of errors in visual search tasks. J Exp Psychol Gen. 2007;136:623–8.

187. Venkatanarasimha N, Damodharan K, Gogna A, et al. Diagnosis and management of complications from percutaneous biliary tract interventions. Radiographics. 2017;37:665–80.

188. Desai KR, Pandhi ME, Seedial SM, et al. Retrievable IVC filters: comprehensive review of device-related complications and advanced retrieval techniques. Radiographics. 2017;37:1236–45.

189. Sigakis CJG, Mathai SK, Suby-Long TD, et al. Radiographic review of current therapeutic and monitoring devices in the chest. Radiographics. 2018;38:1027–45.

190. Taljanovic M, Hunter TB, Miller MD, Sheppard JE. Gallery of medical devices. Part 1: orthopedic devices for the extremities and pelvis. Radiographics. 2005;25:859–70.

191. Hunter TB, Yoshino MT, Dzioba R, Light RA, Berger WG. Medical devices of the head, neck, and spine. Radiographics. 2004;24:257–85.

192. Silva AC, Pimenta M, Guimaraes LS. Small bowel obstruction: what to look for. Radiographics. 2009;29:423–39.

193. Nouh MR, Nasr AMS, El-Shebeny MO. Wooden splinter-induced extremity injuries: accuracy of MRI evaluation. Egypt J Radiol Nucl Med. 2013;44:573–9.

194. Onofrio A, Toye LR. MRI web clinic: foreign body imaging with MRI. 2016. www.radsource.us/foreign-body-imaging-mri/. Accessed 2 Mar 2019.

195. Mathew RP, Thomas B, Basti RS, Suresh HB. Gossypibomas, a surgeon's nightmare-patient demographics, risk factors, imaging and how we can prevent it. Br J Radiol. 2017;90:20160761.

196. Roldan CJ, Paniagua L. Central venous catheter intravascular malpositioning: causes, prevention, diagnosis, and correction. West J Emerg Med. 2015;16:658–64.

197. Katsinelos P, Kountouras J, Paroutoglou G, et al. Migration of plastic biliary stents and endoscopic retrieval: an experience of three referral centers. Surg Laparosc Endosc Percutan Tech. 2009;19:217–21.

198. Saravanan MN, Mathai V, Kapoor D, Singh B. Fractured metallic biliary stent causing obstruction and jejunal perforation. Asian J Endosc Surg. 2013;6:234–6.

199. Hjorth MH, Mechlenburg I, Soballe K, Roemer L, Jacobsen SS, Stilling M. Higher prevalence of mixed or solid pseudotumors in metal-on-polyethylene total hip arthroplasty compared with metal-on-metal total hip arthroplasty and resurfacing hip arthroplasty. J Arthroplasty. 2018;33:2279–86.

200. Lum TE, Fairbanks RJ, Pennington EC, Zwemer FL. Profiles in patient safety: misplaced femoral line guidewire and multiple failures to detect the foreign body on chest radiography. Acad Emerg Med. 2005;12:658–62.

201. Jager G, Futterer JJ, Rutten M. Cognitive errors in radiology: "thinking fast and slow". ECR 2014 poster C-0899. 2014. http://posterng.netkey.at/esr/viewing/index.php?module=viewing_poster&doi=10.1594/ecr2014/C-0899. Accessed 22 Feb 2019.

202. Busby LP, Courtier JL, Glastonbury CM. Bias in radiology: the how and why of misses and misinterpretations. Radiographics. 2018;38:236–47.

203. Lee A, Lau K, Stuckey S. Case report. An endless line on the chest radiograph. BMJ Case Rep. 2014;2014:bcr2014204540.

204. Standards for the reporting and interpretation of imaging investigations. This document was last reviewed in 2014 by the Clinical Radiology Professional Support and Standards Board and the Clinical Radiology Faculty Board. Last update September 2015. https://www.rcr.ac.uk/publication/standards-reporting-and-interpretation-imaging-investigations. Accessed 25 Oct 2016.

205. Kaewlai R, Jackson VP, Abujudeh HH. Peer review in radiology. In: Abujudeh HH, Bruno MA, editors. Quality and safety in radiology. New York: Oxford University Press; 2012. p. 117–25.

206. Itri JN, Krishnaraj A. Do we need a national incident reporting system for medical imaging? J Am Coll Radiol. 2012;9:329–35.

207. Errors in radiology. The Royal College of Radiologists. www.rcr.ac.uk/audit/errors-radiology. Accessed 25 Oct 2016.

208. Standards for learning from discrepancies meetings. London: Faculty of Clinical Radiology, The Royal College of Radiologists; 2014. https://www.rcr.ac.ul/publication/standards-learning-discrepancies-meetings. Accessed 25 Oct 2016.

209. Kaewlai R, Abujudeh H. Peer review in clinical radiology practice. AJR. 2012;199:W158–62.

210. Mahgereteh S, Kruskal JB, Yam CS, Blachar A, Sosna J. Quality initiatives. Peer review in diagnostic radiology: current state and a vision for the future. Radiographics. 2009;29:1221–31.

211. Lee JK. Quality: a radiology imperative-interpretation accuracy and pertinence. J Am Coll Radiol. 2007;4:162–5.

212. Harvey BH, Alkasab TK, Prabhakar AM, et al. Radiologist peer review by group consensus. J Am Coll Radiol. 2016;13:656–62.

213. Soffa DJ, Lewis RS, Sunshine JH, Bhargavan M. Disagreement in interpretation: a method for the

development of benchmarks for quality assurance in imaging. J Am Coll Radiol. 2004;1:212–7.

214. Borgstede JP, Lewis RS, Bhargavan M, Sunshine JH. RADPEER quality assurance program: a multifacility study of interpretive disagreement rates. J Am Coll Radiol. 2004;1:59–65.

215. Ruutiainen AT, Scanlon MH, Itri JN. Identifying benchmarks for discrepancy rates in preliminary interpretations provided by radiology trainees at an academic institution. J Am Coll Radiol. 2011;8:644–8.

216. American College of Radiology Peer Review. www.acr.org/Quality-Safety/RADPEER. Accessed 25 Oct 2016.

217. Brooke OR, Romero J, Brook A, Kruskal JB, Yam CS, Levine D. The complementary nature of peer review and quality assurance data collection. Radiology. 2015;274:221–9.

218. Harvey HB, Sotardi ST. Peer learning and preserving the physician's right to learn. J Am Coll Radiol. 2018;15:444–5.

219. Sharpe RE Jr, Huffman RI, Congdon RG, et al. Implementation of a peer learning program replacing score-based peer review in a multispecialty integrated practice. AJR. 2018;211:949–56.

220. Itri JN, Donithan A, Patel SH. Random versus nonrandom peer review: a case for more meaningful peer review. J Am Coll Radiol. 2018;15:1045–52.

221. Donnelly LF, Dorfman SR, Jones J, Bisset GS. Transition from peer review to peer learning: experience in a radiology department. J Am Coll Radiol. 2018;15:1143–9.

222. Donnelly LF, Larson DB, Heller RE III, Kruskal JB. Practical suggestions on how to move from peer review to peer learning. AJR. 2018;210:578–82.

223. https://www.rcr.ac.uk/audit/learning-errors-and-discrepancies-clinical-radiology. Accessed 3 Mar 2019.

224. https://seram.es/images/site/quality_radiology_report_rcr.pdf. Accessed 3 Mar 2019.

225. European Society of Radiology (ESR). ESR communication guidelines for radiologists. Insights Imaging. 2013;4:143–6.

226. White C. Doctors mistrust systems for reporting medical mistakes. BMJ. 2004;329:12–3.

227. Larson DB, Donnelly LF, Podberesky DJ, Merrow AC, Sharpe RE Jr, Kruskal JB. Peer feedback, learning, and improvement: answering the call of the Institute of Medicine Report on Diagnostic Error. Radiology. 2016. https://doi.org/10.1148/radiol.2016161254.

228. Butler GJ, Forghani R. The next level of radiology peer review: enterprise-wide education and improvement. J Am Coll Radiol. 2013;10:349–53.

229. Halsted MJ. Radiology peer review as an opportunity to reduce errors and improve patient care. J Am Coll Radiol. 2004;1:984–7.

230. Griffith KS, Marx D. Just culture: a shared commitment. In: Abujudeh HH, Bruno MA, editors. Quality and safety in radiology. New York: Oxford University Press; 2012. p. 52–8.

231. Web M & M Cases and Commentaries. Agency for Healthcare Research and Quality (AHRQ). Patient safety network. https://psnet.ahrq.gov/Webmm. Accessed 3 Mar 2019.

232. Shaw CM, Flanagan FL, Fenlon HM, McNicholas MM. Consensus review of discordant findings maximizes cancer detection rate in double-reader screening mammography: Irish National Breast Screening program experience. Radiology. 2009;250:354–62.

233. Sadigh G, Loehfelm T, Applegate KE, Tridandapani S. Evaluation of near-miss wrong-patient events in radiology reports. AJR. 2015;205:337–43.

234. Muchantef K, Forman HP. Professional resource cost of body CT examinations: analysis of interpretation costs in different patient populations. J Am Coll Radiol. 2004;1:652–8.

235. Seidelmann FE, Ward DC. Radiology Quality Institute White Paper. A new methodology for evaluating radiologist error rates: factoring in the complexity of study and potential for significant pathology. 2013. https://docplayer.net/18980530-A-new-methodology-for-evaluating-radiologist-error-rates-factoring-in-the-complexity-of-study-and-potential-for-significant-pathology.html. Accessed Apr 2019.

236. Lauritzen PM, Stavem K, Andersen JG, et al. Double reading of current chest CT examinations: clinical importance of changes to radiology reports. Eur J Radiol. 2016;85:199–204.

237. Lauritzen PM, Andersen JG, Stokke MV, et al. Radiologist-initiated double reading of abdominal CT: retrospective analysis of the clinical importance of changes to radiology reports. BMJ Qual Saf. 2016;25:595–603.

238. Duijim LE, Groenewoud JH, Hendicks JH, de Koenig HJ. Independent double reading of screening mammograms in the Netherlands: effect of arbitration following reader disagreement. Radiology. 2004;231:654–570.

239. Ciatto S, Ambrogetti D, Bonardi R, et al. Second reading of screening mammograms increases cancer detection and recall rates: results in the Florence screening program. J Med Screen. 2005;12:103–6.

240. Liston JC, Dall BJ. Can the NHS breast screening programme afford not to double read screening mammograms? Clin Radiol. 2003;58:474–7.

241. Lian K, Bharatha A, Aviv RI, Symons SP. Interpretation errors in CT angiography of the head and neck and the benefit of double reading. Am J Neuroradiol. 2011;32:2132–5.

242. Wolf M, Krause J, Carney PA, Bogart A, Kurvers RHJM. Collective intelligence meets medical decision-making: the collective outperforms the best radiologist. PLoS One. 2015;10:e0134269.

243. Yates T. The antidote for radiology errors. Imag Technol News. 2012. http://www.itnonline.com/article/antidote-radiology-errors. Accessed 18 Jan 2018.

244. Kahlben CL, Yetter EM, Olson MC, Posniak HV, Aranha GV. Assessing the resectability of pancreatic carcinoma: the value of re-interpreting

abdominal CT performed at other institutions. AJR. 1998;171:1571–6.

245. La L, Sonners AI, Schulman BJ, et al. Reinterpretation of cross-sectional images in patients with head and neck cancer in the setting of a multidisciplinary cancer center. Am J Neuroradiol. 2002;23:1622–6.

246. Tilleman EHBM, Phoa SSKS, van Delden OM, et al. Reinterpretation of radiological imaging in patients referred to a tertiary referral centre with a suspected pancreatic or hepatobiliary malignancy: impact on treatment strategy. Eur Radiol. 2003;13:1095–9.

247. Shetty AS, Mittal A, Salter A, Narra VR, Fowler KJ. Hepatopancreaticobiliary imaging second-opinion consultations: is there value in the second reading? AJR. 2018;211:1264–72.

248. Chang Sen LQ, Mayo RC, Lesslie MD, Yang WT, Leung JWT. Impact of second-opinion interpretation of breast imaging studies in patients not currently diagnosed with breast cancer. J Am Coll Radiol. 2018;15:980–7.

249. Garcia D, Spruill LS, Irshad A, Wood J, Kepecs D, Klauber-DeMore N. The value of a second opinion for breast cancer patients referred to a National Cancer Institute (NCI)-designated cancer center with a multidisciplinary breast tumor board. Ann Surg Oncol. 2018;25:2953–7.

250. Rosenkrantz AB, Duszak R Jr, Babb JS, Glover MK, Kang SK. Discrepancy rates and clinical impact of imaging secondary interpretations: a systematic review and meta-analysis. J Am Coll Radiol. 2018;15:1222–31.

251. Bosmans JM, Peremans L, De Schepper AM, Duyck PO, Parizel PM. How do referring clinicians want the radiologists to report? Suggestions from the COVER survey. Insights Imaging. 2011;2:577–84.

252. Abujudeh HH, Kaewlai R, Asfaw BA, Thrall JH. Quality initiatives: key performance indicators for measuring and improving Radiology Department performance. Radiographics. 2010;30:571–83.

253. Paushter DM, Baron RL. Practical quality assurance. In: Abujudeh HH, Bruno MA, editors. Quality and safety in radiology. New York: Oxford University Press; 2012. p. 29–38.

254. Kaewlai R, Abujudeh HH. Root cause analysis (RCA) and health care failure mode and effect analysis (HFMEA). In: Abujudeh HH, Bruno MA, editors. Quality and safety in radiology. New York: Oxford University Press; 2012. p. 38–51.

255. Sardanelli F. Evidence-based radiology and its relationship to quality. In: Abujudeh HH, Bruno MA, editors. Quality and safety in radiology. New York: Oxford University Press; 2012. p. 255–90.

256. Bruno MA, Flemming DJ. Teaching quality and safety to radiology residents and fellows. In: Abujudeh H, Bruno MA, editors. Quality and safety in radiology. New York: Oxford University Press; 2012. p. 241–4.

257. Ludmerer KM. Learning to heal: the development of American Medical Education. Baltimore: Johns Hopkins University Press; 1996.

258. Ludmerer KM. Let me heal: the opportunity to preserve excellence in American Medicine. New York: Oxford University Press; 2015.

259. Broder JC, Cameron SF, Korn WT, Baccei SJ. Creating a radiology quality and safety program: principles and pitfalls. Radiographics. 2018;38:1786–98.

260. Sarkany DS, Shenoy-Bhangle AS, Catanzano TM, Fineberg TA, Eisenberg RL, Slanetz PJ. Running a radiology residency program: strategies for success. Radiographics. 2018;38:1729–43.

261. Gunderman R, Chan S. Knowledge sharing in radiology. Radiology. 2003;229:314–7.

262. Graber M. Introduction to diagnostic error. The Society to Improve Diagnosis in Medicine. Diagnostic error resources. Video presentation. www.improvediagnosis.org/page/Education. Accessed 24 Oct 2016.

263. Penn curriculum in cognitive bias and diagnostic error for medical residents. In Society to improve diagnosis in medicine. Clinical reasoning toolkit: education. www.improvediagnosis.org/?ClinicalEducation. Accessed 6 Dec 2016.

264. Croskerry P. Dalhousie University critical thinking curriculum. In Society to improve diagnosis in medicine. Clinical reasoning toolkit: education. www.improvediagnosis.org/?ClinicalEducation. Accessed 6 Dec 2016.

Epilogue: Conclusions and Personal Thoughts About Our Education

Abstract

Multiple articles in the literature and my personal experience indicate that the topic of errors is not addressed to satisfaction in our training. In this chapter I propose ways to investigate and correct any deficiencies in our education, so that we can serve and honor the current demands of the medical profession.

General Remarks

Extensive research has been performed over several years on radiological errors and on raising defenses against them. Yet many radiologists first encounter this knowledge at a late stage, after they have formed their "radiologic personality." Thus many of us need to unlearn our default mode of operation and recalibrate to an error resistant version. This process clearly is not efficient, yet many young radiologists are still trained the "old" way.

Multiple voices have raised concerns about the effectiveness of medical undergraduate, graduate, and postgraduate education [1–12].

I will go one step further. I see a *gap* between our *training* and *real life*. After many years of intensive training and studying, we get the approval of our faculty to try the National Board Examinations. If we pass, we are allowed to work as independent radiologists. Yet, some months or years later, we are told that our knowledge is limited, we are overloaded with biases, we do not know what to look for, we have skewed and distorted personalities, we run a high margin of errors, we have leaky or absent safety mechanisms, and we need to shoulder additional responsibilities [13, 14]. This obvious *contradiction* raises questions about our education, whether it is nourishing and supporting a balanced and successful career.

There is another factor that contributes to the gap between where we are and where we should be. The detail of depiction of normal and pathologic anatomy is astonishing [15]. The amount of information generated is massive and I wonder how many general radiologists can stay up to date. Some days I feel that no matter how much I try I will never know enough.

Albert Einstein said that "Education is not the learning of facts, but the training of the mind to think" [16]. Richard Feynman, in the same spirit, exclaimed that there is "a difference between knowing the name of something and knowing (understanding) something" [17]. Peter Drucker, an advocate of life-long learning insisted that "the most pressing task is to teach people how to learn" [18].

Fahey and Prusak have portrayed 11 major ways of knowledge mismanagement [19]. One of them is the assumption that knowledge is a commodity like data that we can manipulate easily in a number of ways, like capturing it and transmitting it. Instead, Fahey and Prusak believe that "knowledge is about imbuing data and information with decision-and-action-relevant meaning."

H. Chryssikopoulos, *Errors in Imaging*, https://doi.org/10.1007/978-3-030-21103-5

The above statements are echoed in the work of visionary authors and educators, who have reached provocative conclusions about medicine (and radiology): "too often, *information (data) is confused with knowledge, ineffective routines* are *propagated* and *new approaches* are *ignored*." "As a result, some people *do not appreciate what they need to know*, while others *do not recognize the value of the knowledge they possess*" [20]. In a nutshell, *our education is constricted by flaws, biases, and inertia*.

Fortunately, some countries and individual radiology residency programs have restructured their curriculum and training to reflect the increasing need for subspecialists and experts [10, 21–23]. A few medical schools offer courses on medical errors and visual perception (www.artfulperception.com/participants.php) [24–26].

My thesis is that there is still a wide margin for improvement of our education and I present my arguments in the section that follows.

The Author's Key Proposals About Reshaping Our Education

(a) Shift the undergraduate curriculum to *doing* and acquisition of *skills*

This transition can be accomplished via a substitution of a large number of hours of traditional courses with new courses. The revised curriculum should include lectures coupled with workshops about errors, independent thinking, problem solving, creativity, team work, knowledge sharing, as well as interpersonal, expression, management, and leadership skills [27–49]. These courses, tutorials, and seminars could be expanded and refined in the postgraduate years. I believe that people in sensitive positions, including physicians, should have a firm grasp of the skills mentioned above. A particular physician may not be interested in managing or leading other physicians, but he should be able to manage and lead himself and his patients, to collaborate with his colleagues, and to handle difficult situations with grace [32]. Leadership is not a title or a position, but an attitude [41–49].

Leadership is about empowerment and about awakening dormant potential.

(b) Solid preparation of students and residents to attain expertise as subspecialists

The senior year of medical school should be elective time: the students should be granted the option of a focused apprenticeship of 9–12 months in the specialty of their choice. Correspondingly, the last 2 years of radiology residency should be dedicated to subspecialty training.

(c) Mandatory study of teaching files

Exposure of residents to cases during each rotation may not be varied enough to fulfill the training objectives [5, 10]. Any such gaps should be ameliorated with simulations of real life cases, such as standardized, carefully engineered, *interactive* teaching files [50].

(d) Termination of all multiple-choice tests and teaching files

Multiple choice (MC) formats are an artificial situation; no patient shows us a MC list after his physical examination or after his CT scan [51, 52]. I believe that MC templates distort and restrict the cognitive pathways of the learner. MC lists applaud a quick search for Aunt Minnie patterns and encourage immediate gratification for finding the correct answer from the list in front of us. Furthermore, the examinee may just guess or may partially recognize the correct answer; is either scenario the same as knowing and understanding the correct answer? Yes, in the eyes of the examiner, yet no in a moral sense or in a real life situation. No patient would be happy if we just tried to guess the diagnosis or if we quasi-remembered the treatment for his illness.

(e) Update atlases, textbooks, and teaching files

Learning via busy images loaded with lines or arrows connected to tiny sized words is a slow and tedious process. With modern technology, we could construct audio-visual, colorful, movie-like, anatomy modules with interactive quizzes. Teaching files could also be run the same way. I believe that the combination of auditory, visual, and color cues would enhance the pleasure and effectiveness of learning.

(f) Uncover and rectify any shortcomings in our training [30, 53–58]

I propose that medical schools, residency programs, major organizations, and institutions undertake large scale, anonymous surveys of its members, students, residents, fellows, and staff. Multidisciplinary task forces should formulate the survey, evaluate the responses, and suggest actions where indicated. These committees could consist of (but not necessarily limited to) medical school chancellors and deans, radiology department chairmen and section chiefs, directors of residency programs, psychiatrists, psychologists, as well as education, ethics, management, and leadership specialists.

Sample questions could include, but not necessarily limited to the following:

- To what degree are you satisfied with the education/training that you received?
- Did your education/training meet your expectations?
- What expectations did you have?
- What were the weak and strong aspects of your medical school or radiology department?
- What percent of accumulated information (data) during medical school and residency remains useful at your current position?
- Were you taught how to learn and how to "decipher" the medical literature?
- Were you taught how to keep up with the advancements in your field and how to incorporate them in your daily work?

- Were you taught about medical errors and how to manage them?
- Were you taught stress management techniques?
- Did you have any teachers who were not efficient in transferring their knowledge, experience, and expertise?
- Was a mentor assigned to you?
- Did you seek a mentor? If not, why not?
- Were you ever notified of substandard performance or problematic behavior?
- If yes, what help did you receive?
- Did you receive counseling about career choices?
- To what degree were you prepared for private practice?
- Were you informed adequately about academic careers?
- Were you prepared to face the challenges of radiology?
- If not, how do you manage?
- If you moved to another institution as a resident or fellow or faculty, how do you compare the different Institutions?
- What are your suggestions for improvement of teaching and learning?

The ultimate question is: what kind of radiologists do we want?

Radiology and all other medical specialties deserve a bright future. A lot of work has been done and we are ready for the decisive leap forward.

Sincerely Yours,

Haris Chrysikopoulos, MD

Case 1

A 57 year-old female with neck pain and radiculopathy.

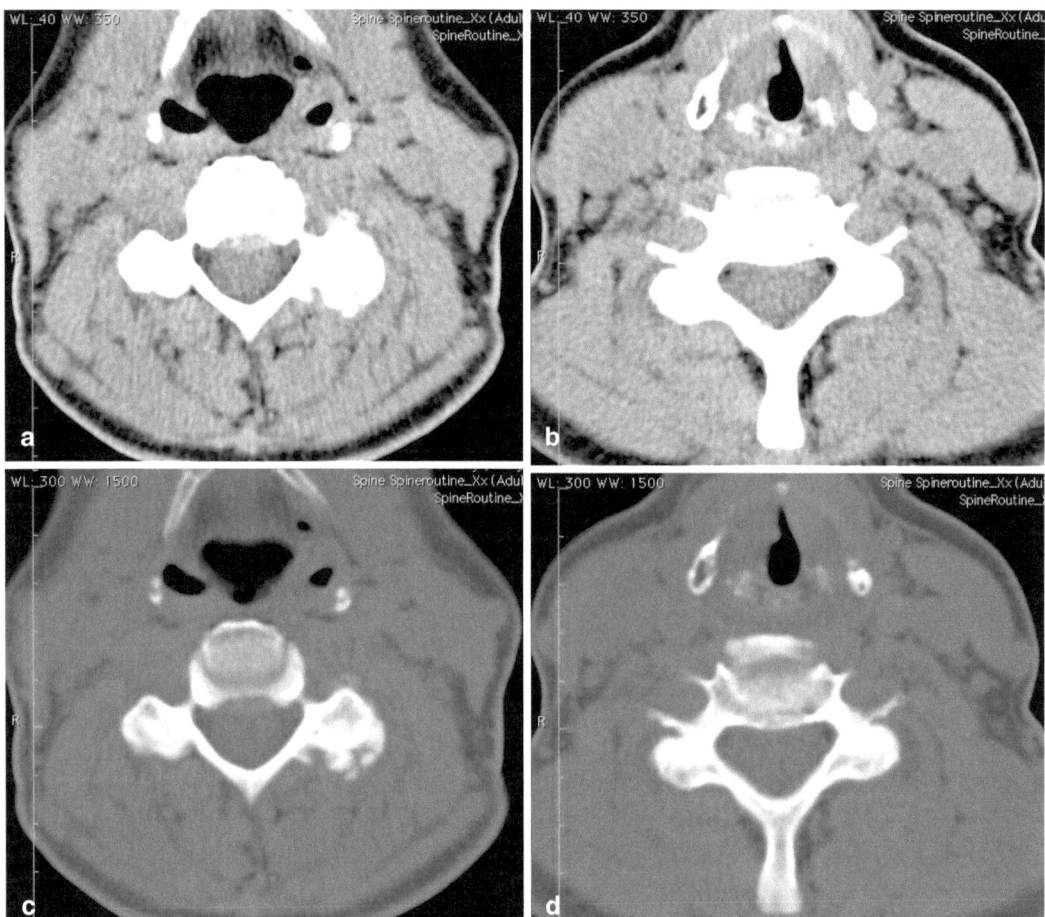

Fig. 1 (**a–d**) Selected slices of a cervical spine CT scan, in pairs of soft tissue and bone windows

Please describe any findings and record them on paper, before proceeding to the next page.

© Springer Nature Switzerland AG 2020
H. Chryssikopoulos, *Errors in Imaging*, https://doi.org/10.1007/978-3-030-21103-3

Discussion

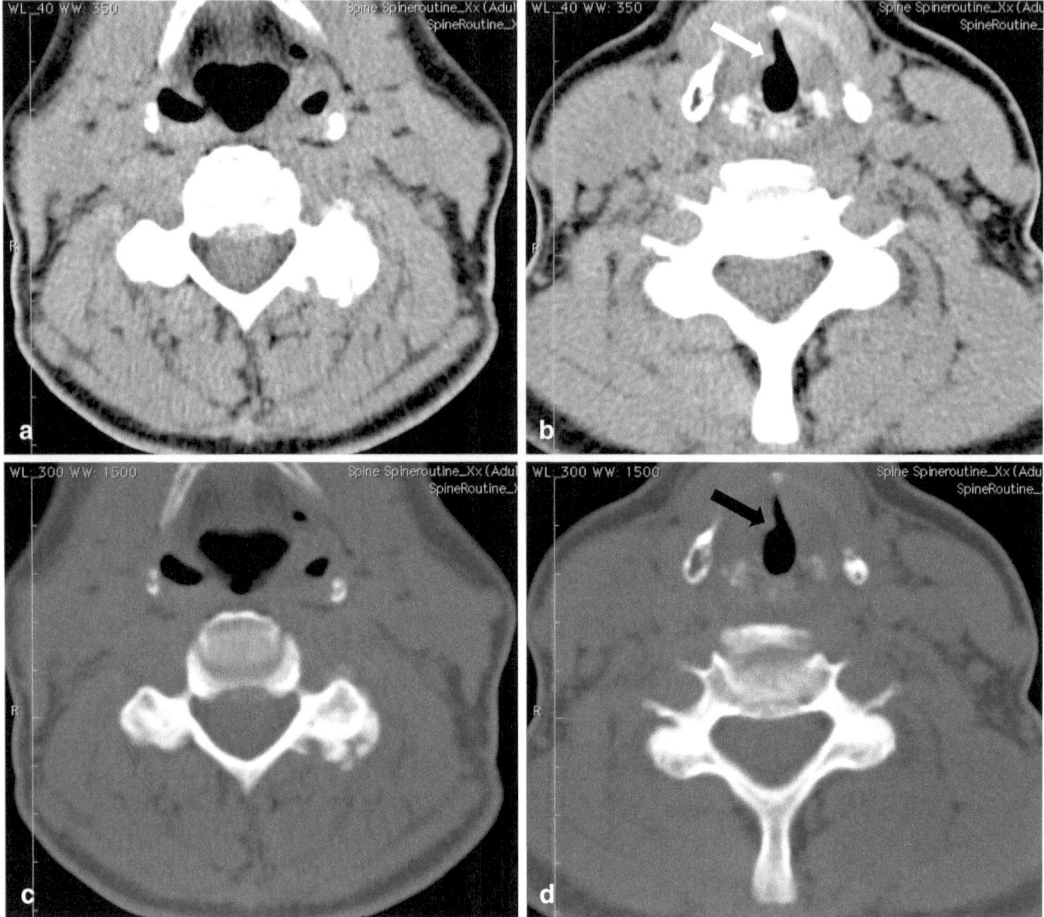

Fig. 2 (**a–d**) There are degenerative changes in the spine. Furthermore, there is an *incidental*, but *important* finding: focal, nodular thickening of the right true vocal cord (arrow) in images (**b, d**). The endoscopist described it as a polyp due to chronic overuse

Teaching Points

This case is a demonstration of two potential pitfalls in detecting a lesion:

(a) satisfaction of search and
(b) suboptimal attention to the "periphery" of the images, beyond the spine and immediate paraspinal soft tissues (or tunnel vision bias).

Please refer to Chap. 3 and 5 for a review of detection errors and biases.

Case 2

A 76-year-old man with recently diagnosed cutaneous melanoma of the neck. Staging included a head CT scan.

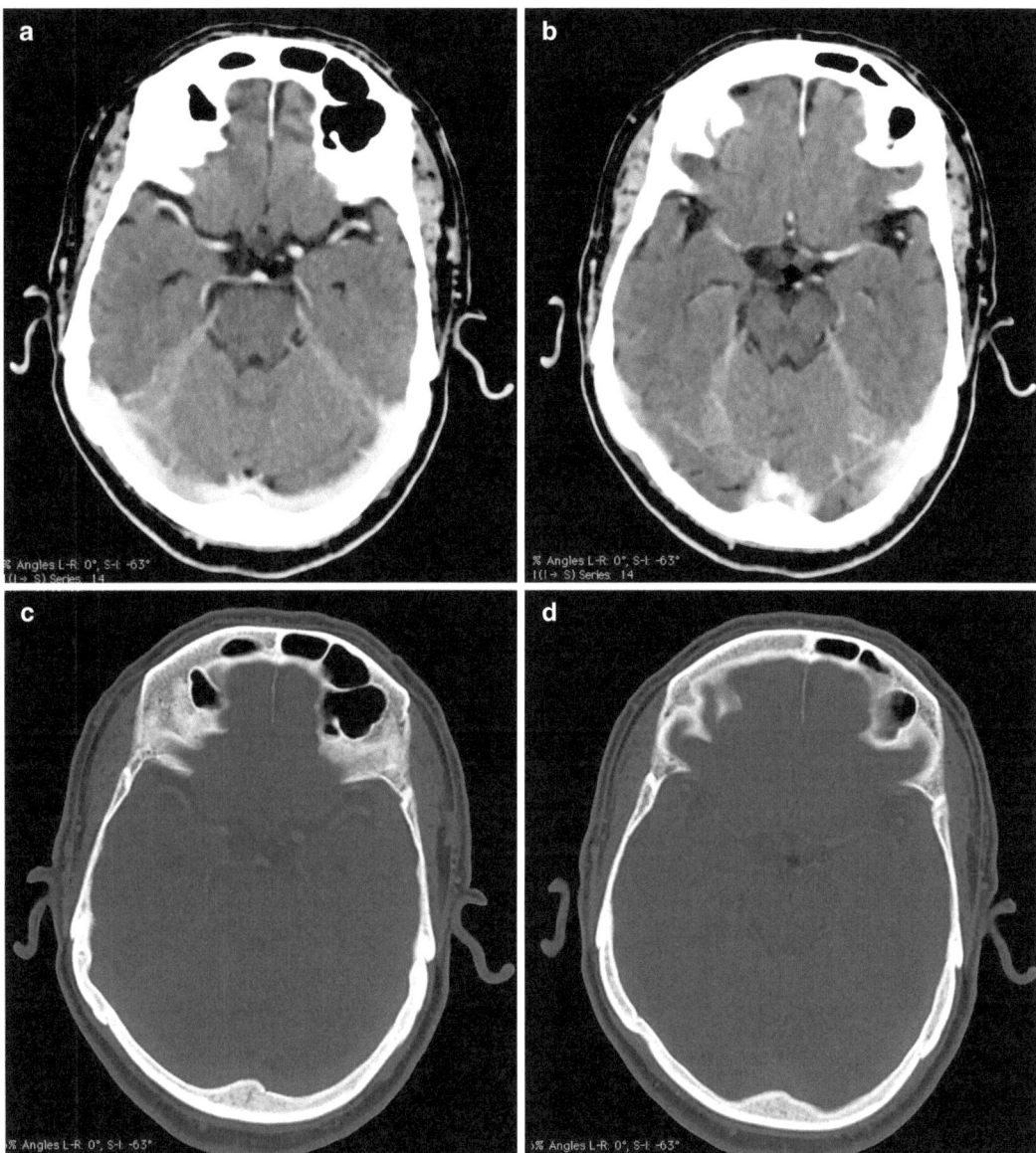

Fig. 1 (**a–d**) Two pairs of consecutive slices after i.v. contrast, displayed in brain and bone "windows."

Please describe any findings and record them on paper before proceeding to the next page

Discussion

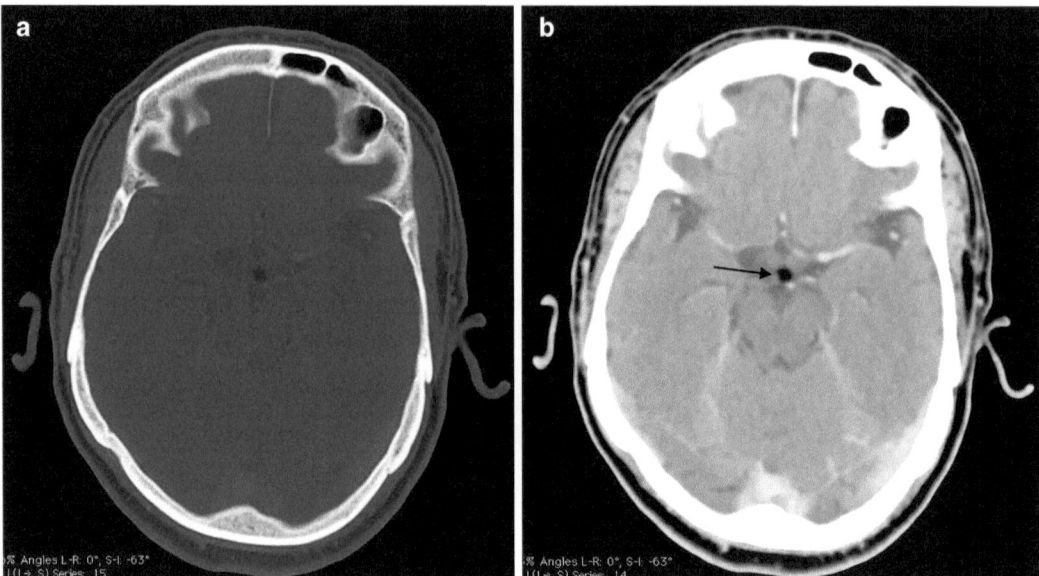

Fig. 2 These images are the same slices as (**d**) and (**b**) of Fig. 1. Image (**b**) of this image pair is displayed at an intermediate window (W 60 L 310)

A small lipoma becomes evident in the midline, between the tip of the basilar artery and the optic chiasm, measuring −80 HU (arrow).

Please revisit Fig. 1, images (b) and (d) and try to discern the lipoma, now that you know where it is.

Teaching Point

Proper selection of windows is crucial to a thorough and correct interpretation of any study. The brain and bone window settings in (a–d) are W100–L50 and W1500–L250 respectively.

You can revisit Chap. 3 if you would like to look up the references on this subject [45, 46].

Case 3

A 72-year-old female with a history of lymphoma, in remission for 6 years. She presents for her annual follow-up. No prior examinations were available. The patient currently appears disease free.

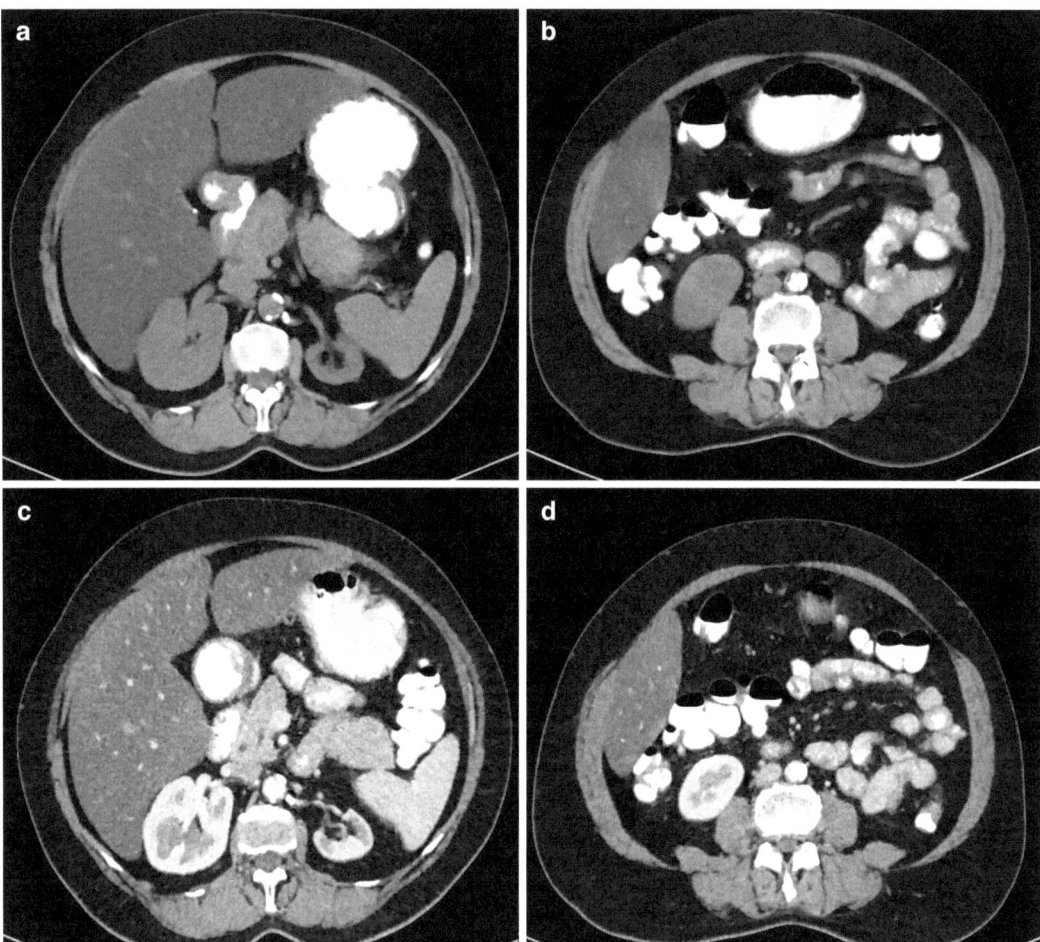

Fig. 1 (**a**, **b**) Two CT slices after administration of oral contrast. (**c**, **d**) Same slices as (**a**) and (**b**), after i.v. contrast administration

Please describe all findings, before proceeding.

Discussion

The patient has an enlarged fatty liver, a small left kidney, and a hypertrophied right kidney. There is no evidence of lymphoma.

The teaching point of this case is the large, heavily calcified plaque of the aorta that completely obliterates its lumen [59].

The plaque is large, nevertheless there is a danger of overlooking it, because it represents a blind spot. However, there is a clue that guides us to look for atherosclerotic plaques: the left kidney is small, with a smooth contour, without scars. There is no hydronephrosis. Could the small size of the left kidney be due to low arterial blood supply, despite good cortico-medullary differentiation? Images (a) and (c) of the prior figure (Fig. 1) show an elongated atherosclerotic plaque at the origin and the initial segment of the left renal artery.

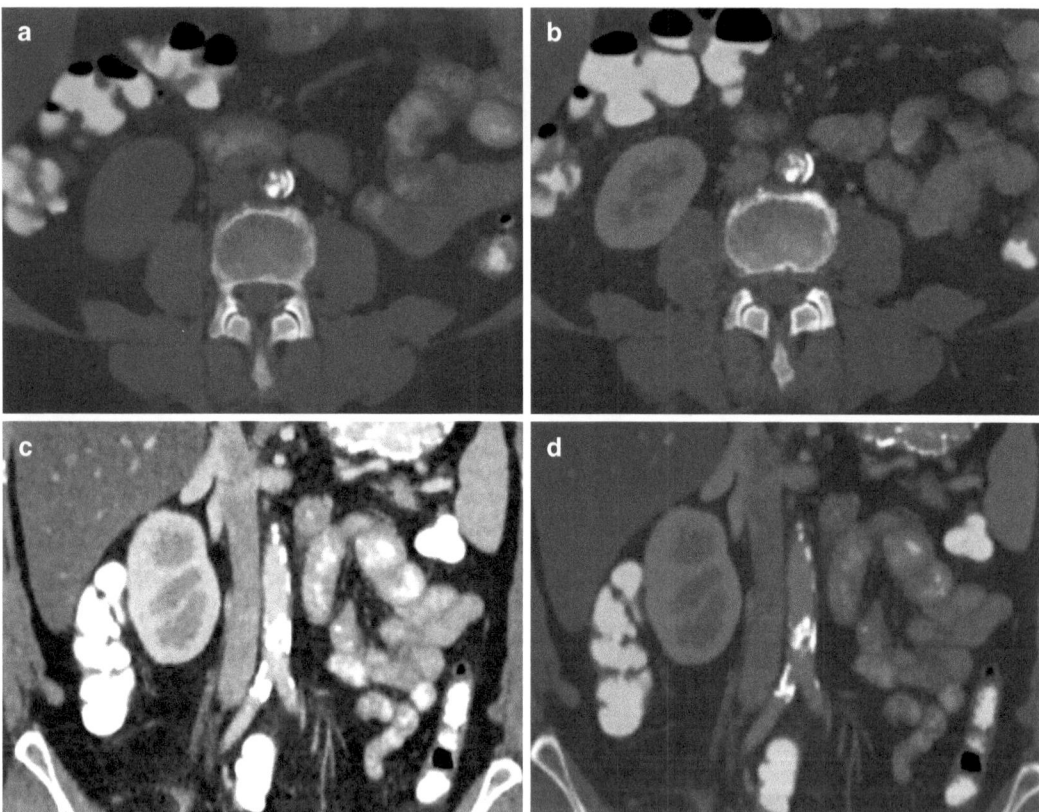

Fig. 2 (**a**, **b**) Magnified views of the aortic plaque, before and after i.v. contrast, same images as in Fig. 1, but filmed with bone windows. (**c**, **d**) Coronal reconstructions post i.v. contrast in soft tissue and bone window settings

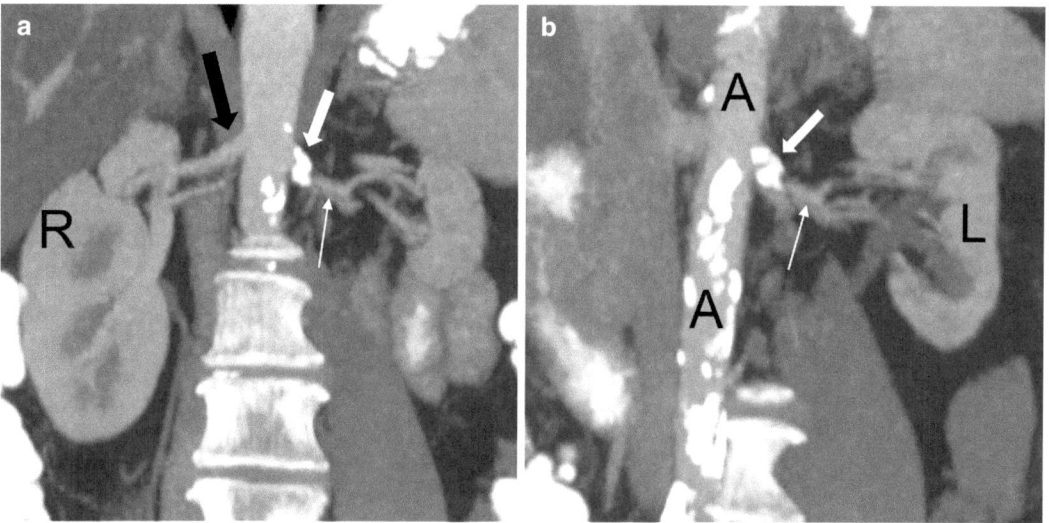

Fig. 3 (**a, b**) Coronal and left oblique coronal thin MIP reconstructions. The right renal artery appears smooth, without atherosclerotic plaques (black arrow). In contrast, heavy calcifications (thick white arrows) obscure the initial segment of the left renal artery (thin white arrows). *A* aorta, *R* right kidney, *L* left kidney

Teaching Point

Blind spots may be quite obvious in retrospect, but they may escape detection in the first reading. We only "see" what we are looking for. Thus we need to examine carefully all "corners" and every single structure that is included in the images. Please see Chap. 1, Sect. 1.3, Chap. 3, Sect. 3.4 and Chap. 6, Sect. 6.2.3.2 for a refreshment of the relevant topics.

   MIP: maximum intensity projection

Case 4

A 67-year-old female with left breast carcinoma, status post mastectomy, undergoing chemotherapy.

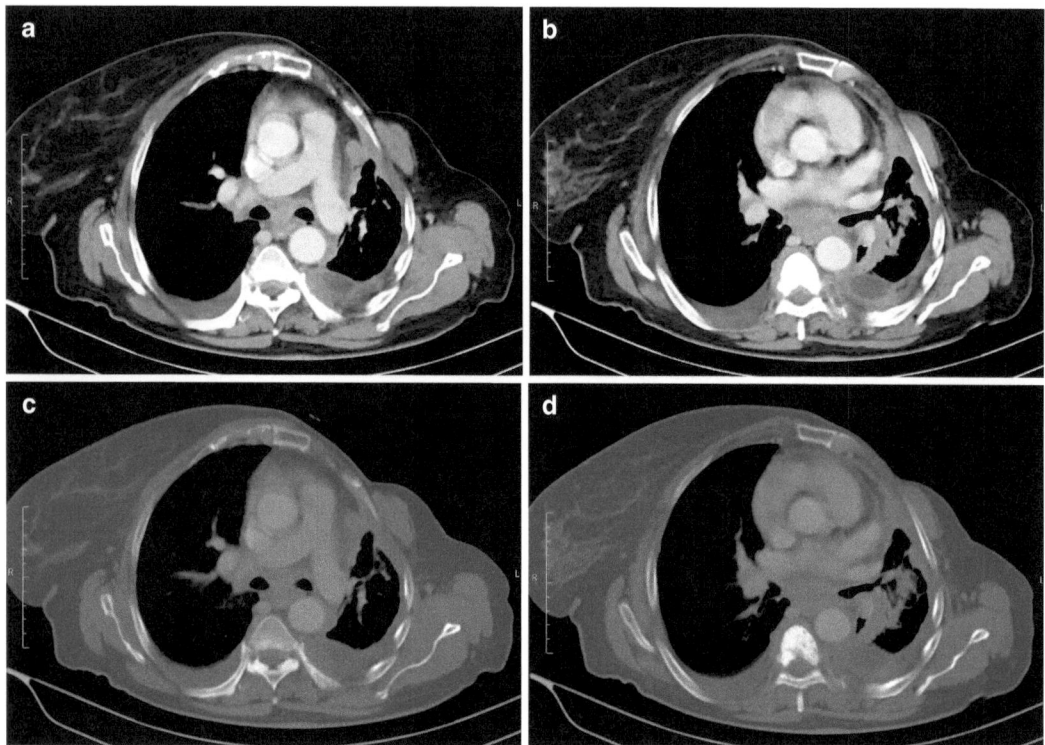

Fig. 1 (**a–h**) Selected images from a restaging CT

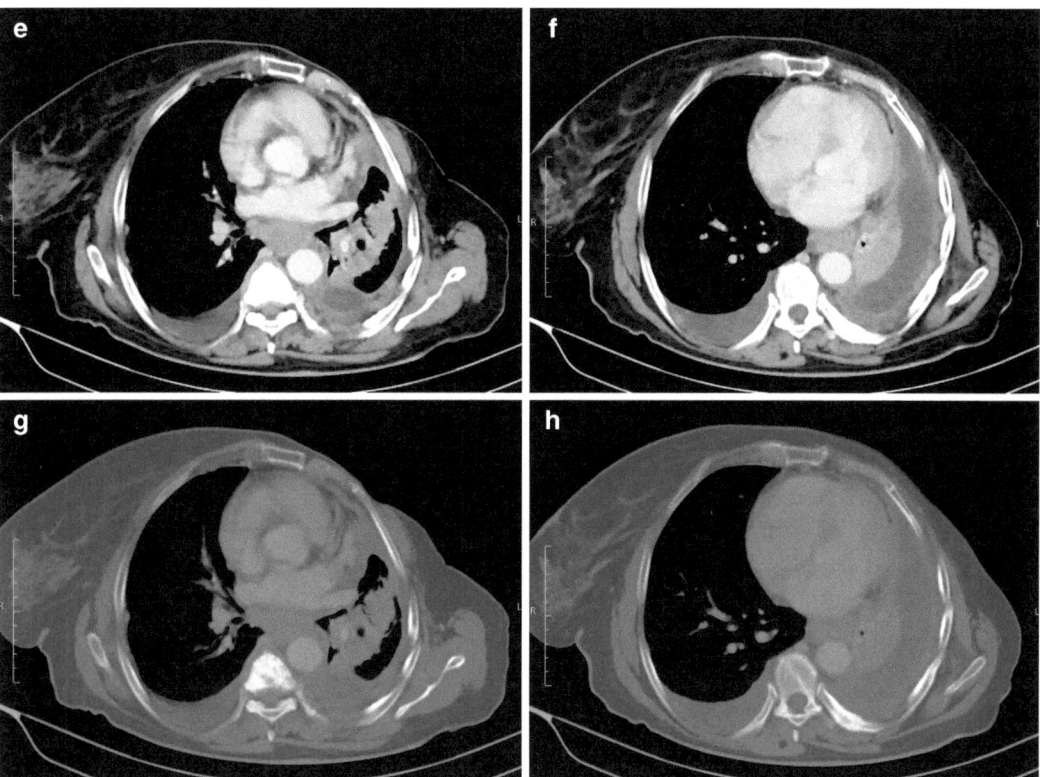

Fig. 1 (continued)

Please record your observations and thoughts on paper before turning the page

Discussion

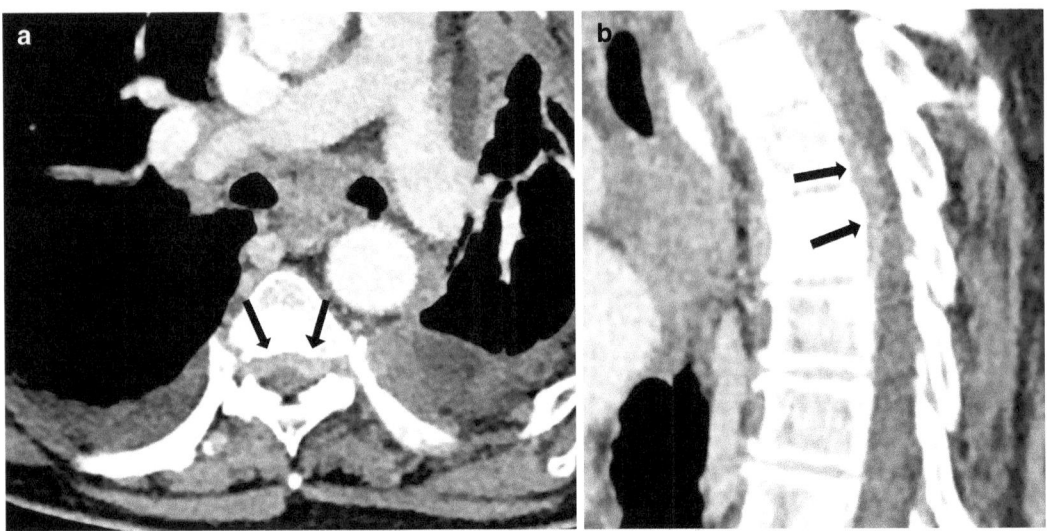

Fig. 2 (**a**)"Cone down" axial image [same as (**a**) of Fig. 1] and (**b**) sagittal reconstruction. Note obliteration of the ventral epidural disease by soft tissue (arrows)

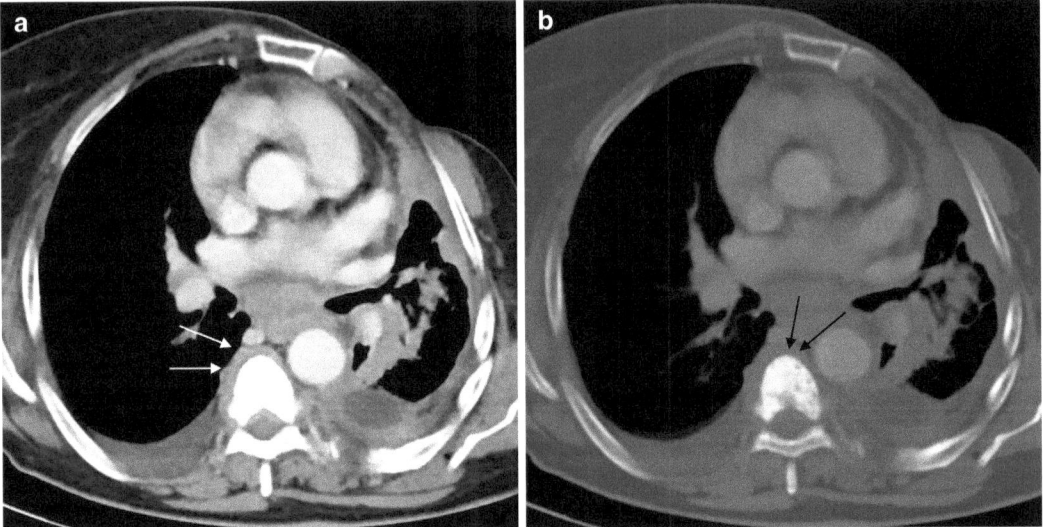

Fig. 3 (**a**, **b**) "Cone down" views of images (**b**) and (**d**) of Fig. 1, provide the clues to searching for intracanalicular extension: note the osseous and paraspinal soft tissue infiltration (arrows)

The images of Fig. 1 are "busy" with a multitude of findings related to the patient's underlying malignancy. Note lymphadenopathy, free and loculated pleural fluid, spine and rib metastases, and infiltration of the pleura, left lung, and paraspinal soft tissues.

The teaching point of this case is the epidural mass that compresses the spinal cord.

Teaching Point

Keep in mind the concept "What can I not afford to miss?" Please see Chap. 7, Sect. 7.2.1.1 and 7.2.1.4 for further elaboration on this topic.

Case 5

A 72-year-old male with metastatic prostate carcinoma. A CT scan was requested because of elevation of PSA despite continuous hormonal therapy.

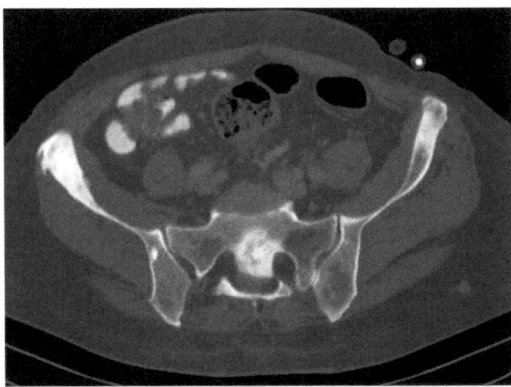

Fig. 1 CT slice through the pelvis photographed in bone window

Please describe the findings. What are your thoughts? Please commit them on paper before proceeding.

Despite an increase in the dose of hormonal therapy, the PSA kept escalating. Furthermore the patient started complaining of new pelvic pain. Thus another CT scan was performed 5 months after the first one.

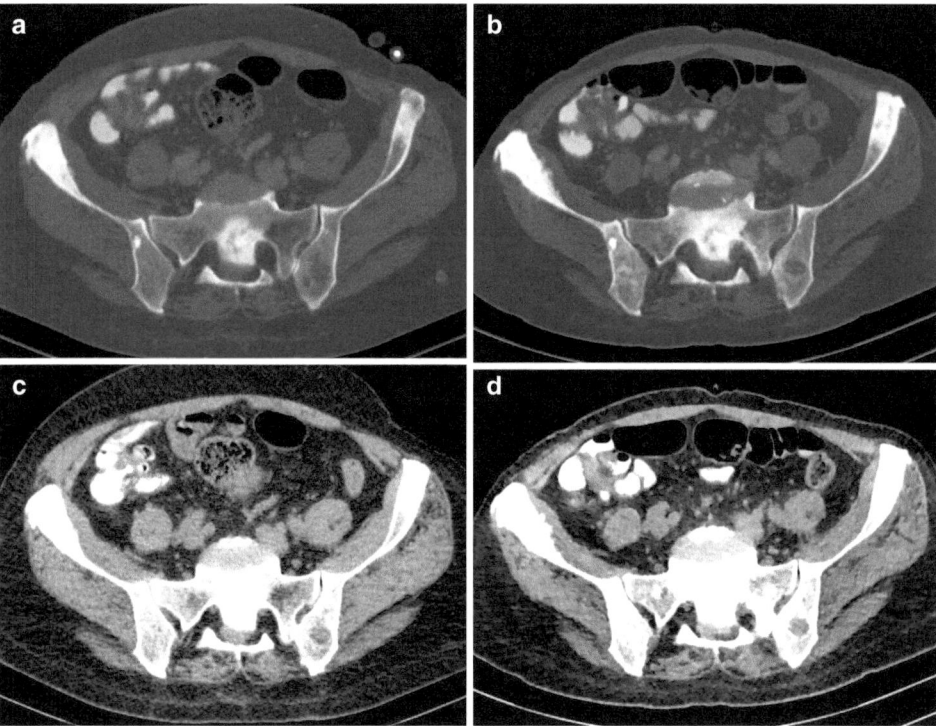

Fig. 2 (**a**, **b**) CT images in pairs (soft tissue and bone windows) from the initial (**a**, **c**) and the subsequent (**b**, **d**) CT scan. Image (**a**) is the same as Fig. 1a

Please compare the two scans. Write your observations and thoughts on paper before proceeding.

Discussion

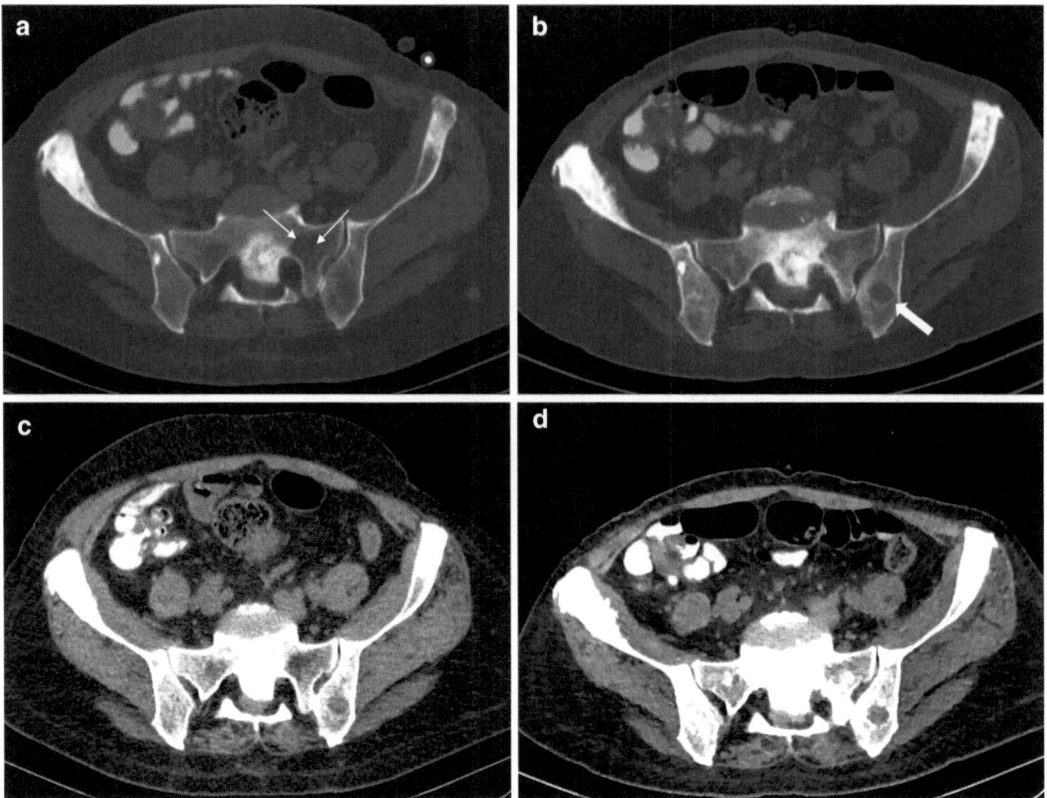

Fig. 3 (**a–d**) Same images as in Fig. 2

New foci of sclerosis have developed in the left sacral wing and in both iliac bones. Note also increased size and increased density of the preexisting sclerotic metastases. "Whiskering" type of periostitis has appeared in the right iliac wing and in the anterior margin of the sacral foramen on the left. The teaching point of this case is a round, lucent area in the left ilium, brought to our attention by the development of a thin, complete sclerotic margin (thick arrow). This finding was subtle in the initial CT scan, and our attention is distracted by the obvious lesions that satisfy our search and expectation biases. In prostate carcinoma we expect to find sclerotic metastases; multiple such lesions are present in this patient, thus our "job" is finished and we do not need to look any further. The nature of the "lucent" lesion in the left ilium could not be ascertained. Perhaps it was not related to the underlying prostatic malignancy. The CT density in its center measured 34 ±16 HU, without detectable interval change. The initial CT scan shows an additional area of diminished bone density due to paucity of trabeculae, in the left sacral wing (thin arrows). It was attributed to an island of fatty marrow, since its density was −79 ± 25 HU. In the follow-up scan it is partly obscured by a new sclerotic metastatic deposit.

Teaching Points

Beware of the satisfaction of search and expectation biases. Please refer to Chap. 5, Sect. 5.2.2.3 for further discussion.

Case 6

A 37-year-old male presenting with progressive right knee pain and "swelling." There was no significant past medical history.

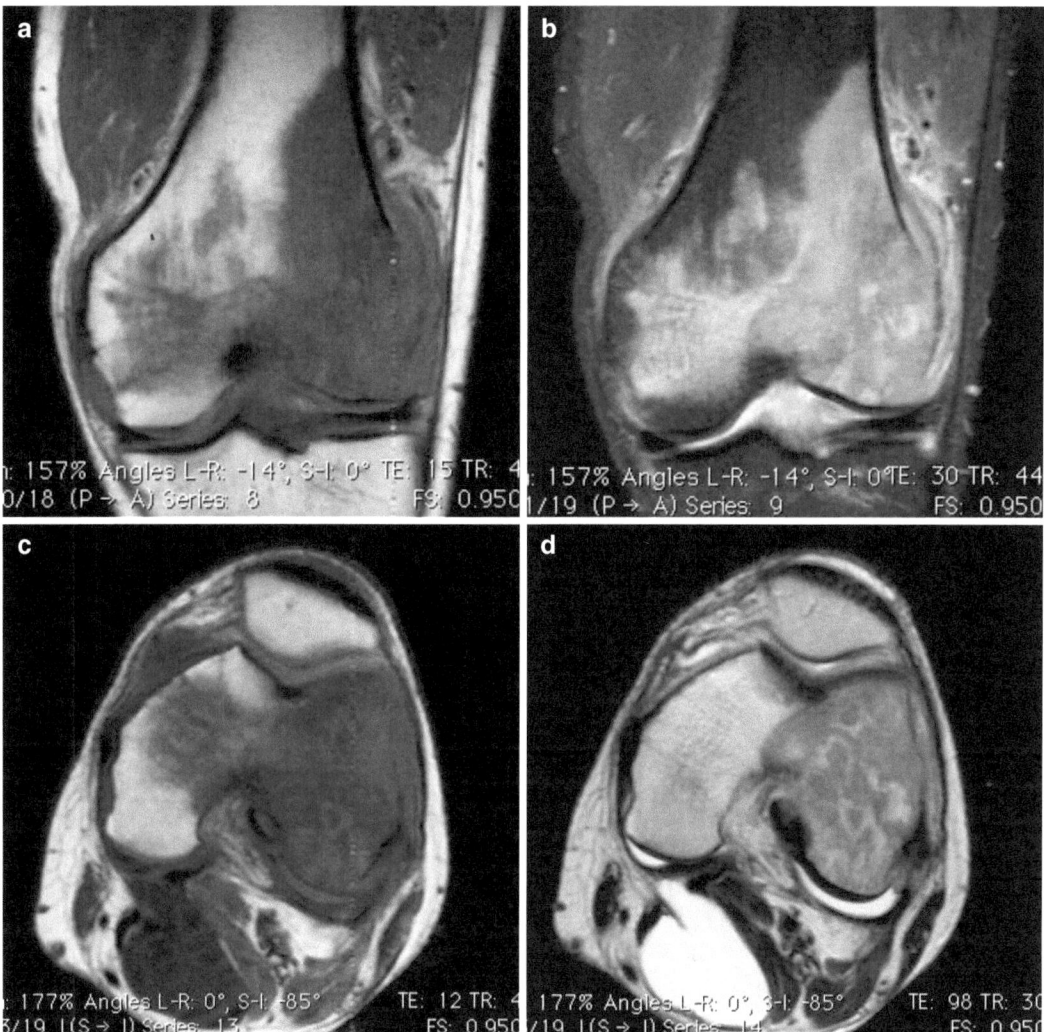

Fig. 1 (**a**, **b**) Coronal T1w and STIR images, (**c**, **d**) axial T1w and T2w images

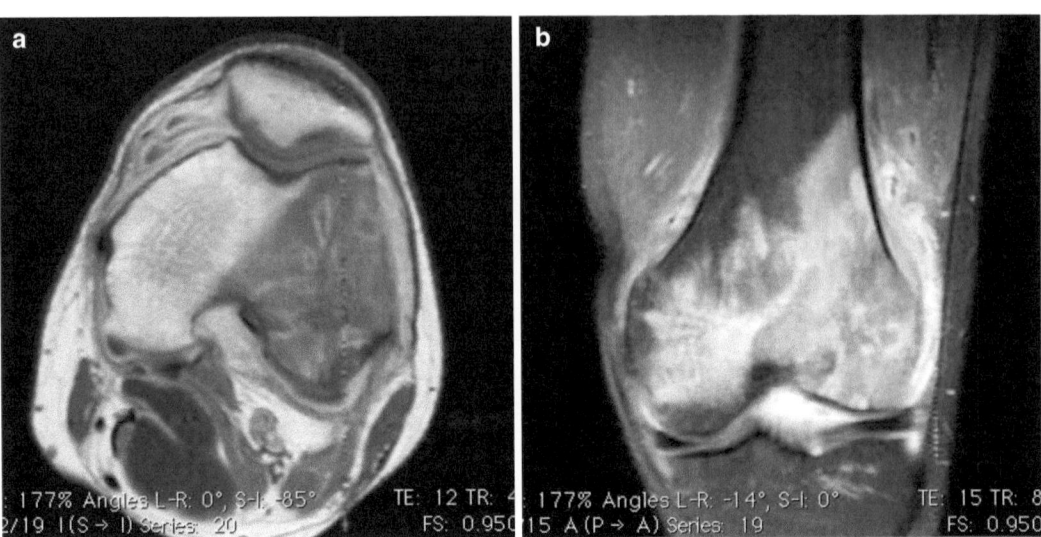

Fig. 2 (**a**, **b**) Contrast enhanced T1w images in the axial and coronal plane without and with fat suppression, respectively

Please describe the findings, formulate a differential, and commit them on paper.

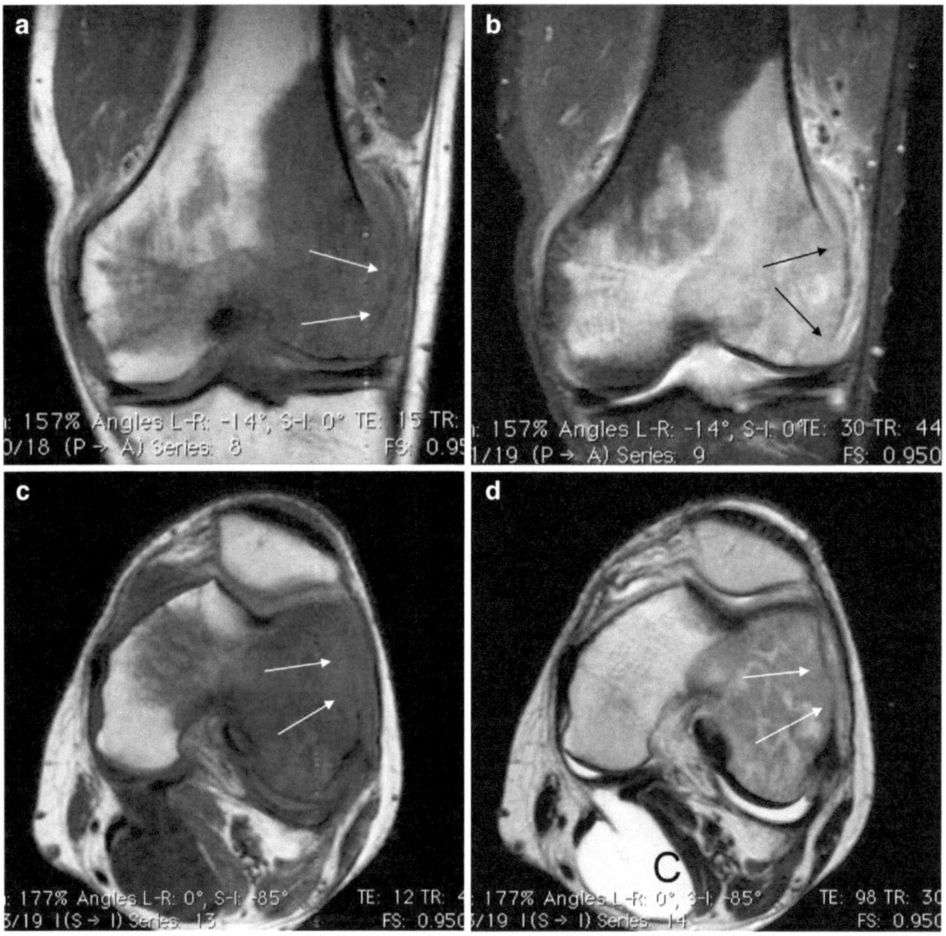

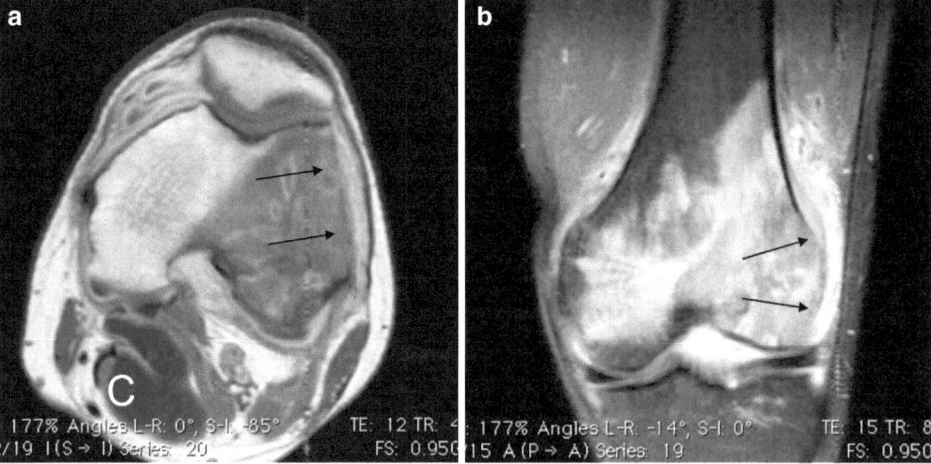

Fig. 3 (**a–d**) Same as Fig. 1a–d

Fig. 4 (**a, b**), same as Fig. 2a, b

Discussion

There is a solid infiltrative lesion of the bone marrow of the right femur. The contrast enhancement is intense and slightly inhomogeneous. Note thinning and breakthrough of the cortex of the lateral condyle (arrows) and extraosseous extension. A popliteal cyst represents an incidental finding (C).

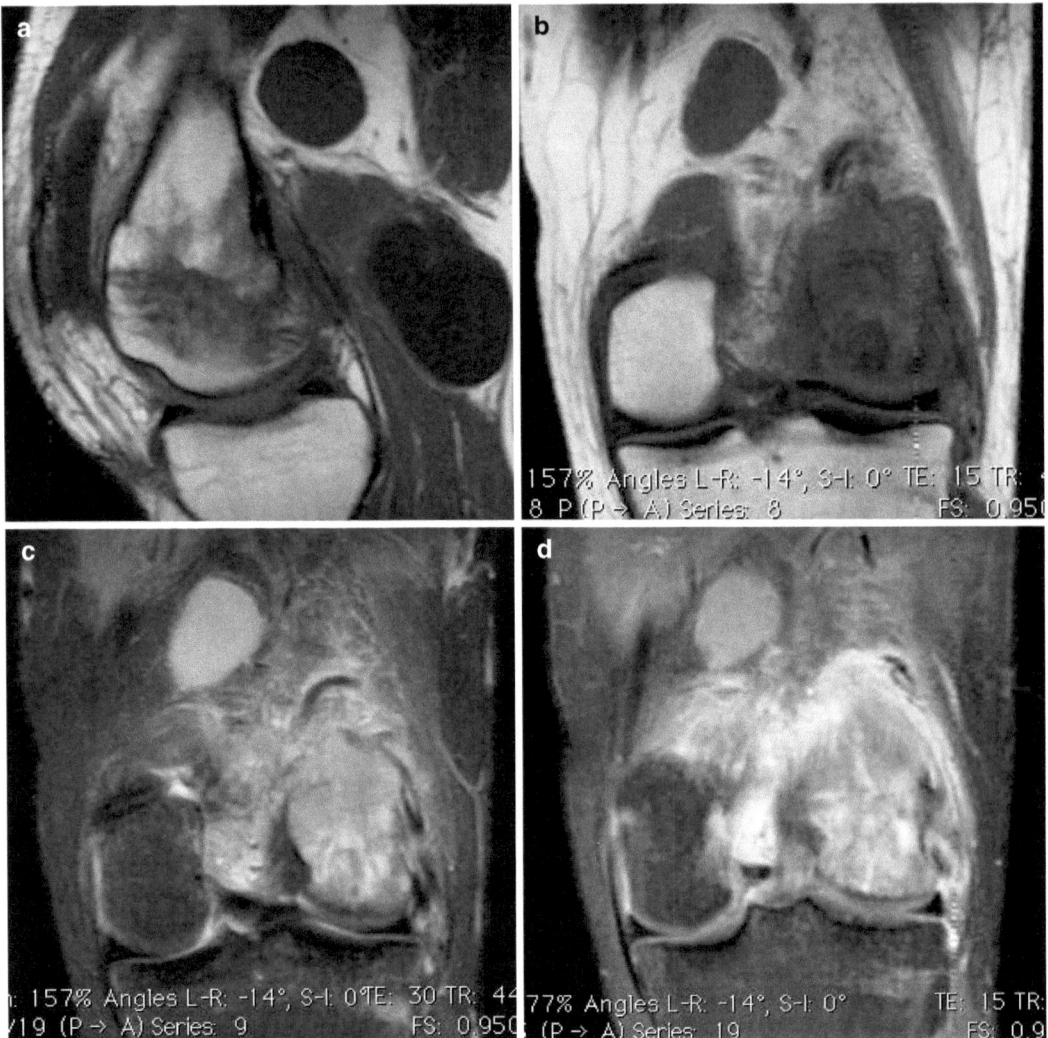

Fig. 5 (**a**, **b**) Sagittal and coronal T1w images; (**c**, **d**) coronal STIR and fat suppression post i.v. contrast T1w images

What additional information can you extract from these images? Can you narrow you differential diagnosis list?

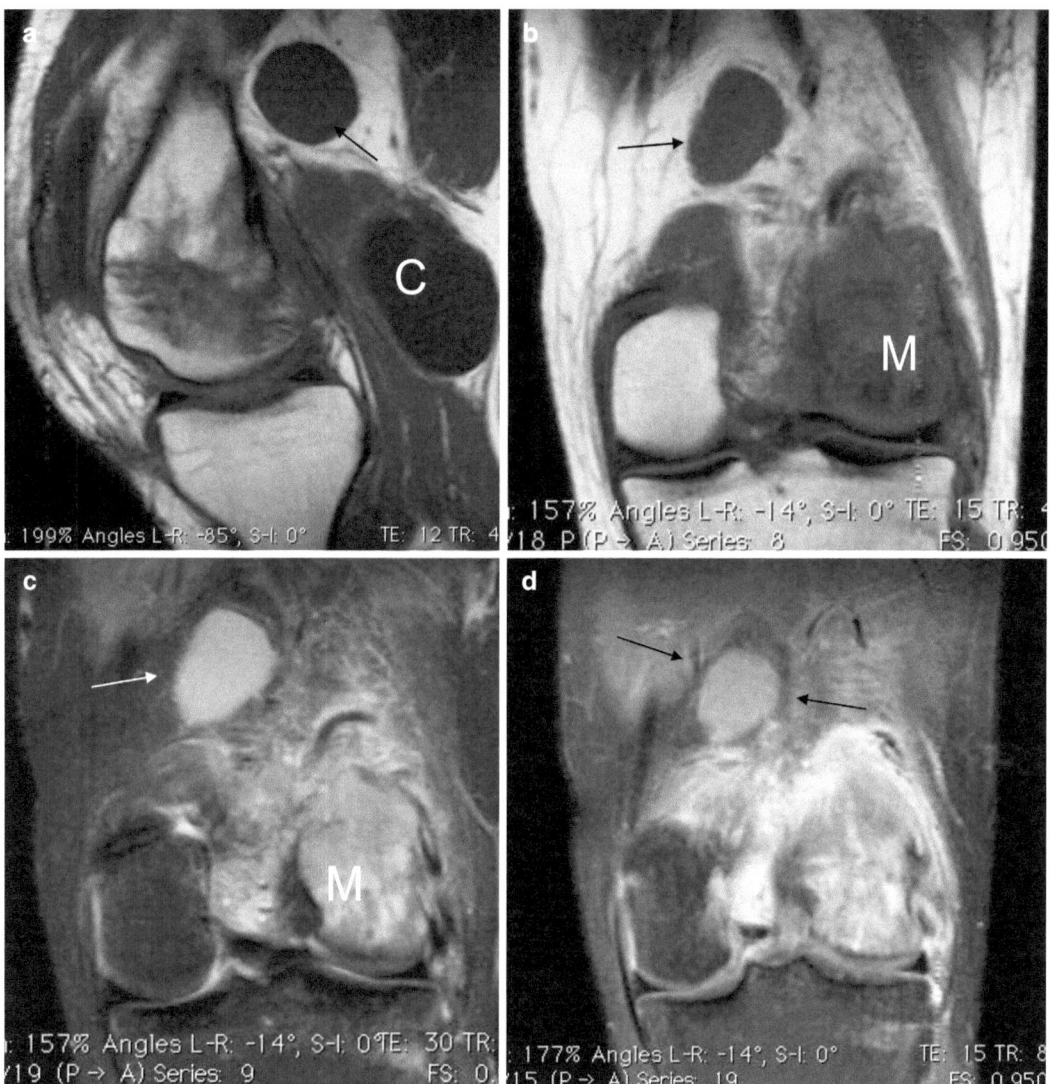

Fig. 6 (**a–d**) Same as Fig. 5a, b

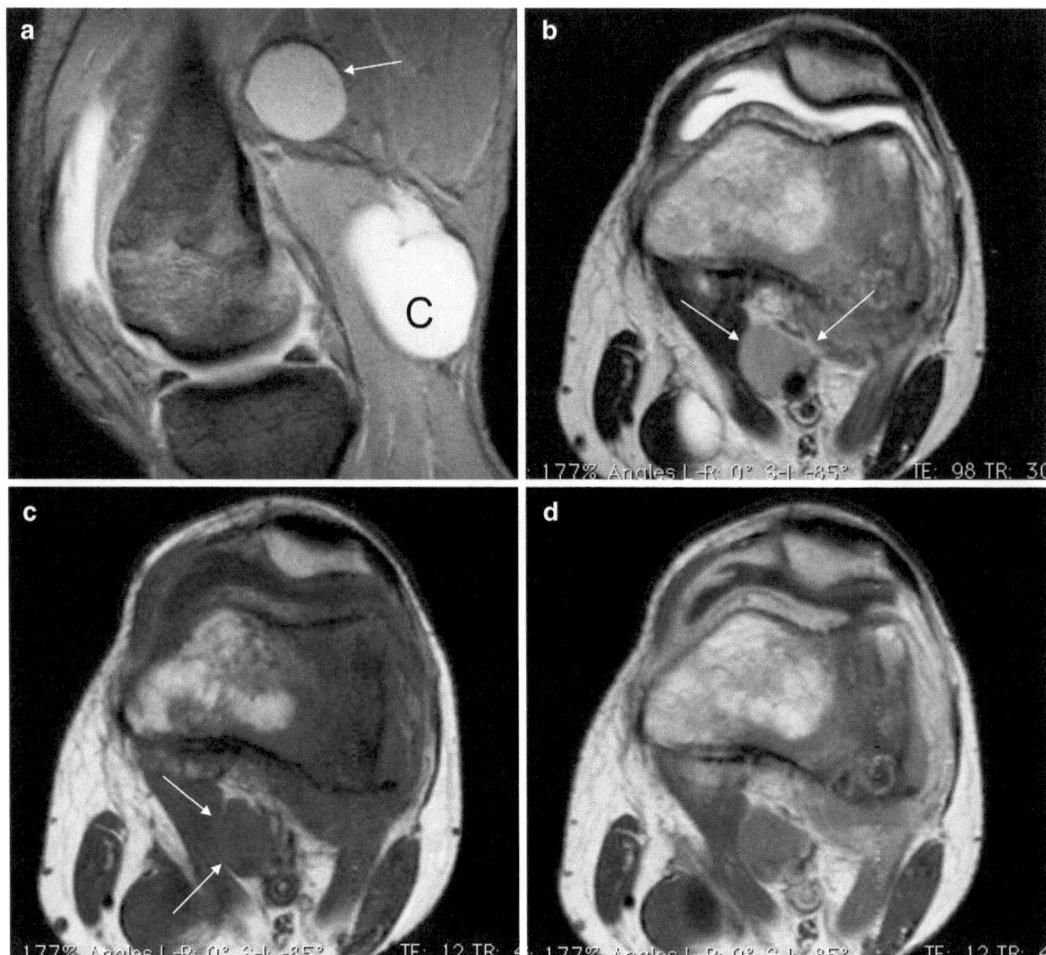

Fig. 7 (**a–d**) Sagittal T2 gradient echo, axial T2w, and axial T1w images pre and post i.v. contrast

There is a large (2.8 cm) lymph node in the popliteal fossa, without necrosis or extracapsular infiltration (arrows). Note again extensive marrow infiltration of the lateral femoral condyle (*M*). A popliteal cyst (*C*) is an incidental finding.

The final diagnosis, following open surgical biopsy, was primary bone lymphoma [60–62].

This case was presented piece by piece, on purpose. Figures 1 and 2 allow one to construct a wide differential list, whereas Fig. 5 guides one to the specific diagnosis of lymphoma.

Teaching Points

Beware of the premature closure bias; please revisit Chap. 5, Sect. 5.2.2.3.

Lymphoma can have a variety of manifestations, addressed in Chap. 7, Sect. 7.2.1.5.

Case 7

A 65-year-old male evaluated for iron deficiency anemia.

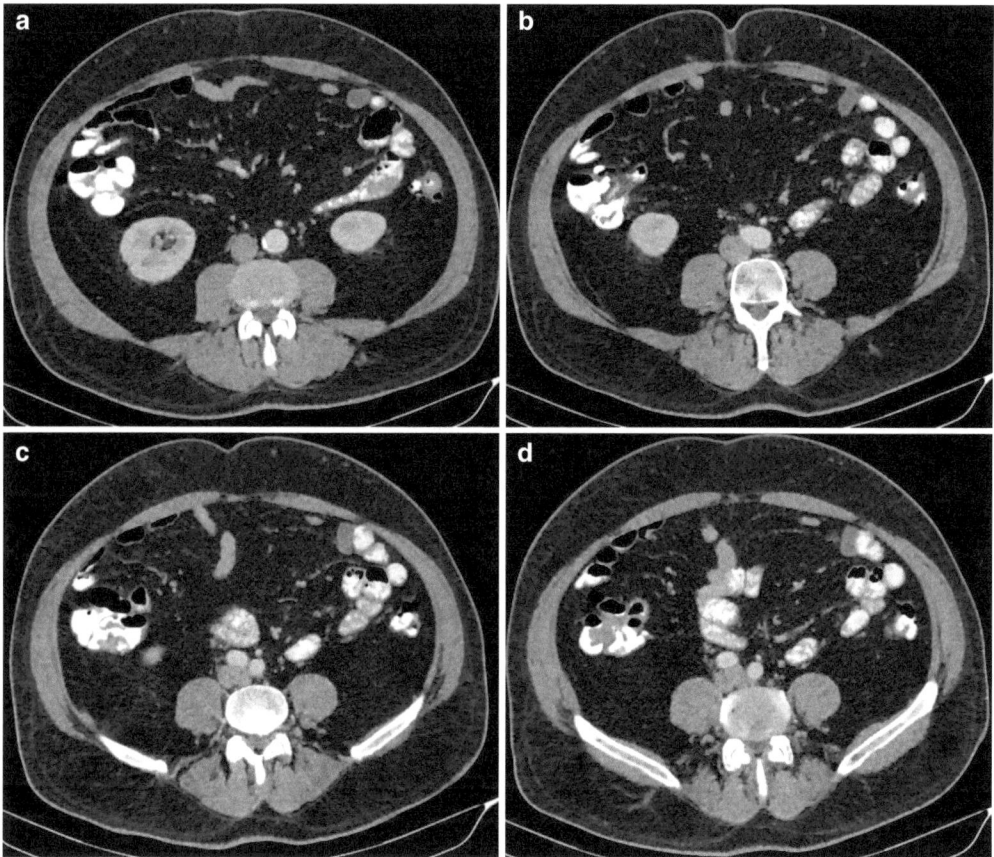

Fig. 1 (**a–d**) Selected CT images after i.v. and oral contrast administration

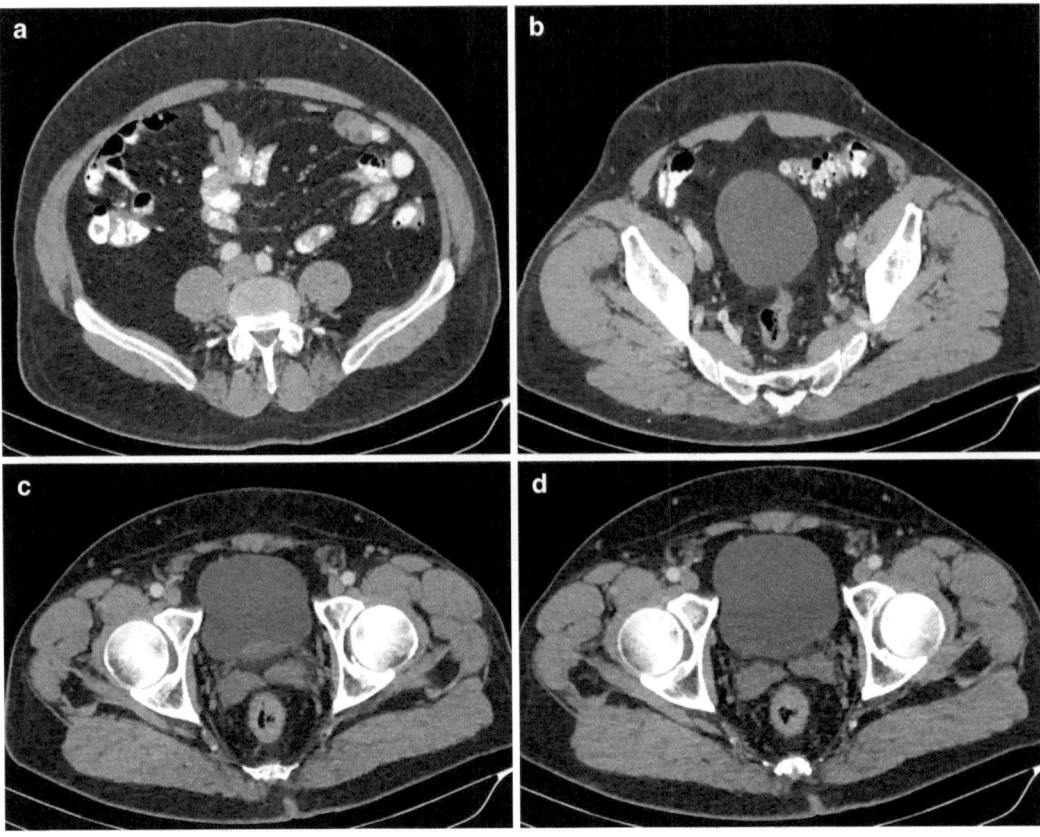

Fig. 2 (**a–d**) Selected CT images after i.v. and oral contrast administration

Please record your findings and your thoughts before proceeding.

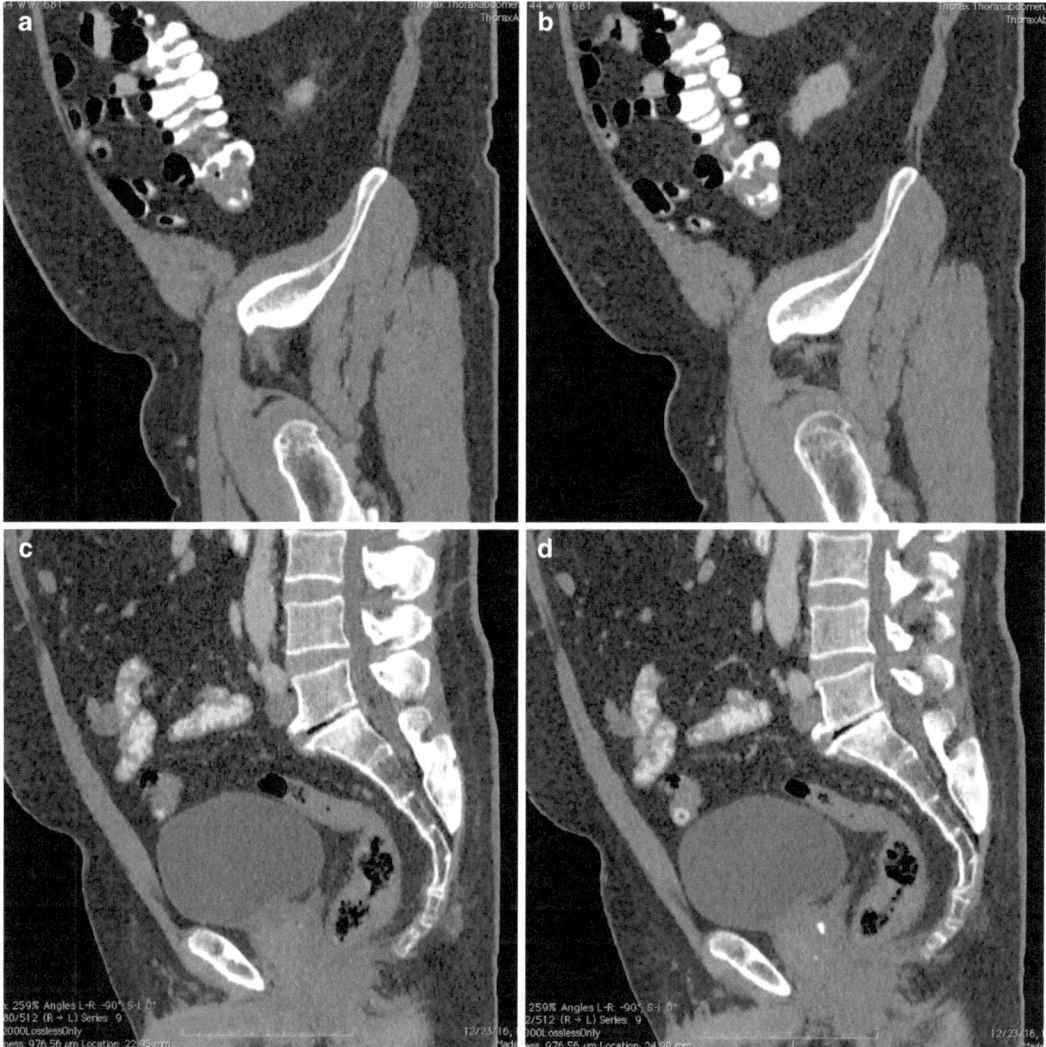

Fig. 3 (**a–d**) Sagittal reconstructions through the right lateral part of the abdomen and through the midline

Do these images add confidence to your diagnosis?

Discussion

Colonoscopy followed by surgical excision and histopathologic examination revealed two neoplasms:

(a) A sessile tubulovillous adenoma covering about half of the cecal floor, containing a dysplastic focus.
(b) An ulcerated rectal adenocarcinoma 5 cm from the anal verge, infiltrating the anterior and left lateral rectal walls.

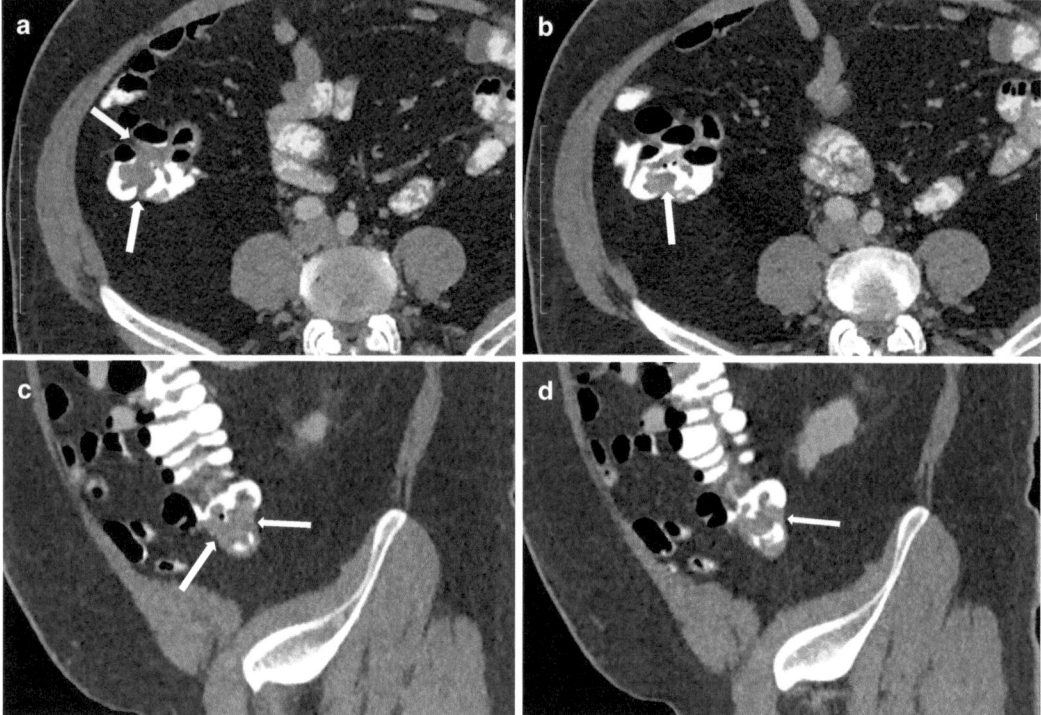

Fig. 4 (**a–d**) Magnified views of the cecum. (**a**) Magnified view of Fig. 1d; (**c, d**) magnified views of Fig. 3a, b

The adenoma (arrows) can be easily misinterpreted as fecal matter or haustral contractions

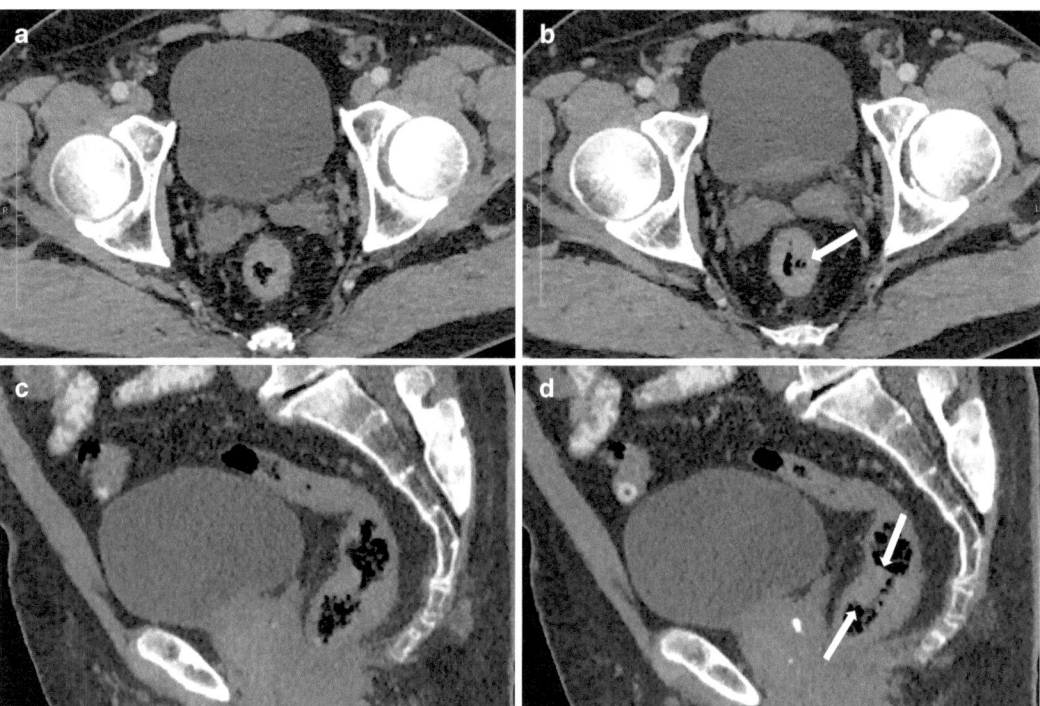

Fig. 5 (**a–d**) Magnified views of the rectum, taken from Figs. 2a, b and 3c, d

The carcinoma is difficult to detect because of nonopacification of the rectal lumen. Careful examination of the borders of the rectum reveals the carcinoma as subtle thickening of the left anterolateral wall, with abrupt "shouldering" (opposing arrows). Note small air bubble in the ulcer crater in the tumor bed (single arrow)

Teaching Points

It is important to pay attention to lobulation, irregularity, or abrupt changes of contours.
    Synchronous related lesions can occur in the same anatomic structure.

Case 8

A 68-year-old male status post partial colectomy 2 years ago, for adenocarcinoma of the colon. He has been disease free since the surgical operation. He presents for his routine surveillance scan.

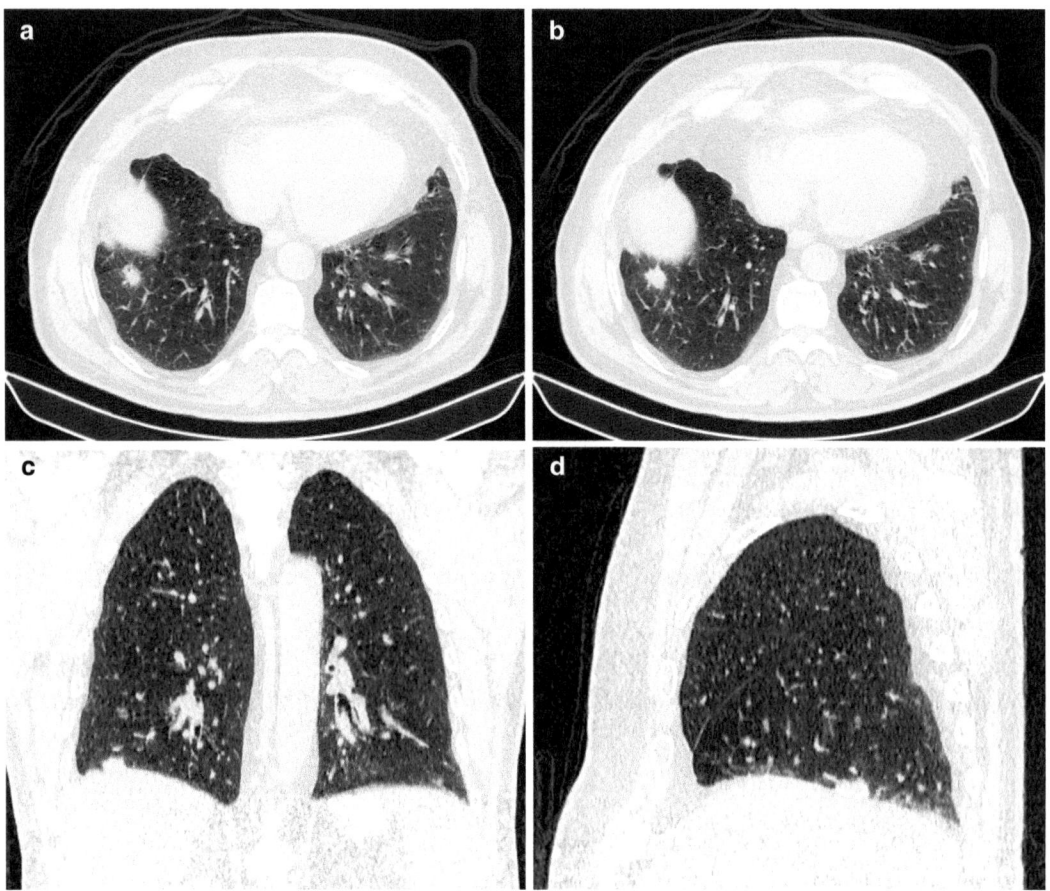

Fig. 1 (**a**, **b**) Axial CT slices; (**c**, **d**) coronal reconstructions, in lung "windows"

Please record your findings and your thoughts before proceeding.

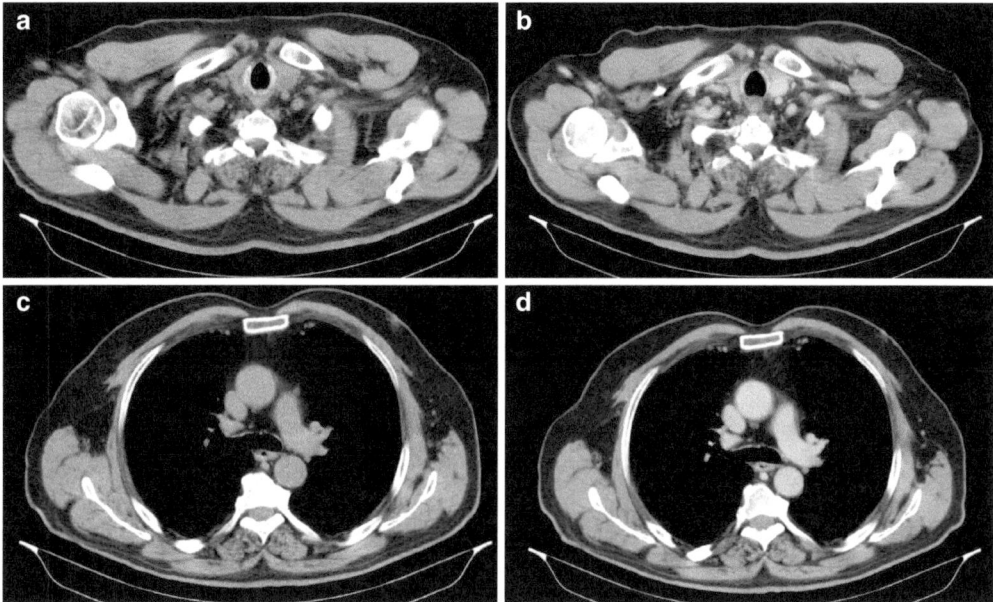

Fig. 2 (**a–d**) Pairs of images in soft tissue windows pre (**a**, **c**) and post i.v. contrast (**b**, **d**)

Please record your findings and your thoughts before proceeding.

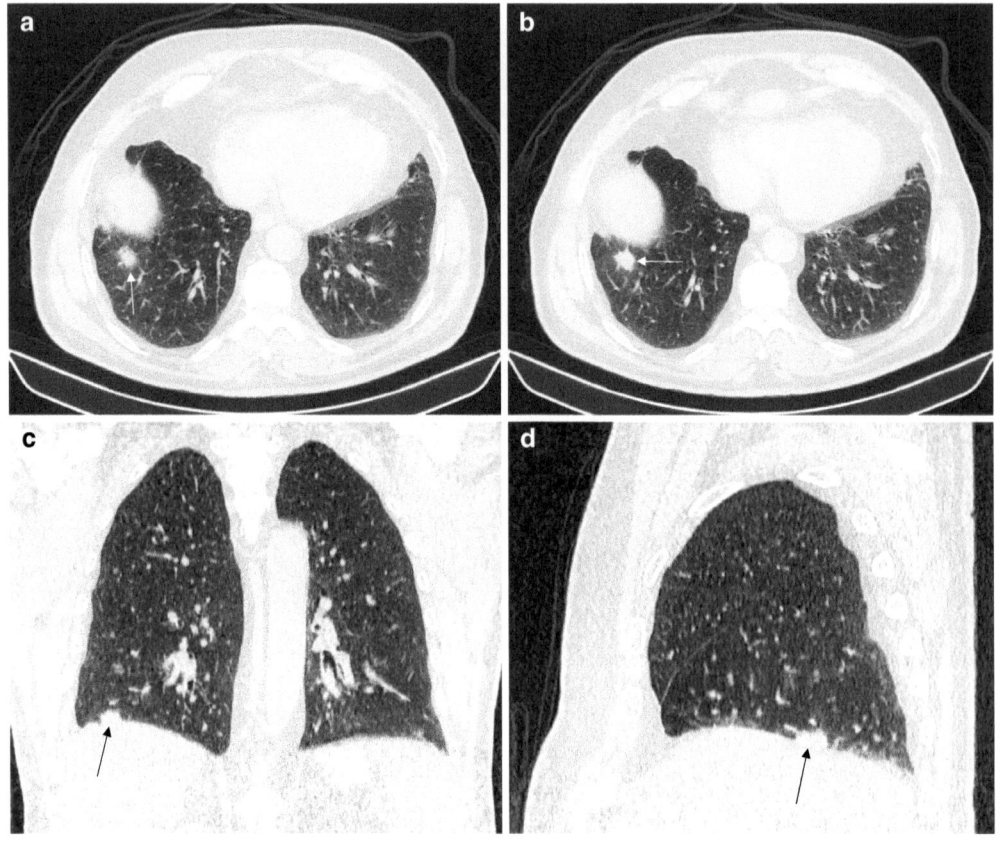

Fig. 3 (**a–d**) Same slices as in Fig. 1a–d

A solid nodule in the right lower lobe abuts the right diaphragm (arrows). The nodule was resected and confirmed to represent a metastasis from the known primary colonic adenocarcinoma.

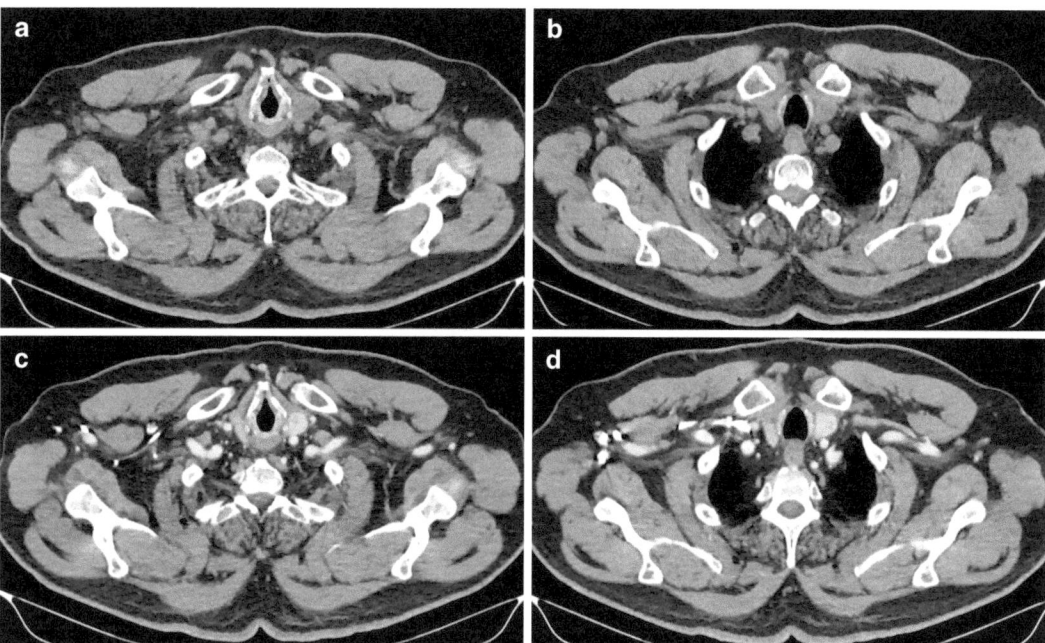

Fig. 4 (**a–d**) Pairs of CT images (s/p resection of the metastatic lung nodule), before (**a**, **b**) and after (**c**, **d**) i.v. contrast enhancement, obtained 3 months after the initial CT (shown in Figs. 1 and 2)

Please write your observations and your thoughts on paper before proceeding.

Discussion

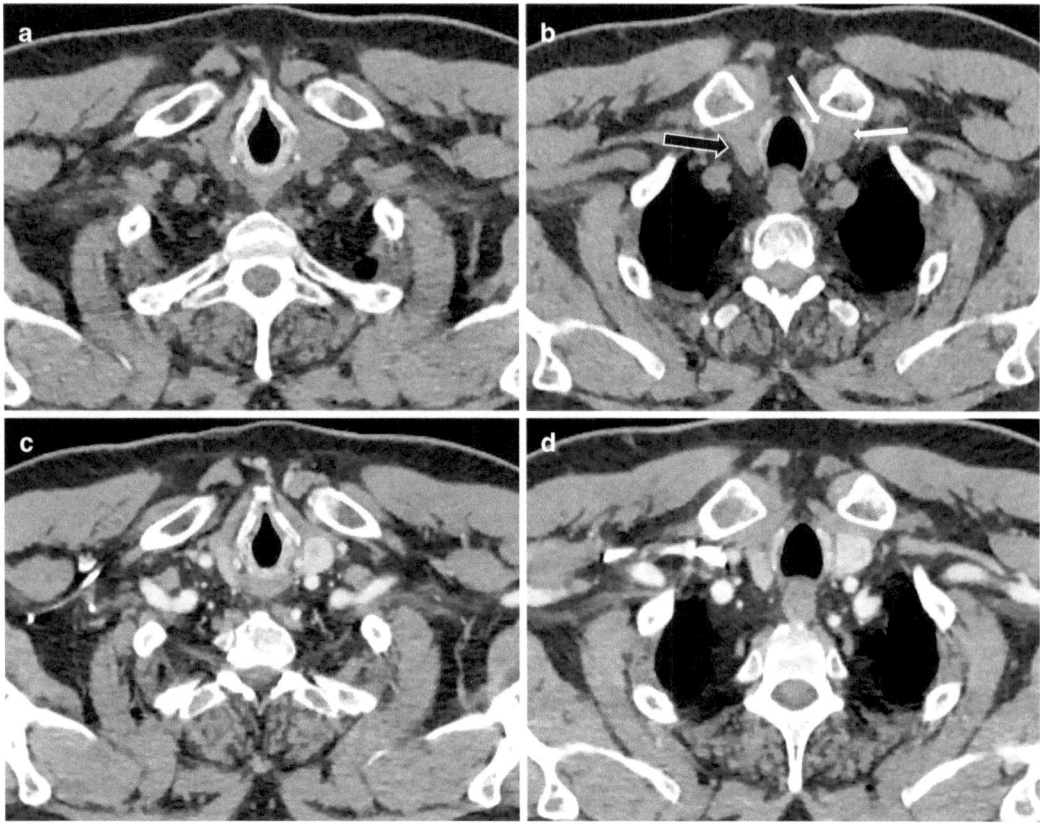

Fig. 5 (a–d) Same images as in previous Fig. 4, "magnified"

A solid nodule with strong enhancement expands the left lobe of the thyroid gland (thin arrows). Compare with the right thyroid lobe (thick arrow).

The nodule was resected and turned out to be a primary medullary carcinoma of the thyroid.

This nodule was overlooked on the initial study, Fig. 2 (**a**) and (**b**), because of suboptimal contrast administration, and because it was included only in the two most cranial slices of the study.

Teaching Points

Do not rush through the most cranial and most caudal slices. Please look up "overload–unload" bias in Chap. 5, Sect. 5.2.2.3.

Two unrelated tumors can coexist in a given patient, a concept presented in Chap. 7, Sect. 7.2.1.8

Case 9

A 58-year-old male presenting after his first epileptic seizure. An MR scan was performed.

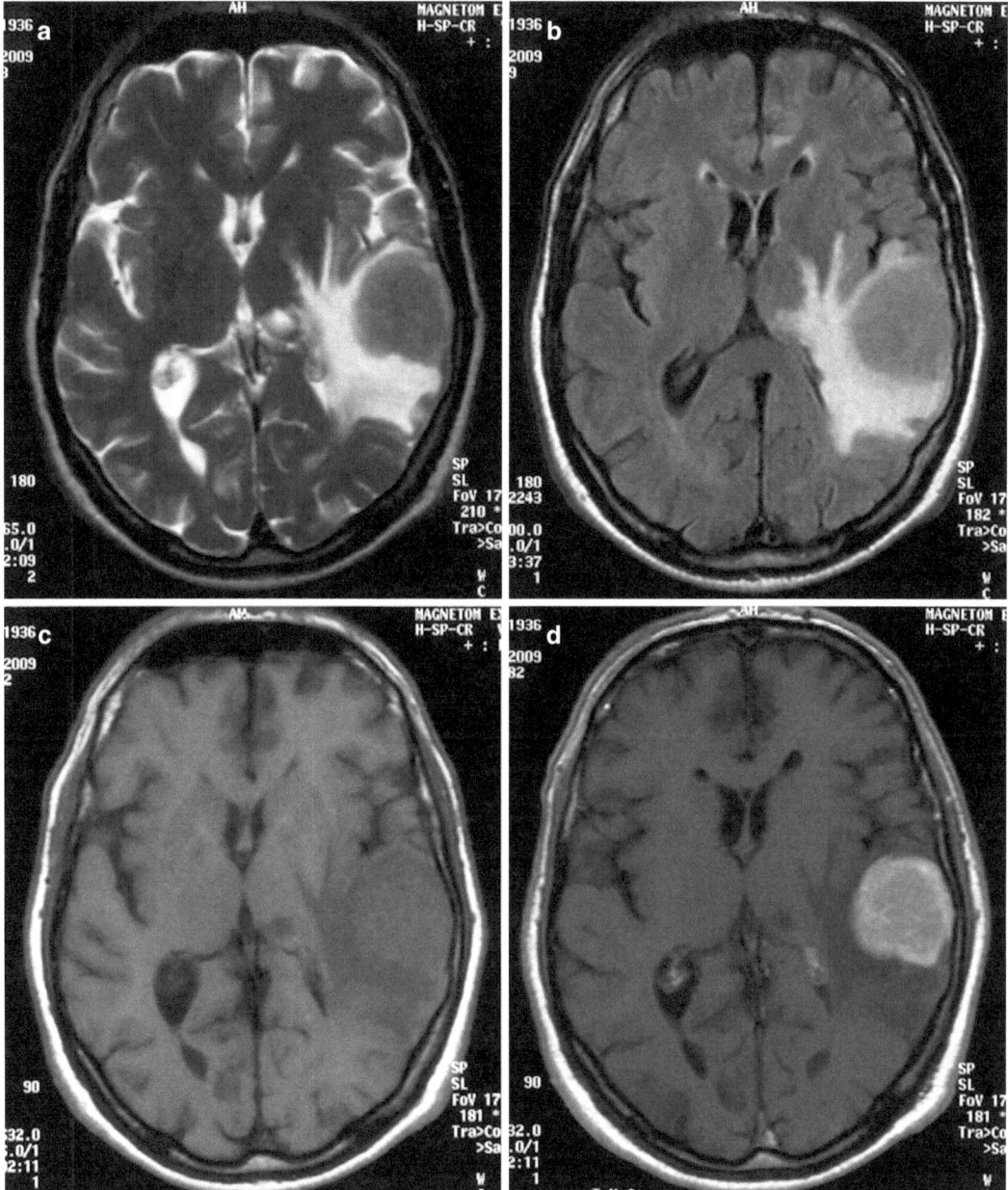

Fig. 1 (**a–d**) T2w, FLAIR, T1w, and contrast enhanced T1w axial images

Please commit your observations and your thoughts on paper before proceeding.

Discussion

A solid mass is present in the left temporal area. *Superficially* it resembles a meningioma with perifocal edema: the mass has solid consistency, signal intensity similar to brain parenchyma, intense and nearly homogeneous contrast enhancement.

However, the mass proved to be an *intra-axial primary brain lymphoma* [62–64]

How can we tell that the mass is intra-parenchymal [65, 66]?

CSF is not interposed between the mass and the inner skull table.

We do not see the cortical ribbon compressed by the mass.

There is no gray-white interface adjacent to the mass.

Teaching Points

Correct and precise anatomic localization of the abnormality is of paramount importance.

Fast decisions based on Aunt Minnie or pseudo Aunt Minnie patterns may lead us to erroneous conclusions. Please look up "Aunt Minnie bias" in Chap. 5, Sect. 5.2.2.3.

Perhaps you were biased by statistical rules, and did not expect to see another case of lymphoma, after seeing an example of primary bone lymphoma in Case 6. Please look up my comments on the use of statistical tools in Chap. 4, Sect. 4.7.

Case 10

A 75-year-old female with insidious onset of dull low back pain, progressing over several months. There was no history of trauma. Past medical history was not significant. An MRI study was requested as the initial evaluation.

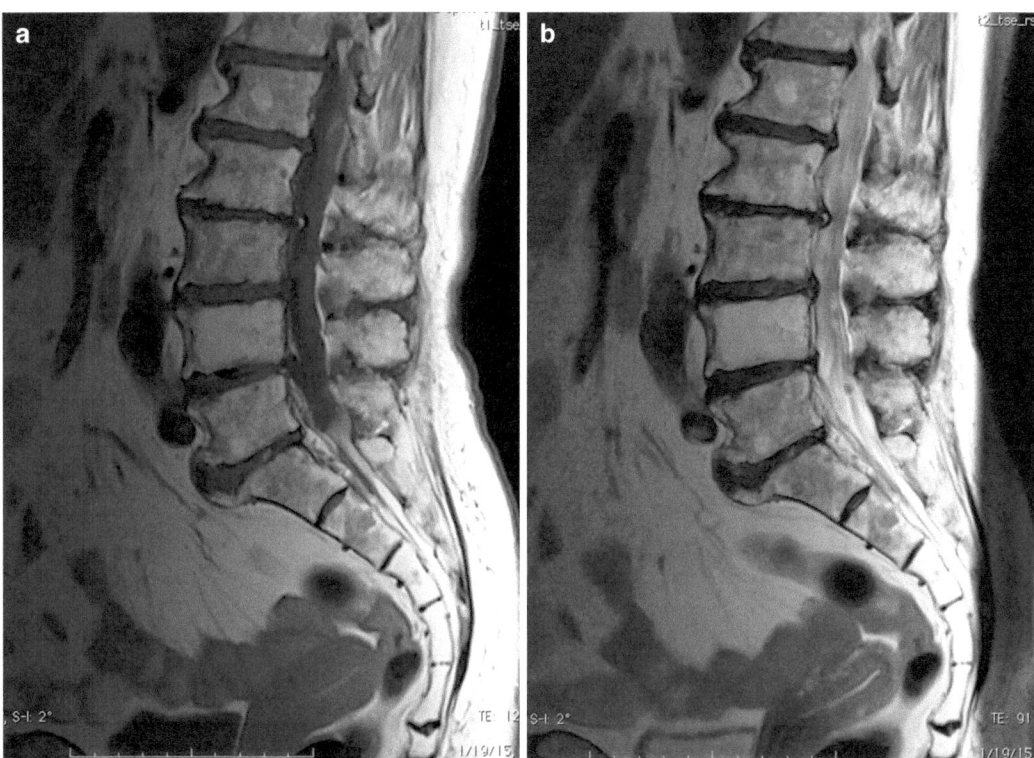

Fig. 1 (**a**, **b**) Sagittal T1w and T2w images

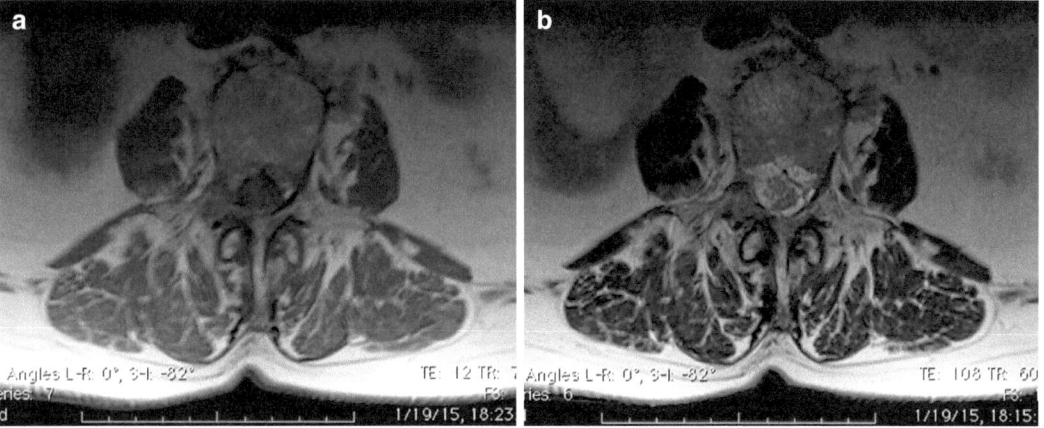

Fig. 2 (**a**, **b**) Axial T1w and T2w images at the L3 level

Please record your findings and your thoughts before proceeding.

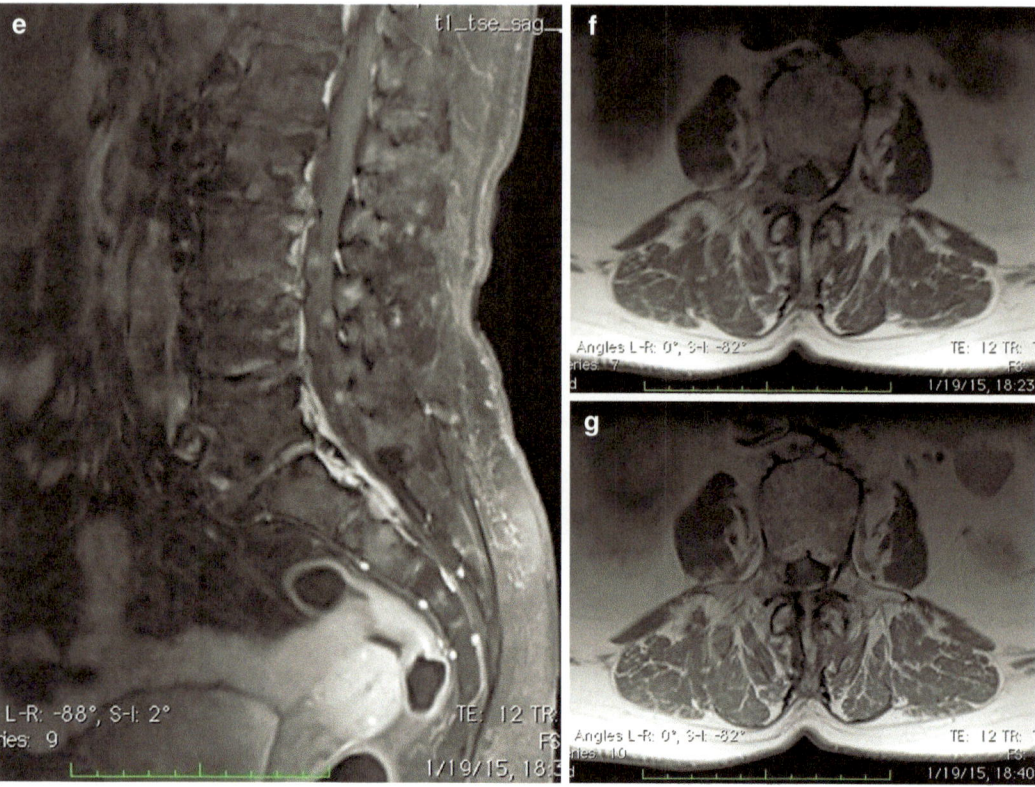

Fig. 3 (**a**) Sagittal fat suppressed T1w image post i.v. contrast; (**b**, **c**) axial T1w images pre and post i.v. contrast, through the L3 level

Are there any changes in your thoughts?

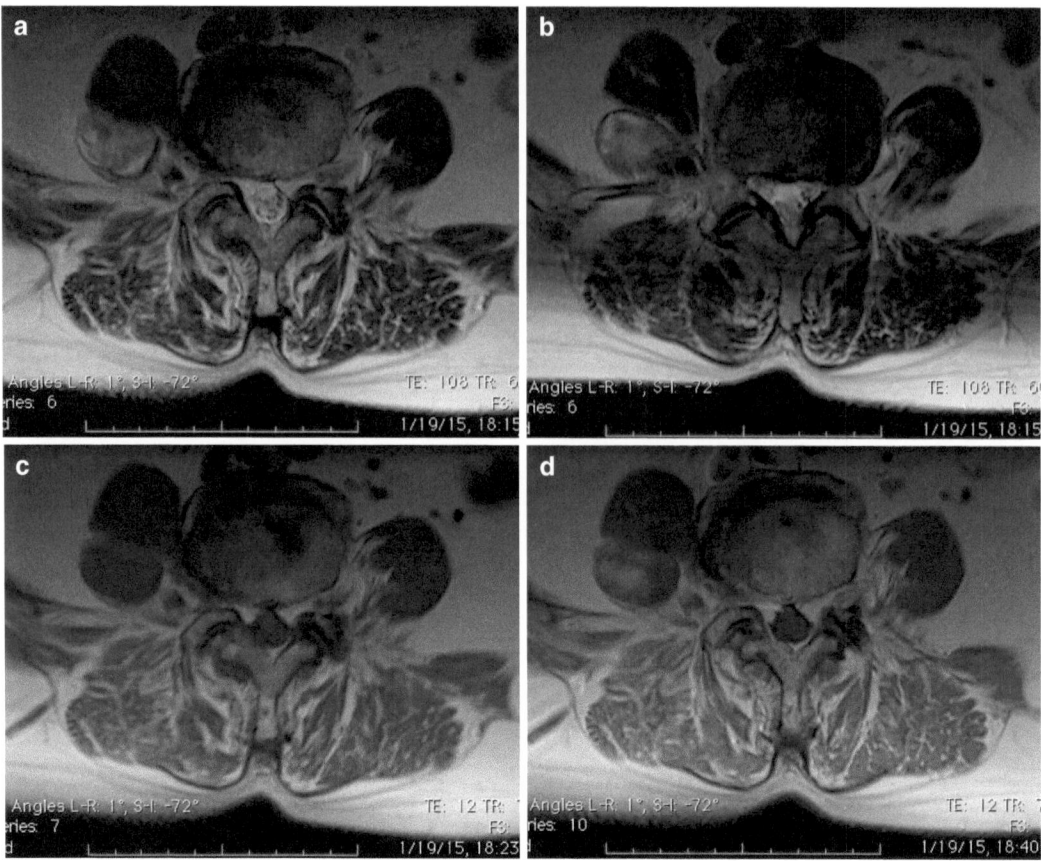

Fig. 4 (**a**, **b**) Consecutive transverse T2w axial images through the L4 level. (**c**, **d**) Axial T1w images, before and after i.v. contrast, at the L3 level, corresponding to image (**a**)

Please establish your final diagnosis or diagnoses, after describing and analyzing these findings.

Discussion

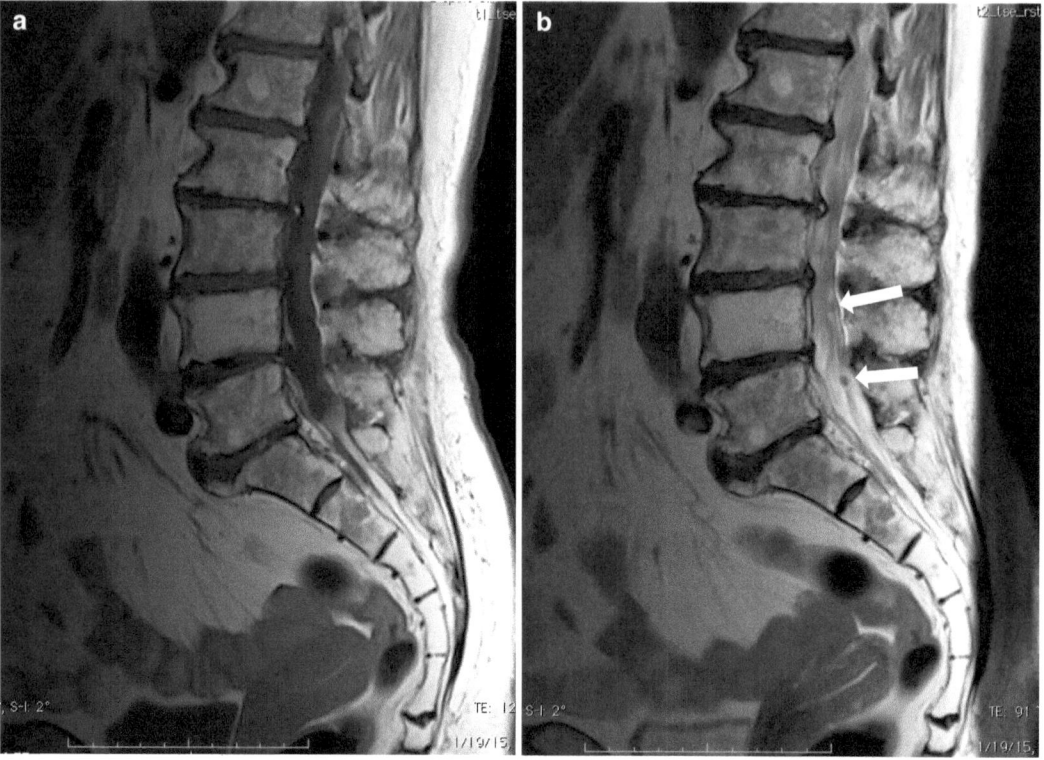

Fig. 5 (**a, b**) Same images as in Fig. 1

There are two small intradural solid nodules at the L4 and L5 levels (arrows), blending in with the roots of the cauda equina

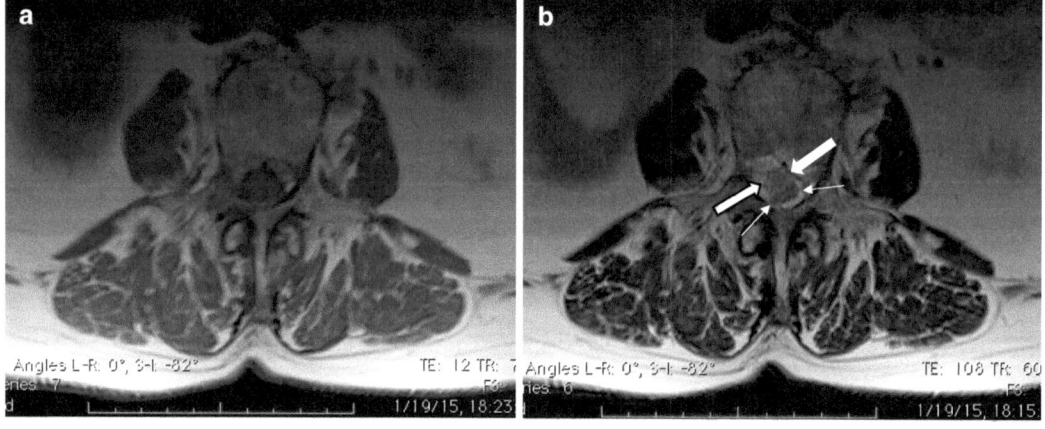

Fig. 6 (**a, b**) Same images as in Fig. 2

A solid nodule (thick arrows) displaces dorsally the cauda equina (thin arrows). Motion artifact in the T1w image precludes easy identification of this nodule

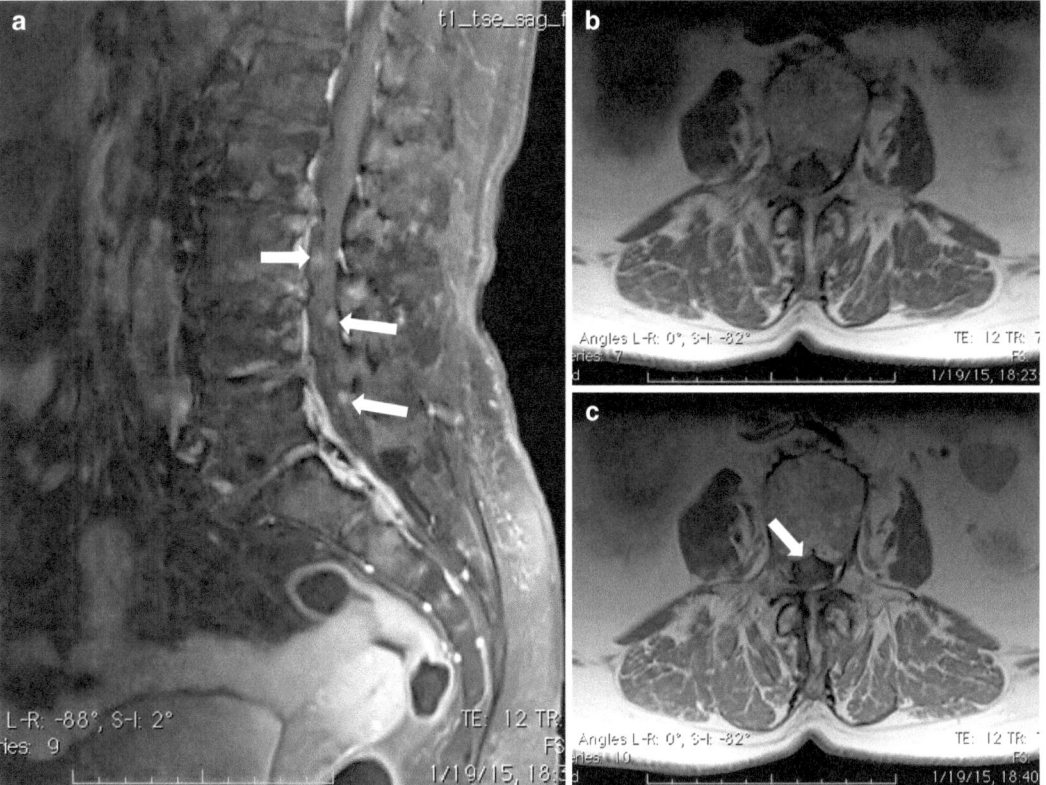

Fig. 7 (**a–c**) Same images as in Fig. 3

The intradural nodules show homogeneous contrast uptake (arrows).

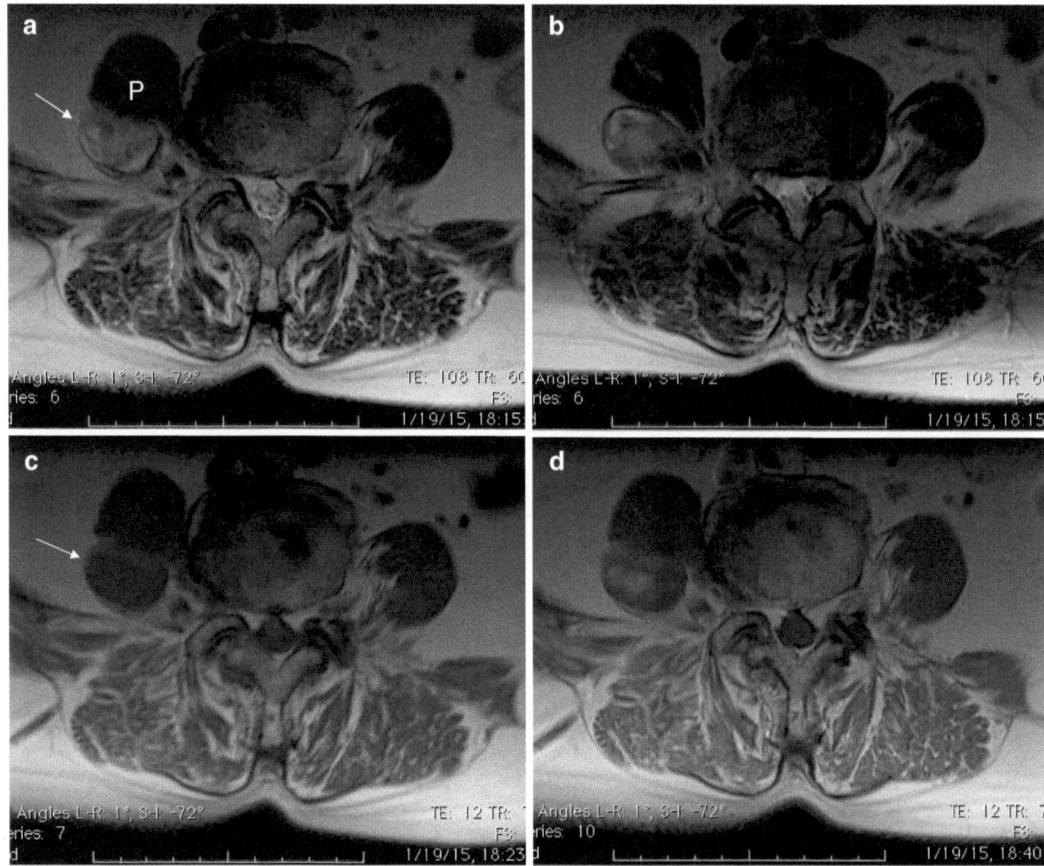

Fig. 8 (a–d) Same images as in Fig. 4

A mass resides just behind the right psoas muscle (arrows). It has smooth, well-defined borders and homogeneous, intermediate T1 signal intensity. Its T2 signal intensity is inhomogeneous, with the "brighter" parts arranged in the periphery. Contrast enhancement is located centrally

Can we tie all these findings under a single diagnosis?

Or do we have to invoke two separate disease entities?

Surgical extirpation confirmed one extraspinal and three intradural *schwannomas*.

The MRI behavior of the extraspinal tumor is characteristic for schwannoma [67, 68]. Thus we ascribe the intradural nodules to schwannomas as well. The patient did not have a history of neurofibromatosis and further evaluation did not reveal any other features of neurofibromatosis.

I purposely showed this case as a piece meal problem: were you flexible enough to change your mind, given additional important evidence? Or did you become "locked" in an Aunt Minnie or premature closure pattern thinking about "drop" metastases?

Teaching Points

Beware of Aunt Minnie and premature closure biases; please revisit Chap. 5, Sect. 5.2.2.3.

If there are multiple lesions, strive for a unifying diagnosis, before you consider multiple coexisting conditions.

Case 11

A 65-year-old female with abdominal pain. An upper abdominal CT was requested.

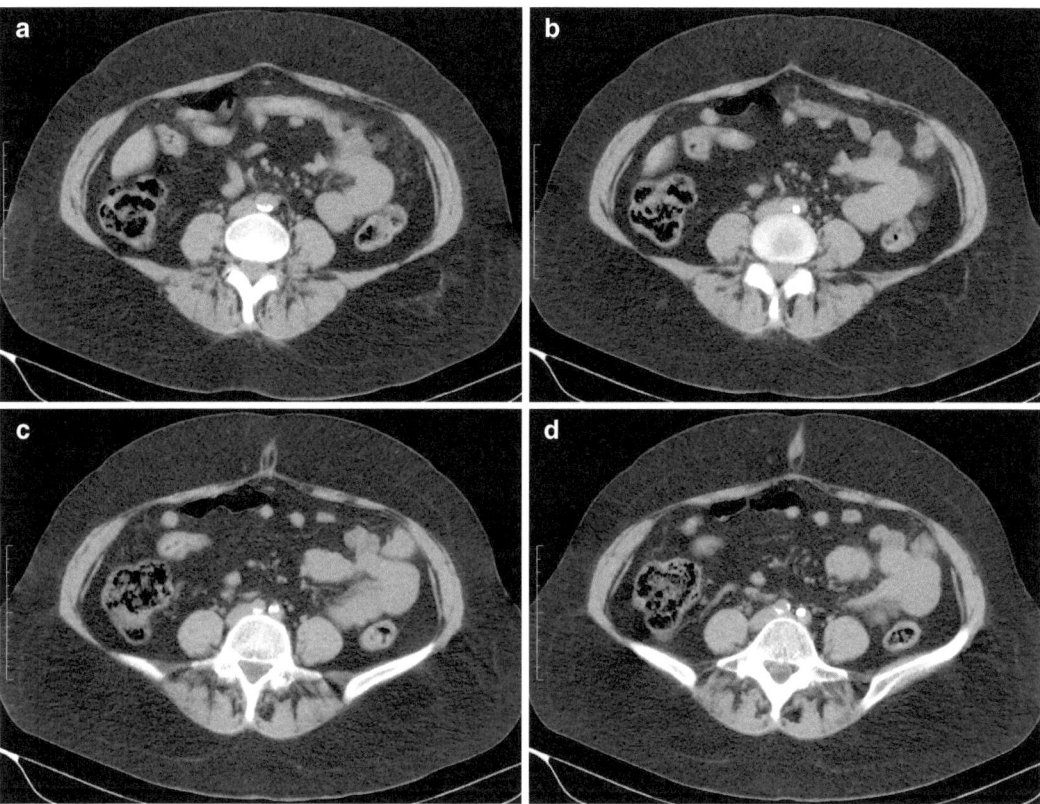

Fig. 1 (**a–d**) Consecutive CT images before i.v. contrast

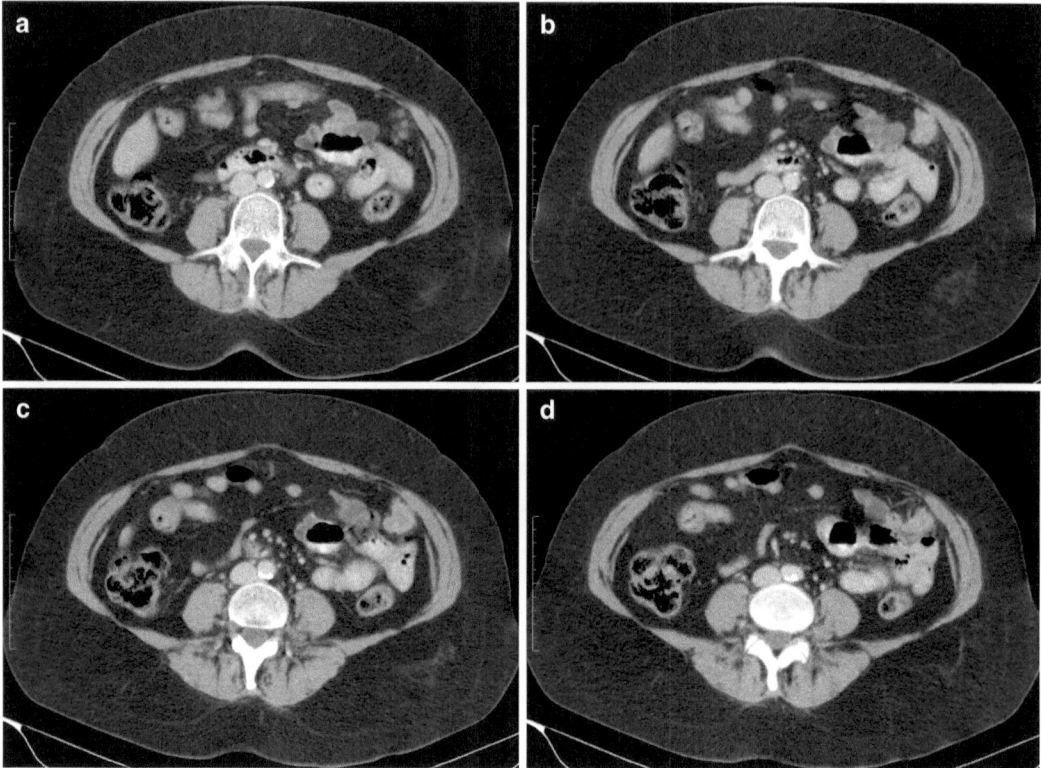

Fig. 2 (**a–d**) same as Fig. 1. Consecutive CT images after i.v. contrast. Oral contrast was also administered

Please write your observations and thoughts on paper before proceeding.

Discussion

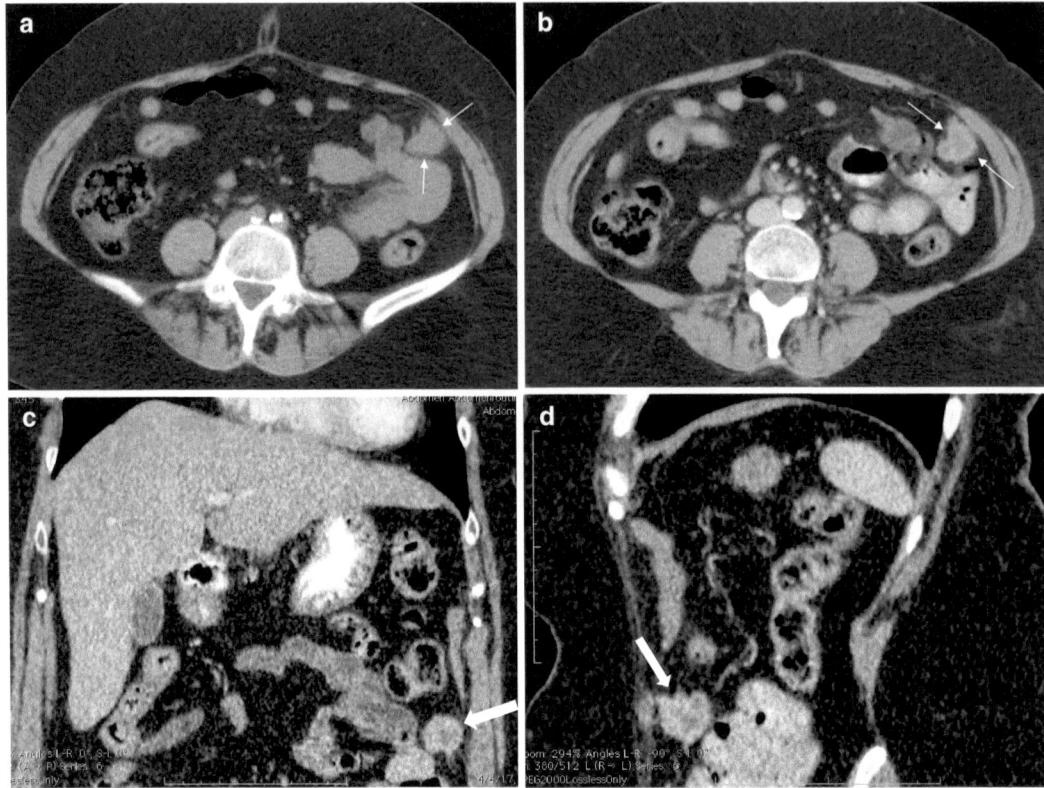

Fig. 3 (**a**, **b**) Two axial slices, before and after i.v. contrast [same as images (**c**) of Figs. 1 and 2, slightly "magnified"]. (**c**, **d**) Coronal and left lateral sagittal reconstructions

A peritoneal nodule is situated close to left anterolateral abdominal wall (arrows). Its detection is difficult, because of its proximity to small bowel loops. Close inspection reveals that the peritoneal implant is not a tubular structure and that it is not continuous with bowel loops. Furthermore, there are some spiculations toward the peritoneal fat and the ring of contrast enhancement is slightly thicker than a normal small bowel wall. Two metastases were also detected in the liver and spleen (not shown). Subsequent imaging of the pelvis with MRI revealed two solid tumors, one in the endometrium and one in the left ovary (not shown). The patient underwent total hysterectomy and oophorectomy. Both tumors were adenocarcinomas. The peritoneal implant shown in this case was confirmed at surgery.

Teaching Points

Beware of blind spots. This case is an example of peritoneal implants hiding amidst bowel loops. Please revisit "Blind Spots" in Chap. 3, Sect. 3.4.

Case 12

A 48-year-old male with dull low back pain of 2 months duration.

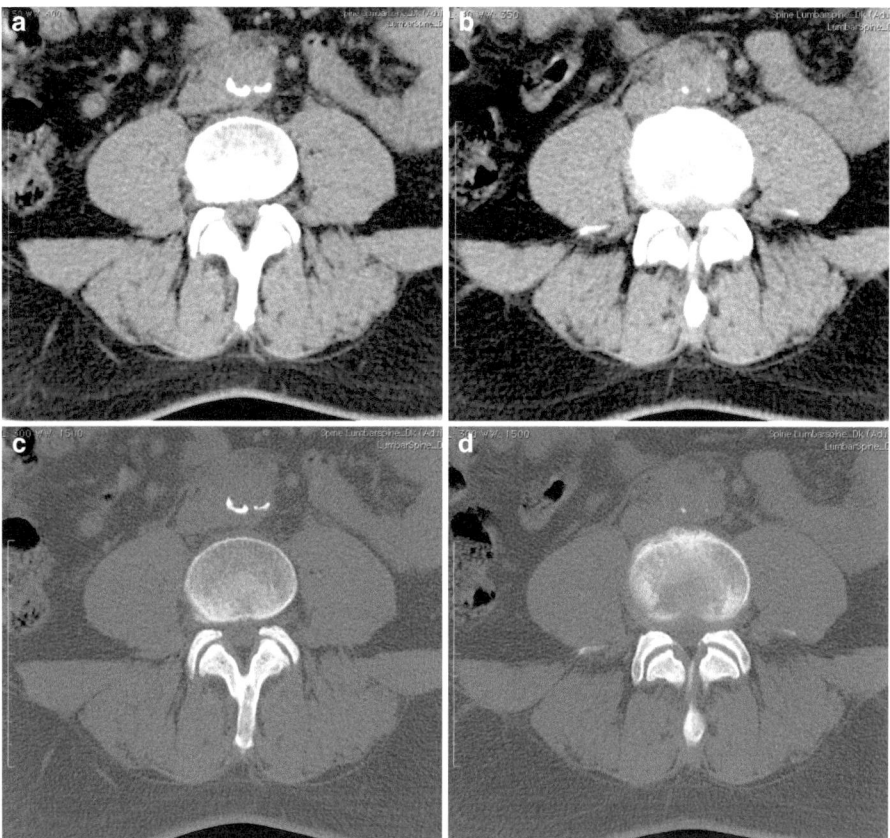

Fig. 1 (**a–d**) Pairs of CT images at the L4–L5 level in soft tissue and bone windows

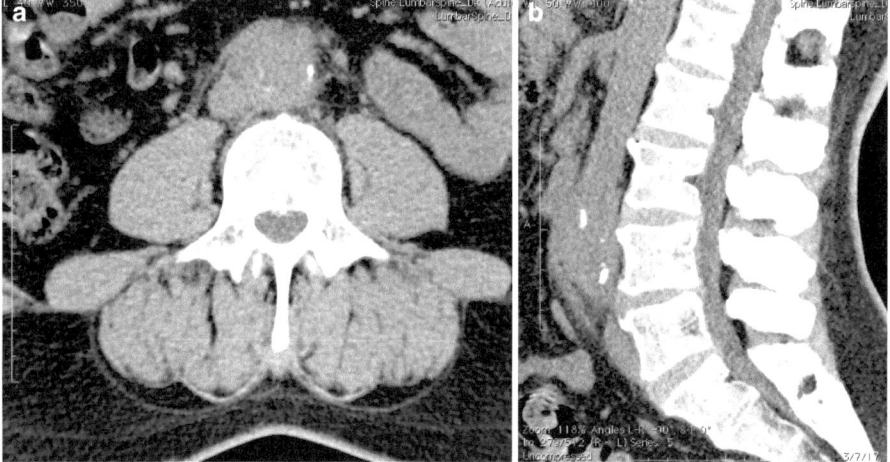

Fig. 2 (**a**) Axial CT slice at the mid L4 level and (**b**) a paramidline sagittal reconstruction

Please write your observations and your thoughts on paper before proceeding.

An MRI was performed 3 months after the CT scan, because of a change in the nature of the pain, radiating anteriorly.

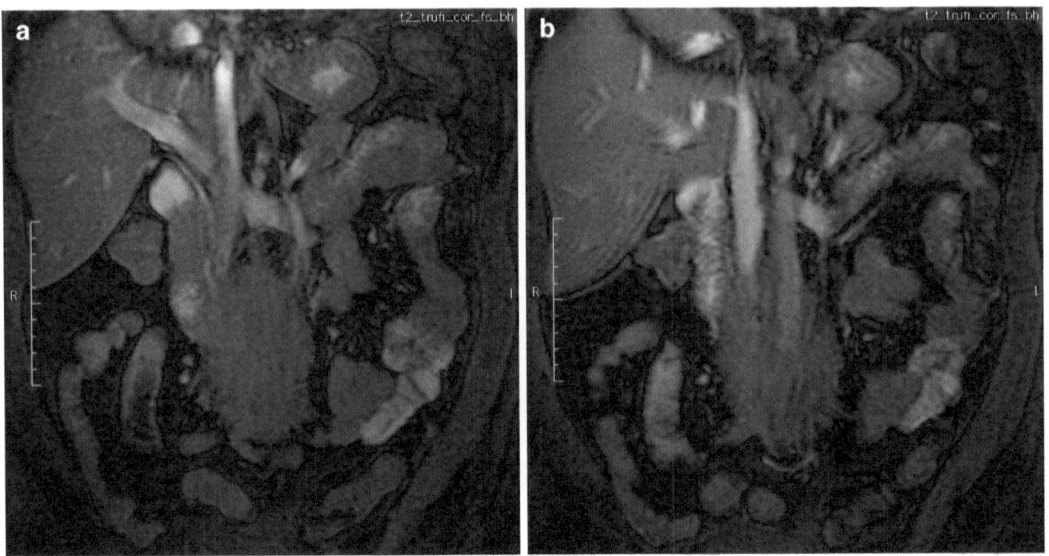

Fig. 3 (**a**, **b**) Two coronal true FISP images with fat suppression

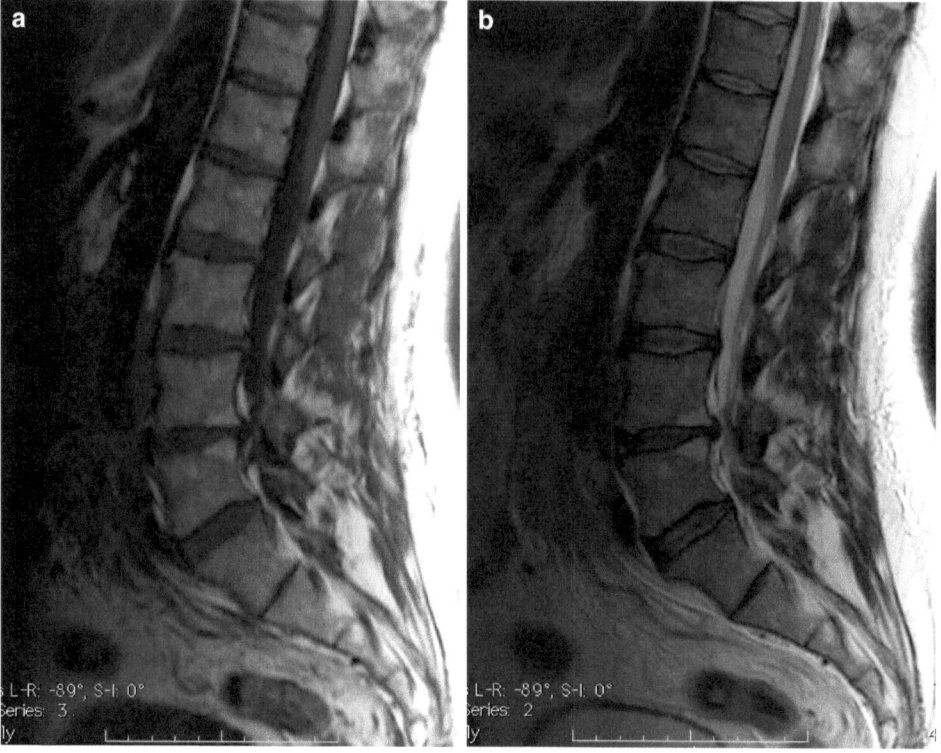

Fig. 4 (**a, b**) Sagittal T1w and T2w slices

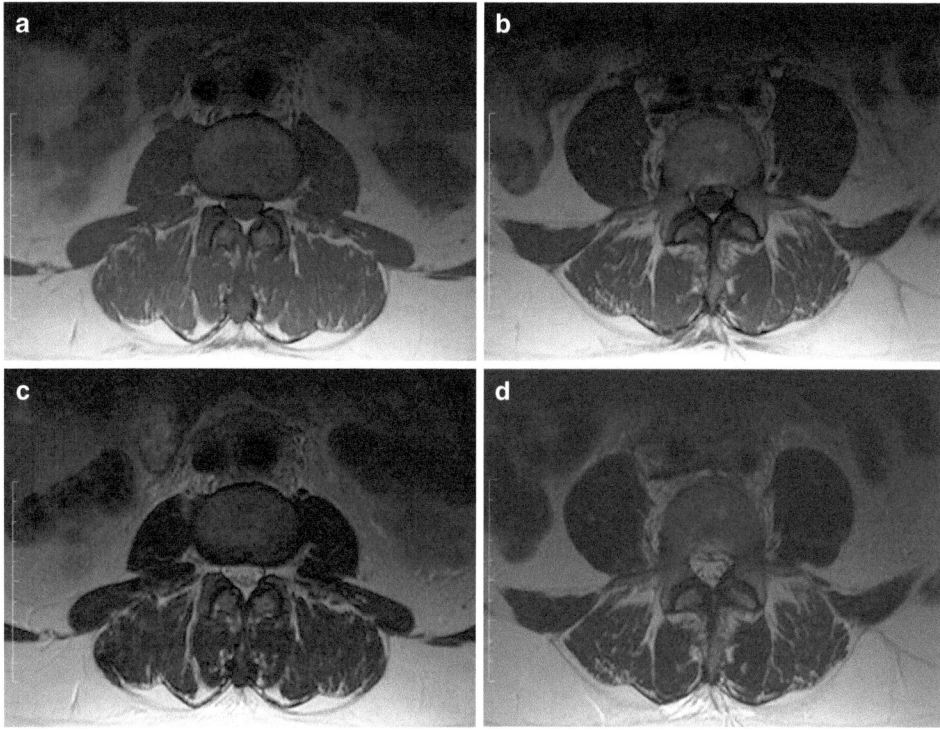

Fig. 5 (**a–d**) Pairs of axial T1w and T2w images at the L4 level

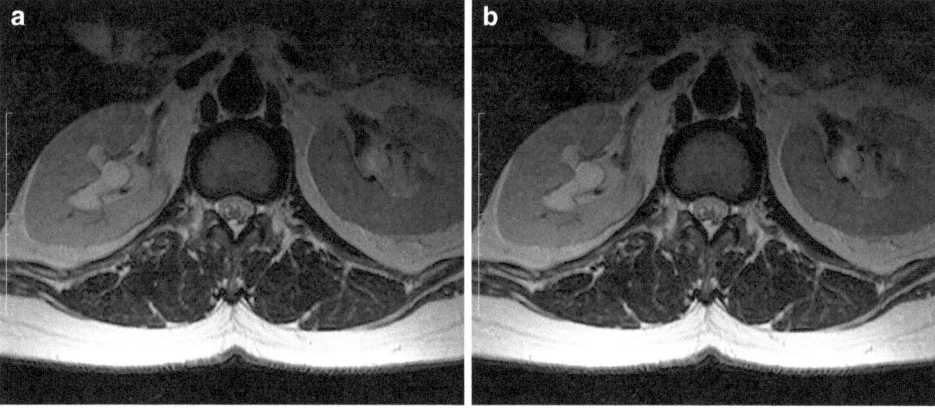

Fig. 6 (**a, b**) Two axial T2w images at the L1–L2 level

Please write your observations and your thoughts on paper before proceeding.

Discussion

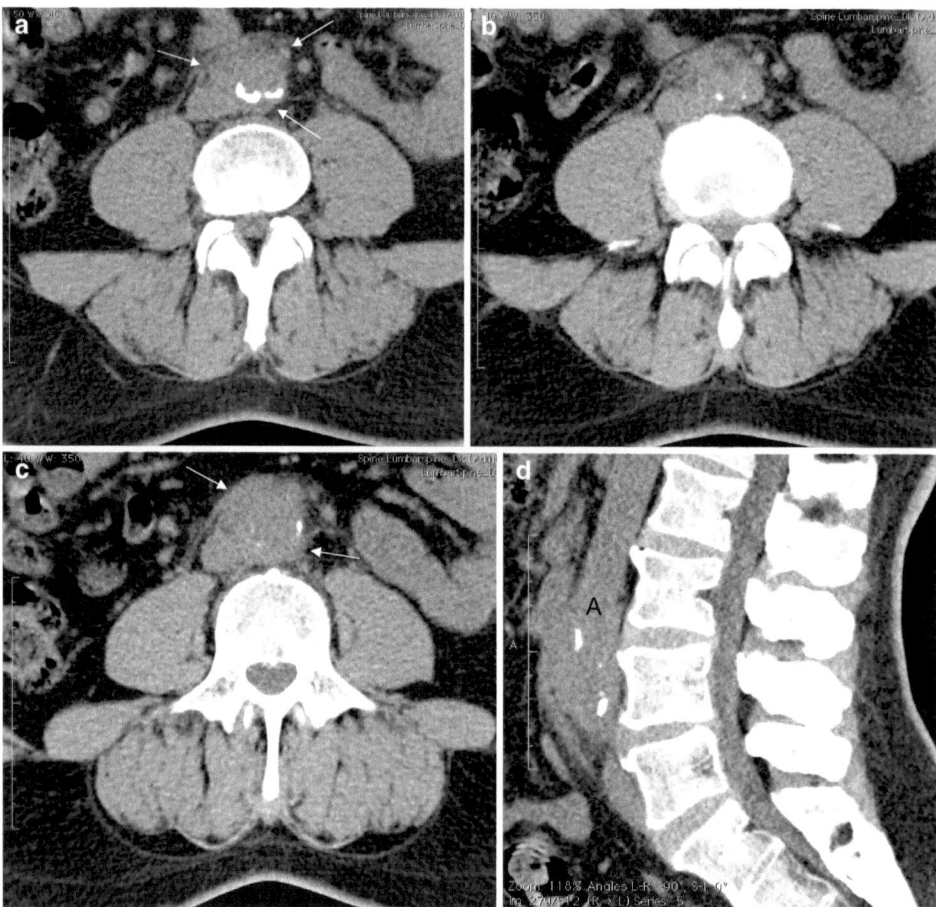

Fig. 7 (**a–c**) axial images and (**d**) a sagittal reconstruction, selected from Figs. 1 and 2

There is degenerative disk disease. However, the salient feature of this case is a thin layer of soft tissue surrounding the calcified walls of the abdominal aorta and common iliac arteries (arrows). Note also the loss of the fat plane between the aorta and the inferior vena cava as well as limited stranding of the retroperitoneal fat. There is neither osseous erosion nor periosteal reaction.

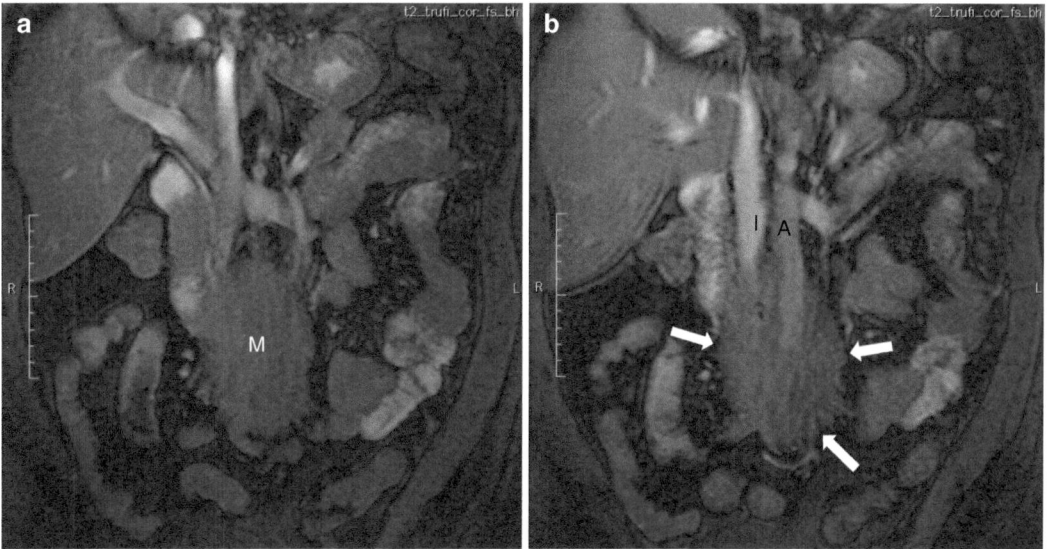

Fig. 8 (**a**, **b**) Two coronal MR images, same as in Fig. 3

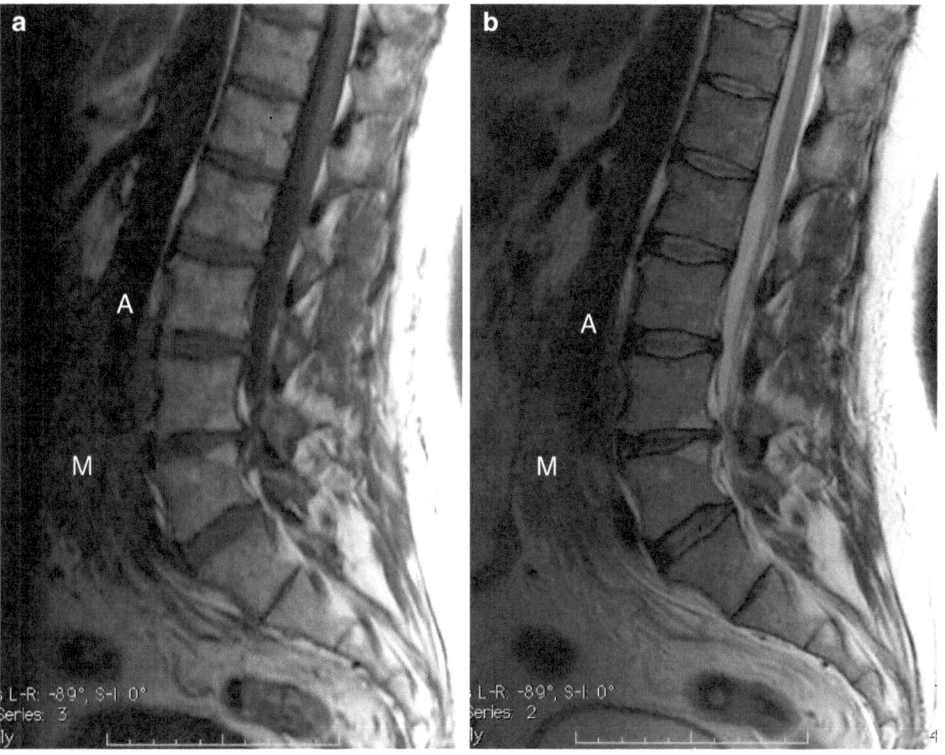

Fig. 9 (**a**, **b**) Two sagittal MR images, same as in Fig. 4

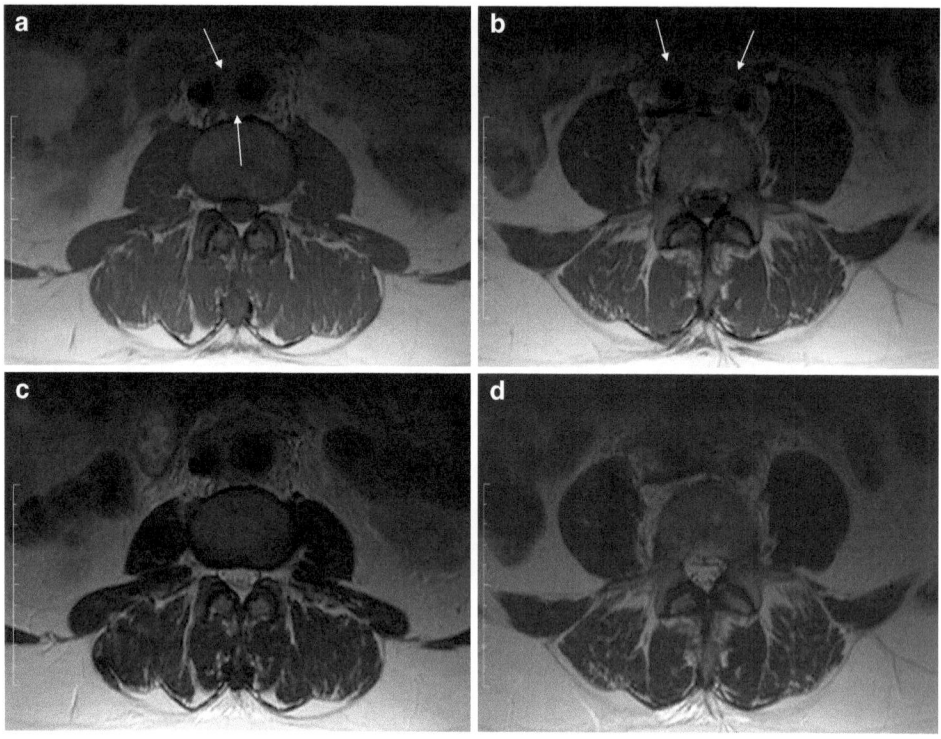

Fig. 10 (**a–d**) Four axial MR images, same as in Fig. 5

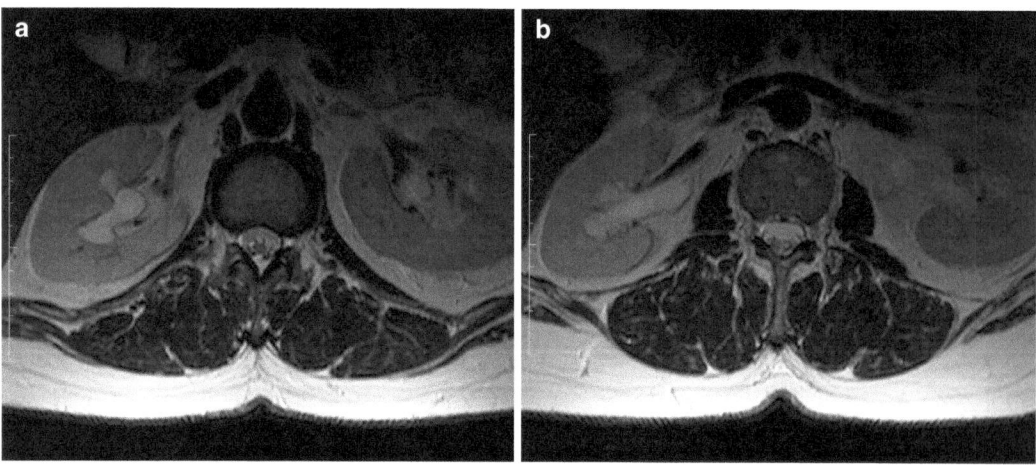

Fig. 11 (**a, b**), Two axial MR images, same as in Fig. 6

The retroperitoneal soft tissue mass (*M*) has intermediate T1 and T2 signal intensity, and it forms a collar around the aorta and proximal common iliac arteries. It is easy to appreciate the exact craniocaudal extent of the abnormality (thick arrows). MRI due to superior contrast resolution compared to CT makes it is easier to differentiate the extraneous soft tissue rind (thin arrows) from nearby vessels. A: aorta, I: inferior vena cava. The T2w images through the kidneys show mild hydronephrosis on the right, attributed to entrapment of the right ureter by the retroperitoneal abnormality. Bilateral hydronephrosis was shown in a subsequent abdominopelvic CT scan.

Final diagnosis: *retroperitoneal fibrosis*.

The patient was treated with corticosteroids with rapid resolution of his pain. He remains pain free at 2-year follow-up. The fibrotic tissue had decreased by about 50% at the 9-month follow-up CT scan, and has remained stable so far (his latest CT scan was performed 2 years after the establishment of the diagnosis).

Teaching Point

Keep in mind the importance of fat planes; please return to Chap. 3, Sect. 3.4. Think of complications, specifically think of hydronephrosis in this case. Please go to Chap. 7, Sect. 7.2.1.6. for further elaboration of the topic of complications.

Case 13

A 53-year-old male with a remote history of seminoma, S/P left orchiectomy, and left nephrectomy–ureterectomy. No other significant medical history. Prior imaging studies or prior imaging reports not available.

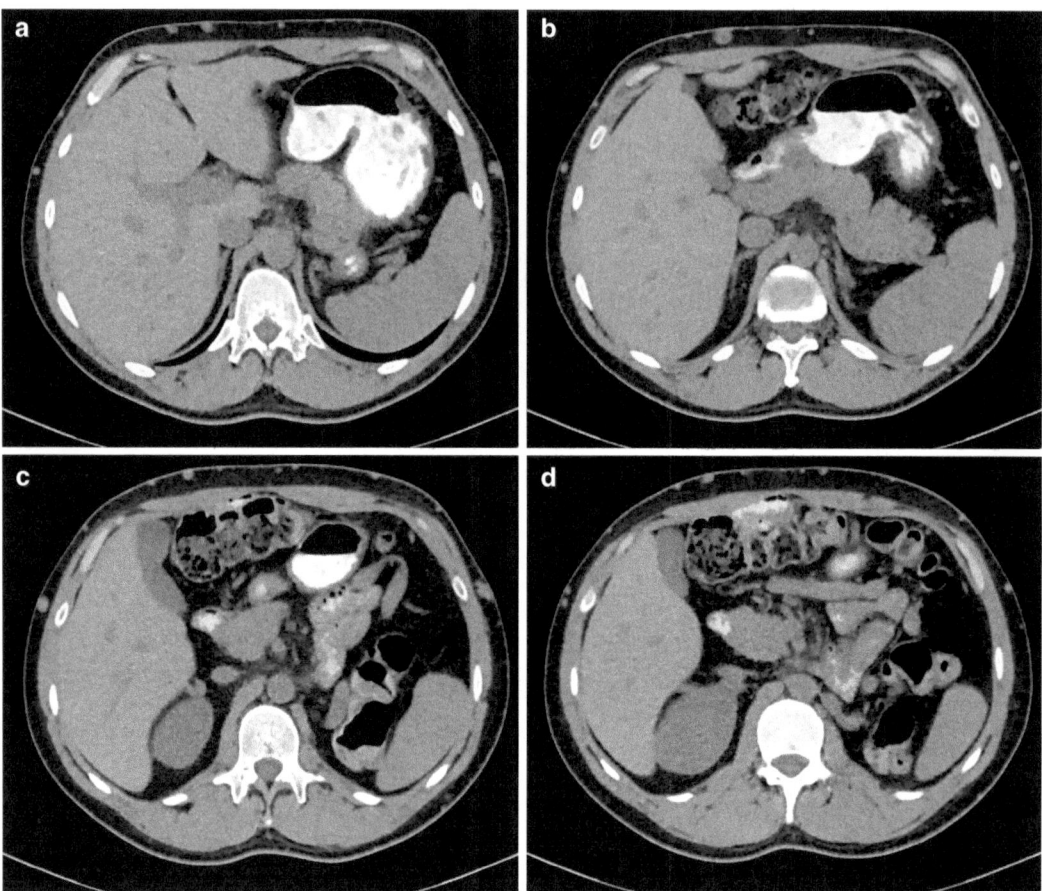

Fig. 1 (a–d) CT images through the upper abdomen, after oral contrast

Please record your findings and your thoughts before proceeding.

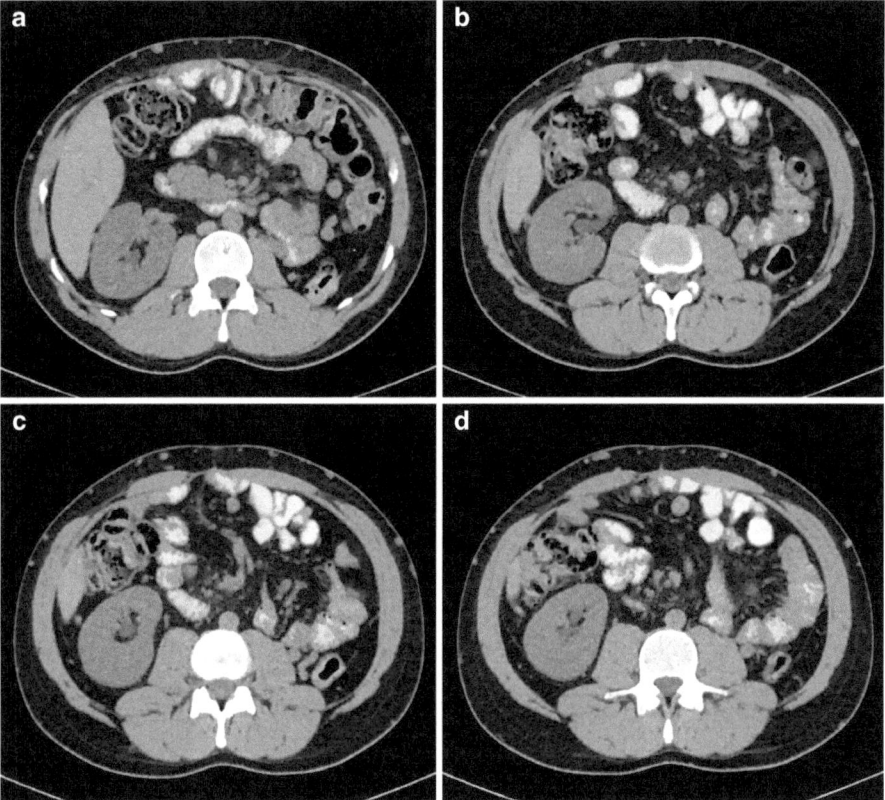

Fig. 2 (**a–d**) Additional CT slices through the abdomen, at more caudal levels.

What additional information can you extract?

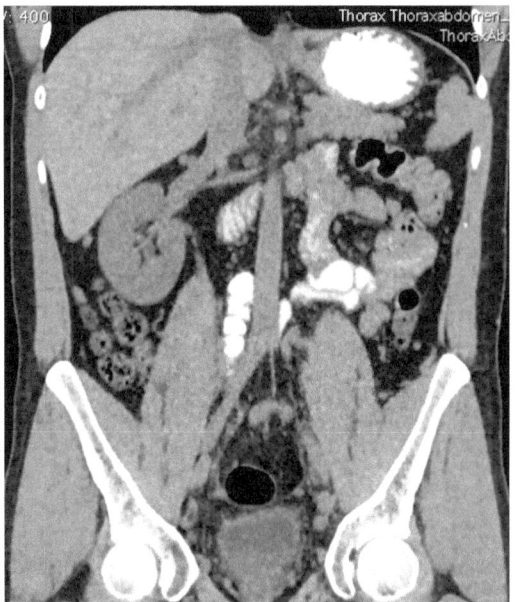

Does this image confirm your diagnosis?

Fig. 3 Coronal CT reconstruction

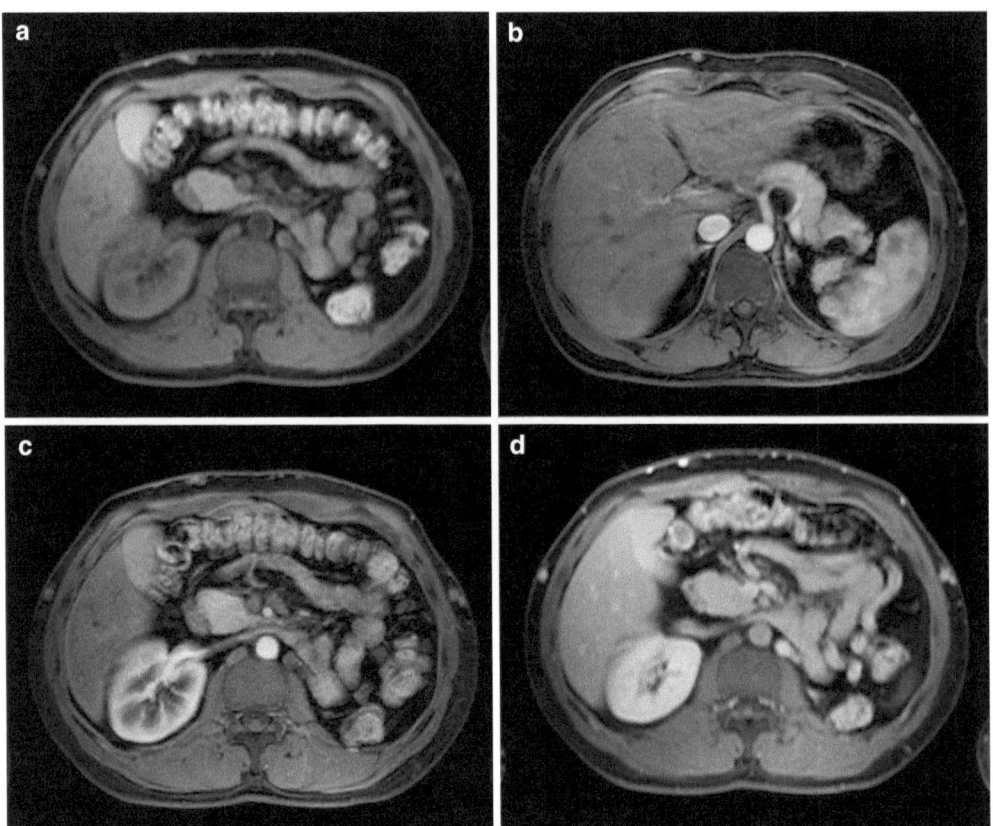

Fig. 4 (**a–d**) four axial MR images: (**a**) T1w TSE image with fat suppression through the right kidney; (**b**, **c**) arterial phase T1 VIBE images with fat suppression, at suprarenal and renal levels; (**d**) delayed phase post contrast, same slice as (**c**). [(**c**, **d**) of this figure are at the same transverse level as Fig. 2a]

Have you reached a diagnosis?

Discussion

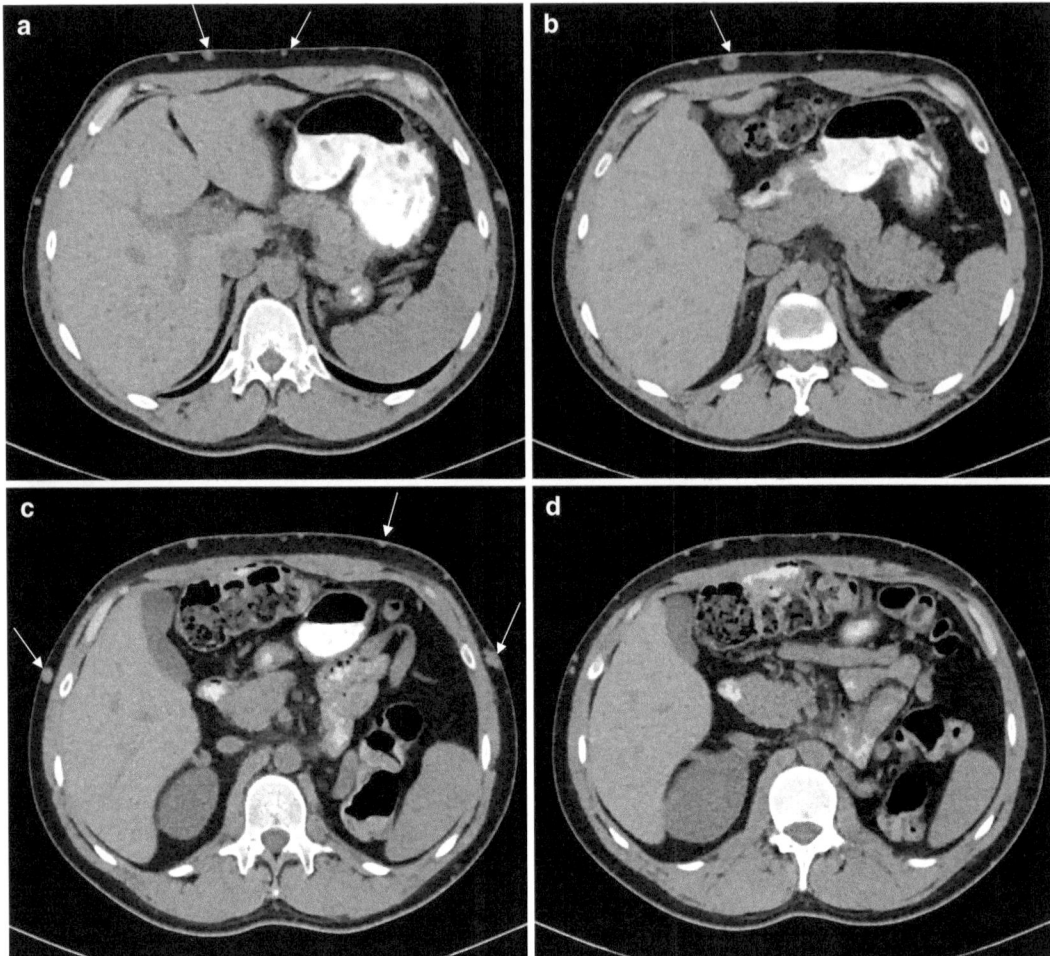

Fig. 5 (**a–d**) Same as Fig. 1. Please also visit Fig. 6 (next page) before reading the caption

This study shows postoperative changes and a congenital anomaly (variant): the left kidney has been removed and there is agenesis of the infrarenal segment of the vena cava.

The obvious findings are: non-visualization of the left kidney and compensatory hypertrophy of the right kidney. No stump of the left renal artery or left ureter was visualized. No lesions were detected in the left renal fossa, or in the course of the left ureter.

The partial agenesis of the vena cava can be difficult to detect. The hypertrophic crus of the right diaphragm (solid black arrow) mimics the aplastic part of the vena cava. At a more caudal level, below the diaphragmatic crura, we note that the space of the cava is occupied by fat and the duodenum (open arrow). Clues to this vascular variation are the numerous collaterals in the subcutaneous fat and within the abdominal cavity (white arrows).

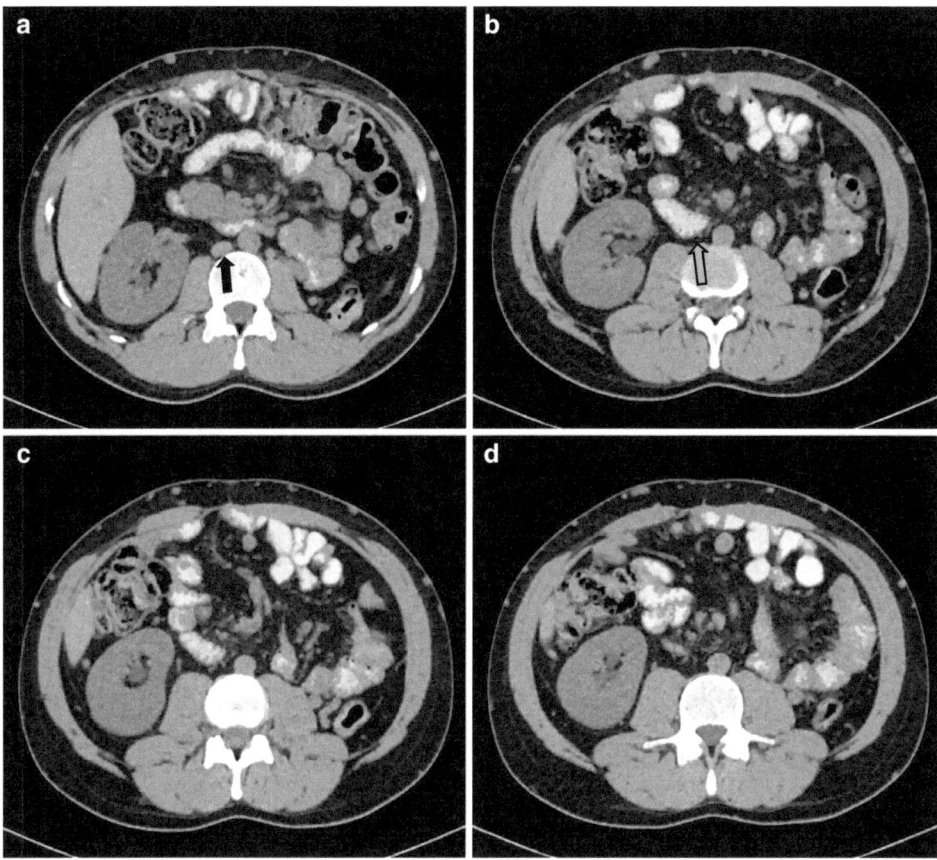

Fig. 6 (**a–d**) Same as Fig. 2

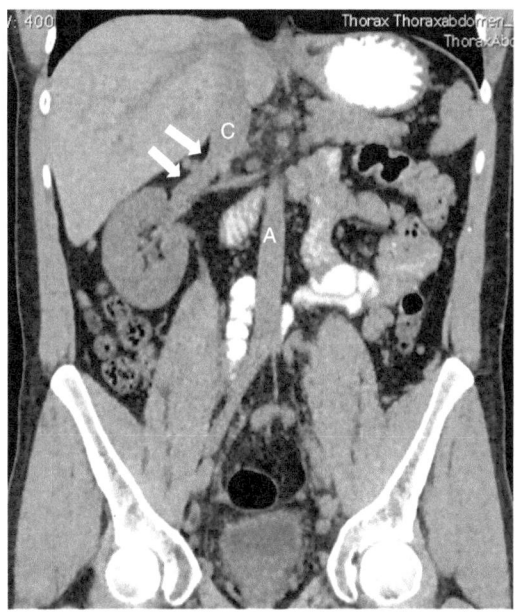

Non-visualization of infrarenal vena cava. Note the right renal vein (arrows) coursing to the formed segment of the inferior vena cava (C). The aorta is indicated by A.

Fig. 7 Same as Fig. 4

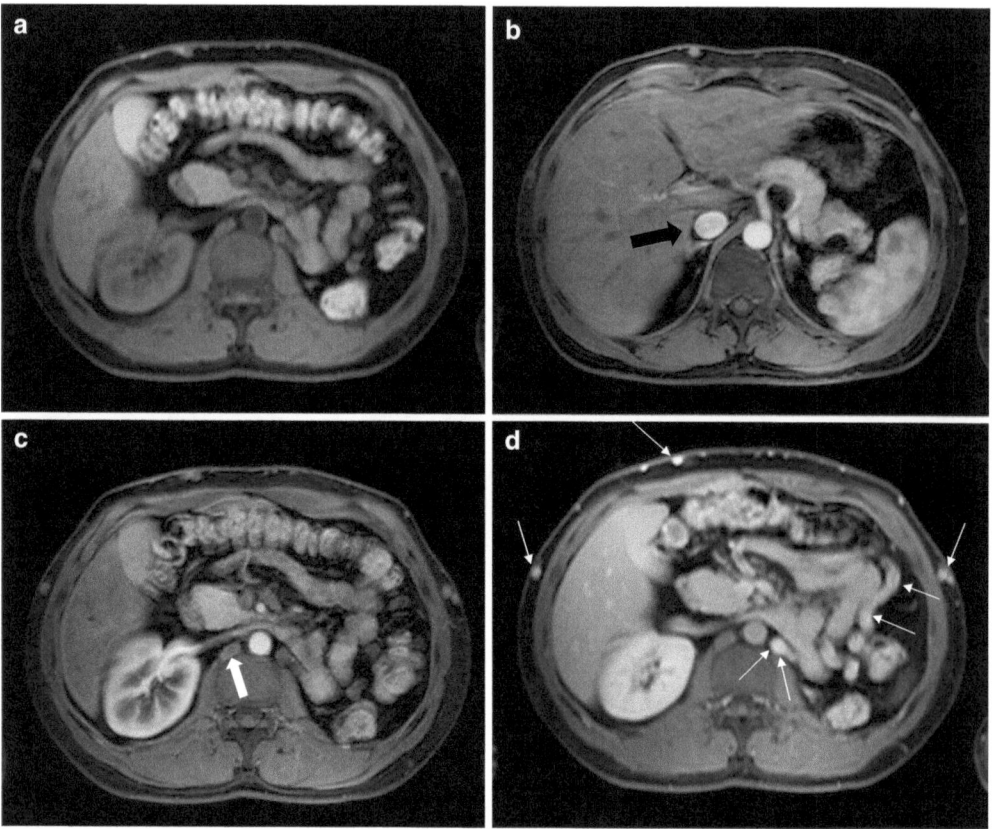

Fig. 8 (**a–d**) Same as Fig. 3

There is intense enhancement of the lumen of the suprarenal segment of the inferior vena cava (black arrow), and no obvious enhancement of the right diaphragmatic crus (thick white arrow). Note also the multiple venous collaterals in the abdominal cavity and the subcutaneous fat (thin white arrows)

Now we have to go a step further and ask: what spectrum of pathologies is associated with this congenital abnormality, specifically caval aplasia [69, 70]?

Teaching Points

Ensure the presence of all normal structures.

Do not stop at the findings, go a step further and search for the underlying cause.

In the appropriate setting, think of associated syndromes or congenital malformations. To revisit these conditions, please go to Chap. 7, Sect. 7.2.1.4.

Case 14

A 70-year-old male s/p total right nephrectomy for stage I renal clear cell carcinoma. He did not receive chemotherapy or radiation therapy.

A follow-up CT scan was obtained 6 months after the nephrectomy. The patient was asymptomatic.

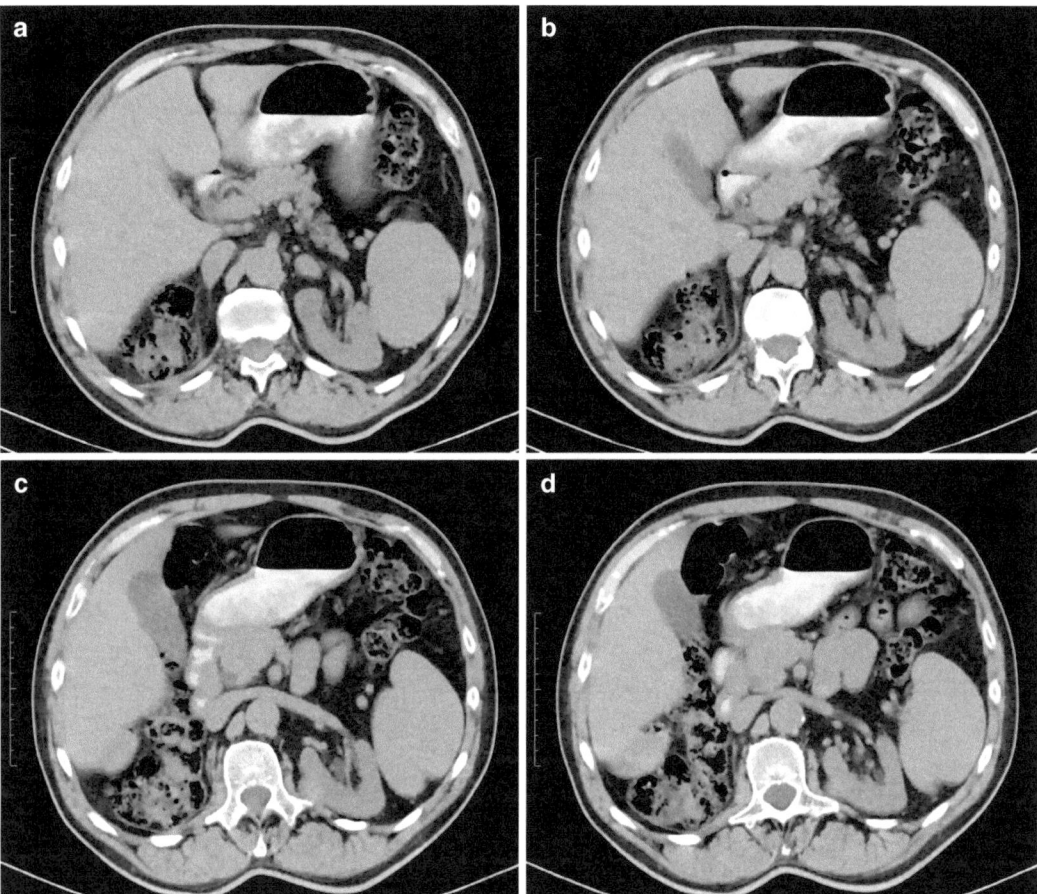

Fig. 1 (**a–d**) CT slices through the upper abdomen. Contrast material was not administered because of renal impairment

Please record your findings and your thoughts before proceeding.

Discussion

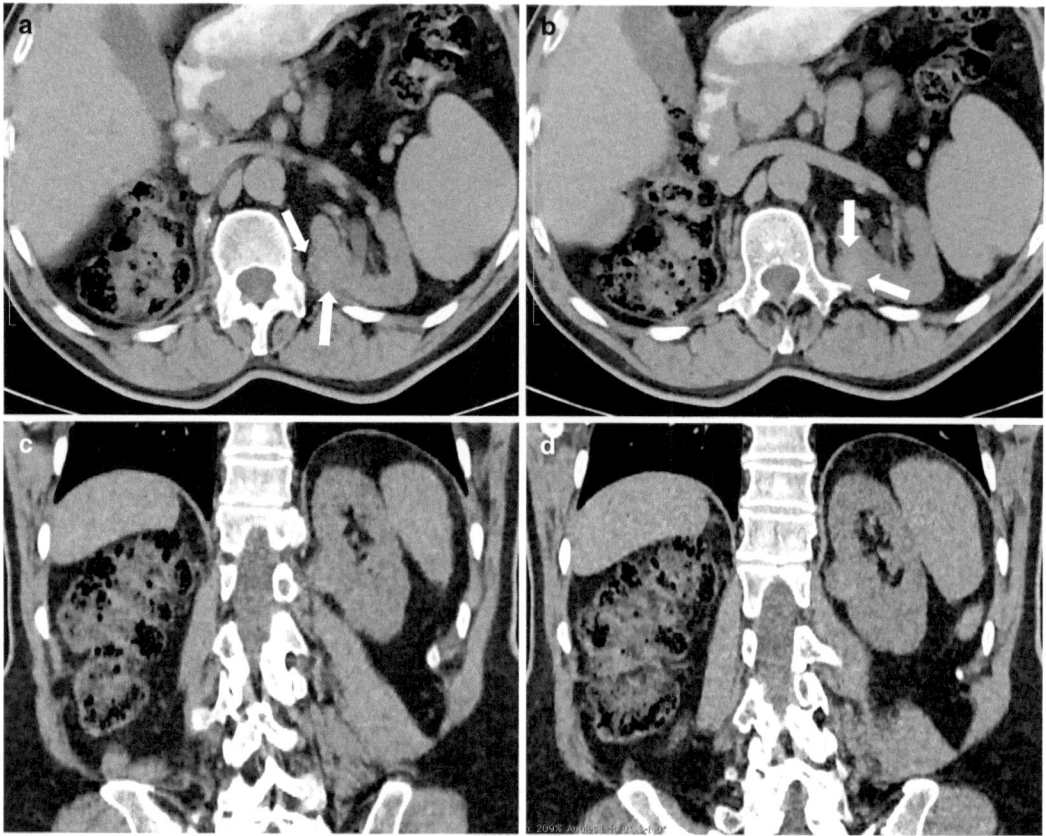

Fig. 2 (**a**, **b**) Two axial CT slices [same as Fig. 1b, c], and (**c**, **d**) two coronal CT reconstructions

There are no signs of local recurrence in the surgical bed. There is focal lobulation and apparent thickening of cortex of the medial aspect of the left kidney (arrows). These findings are due to an iso- to borderline hyper-dense nodule that projects partly beyond the confines of the kidney. The coronal reconstructions confirm the presence of an exophytic nodule of the left kidney. This mass was resected and microscopically was composed of clear cells. It was considered to represent a metastatic focus from the original malignancy in the right kidney. An additional metastasis was found in the left adrenal gland (not shown).

Teaching Point

Contour and density deviations may be the only clue to significant abnormalities; please go to Chap. 3, Sect. 3.4 for further elaboration.

Case 15

A 48-year-old male with transitional cell carcinoma of the urinary bladder, complaining of new onset headaches. The initial imaging evaluation consisted of a head CT scan.

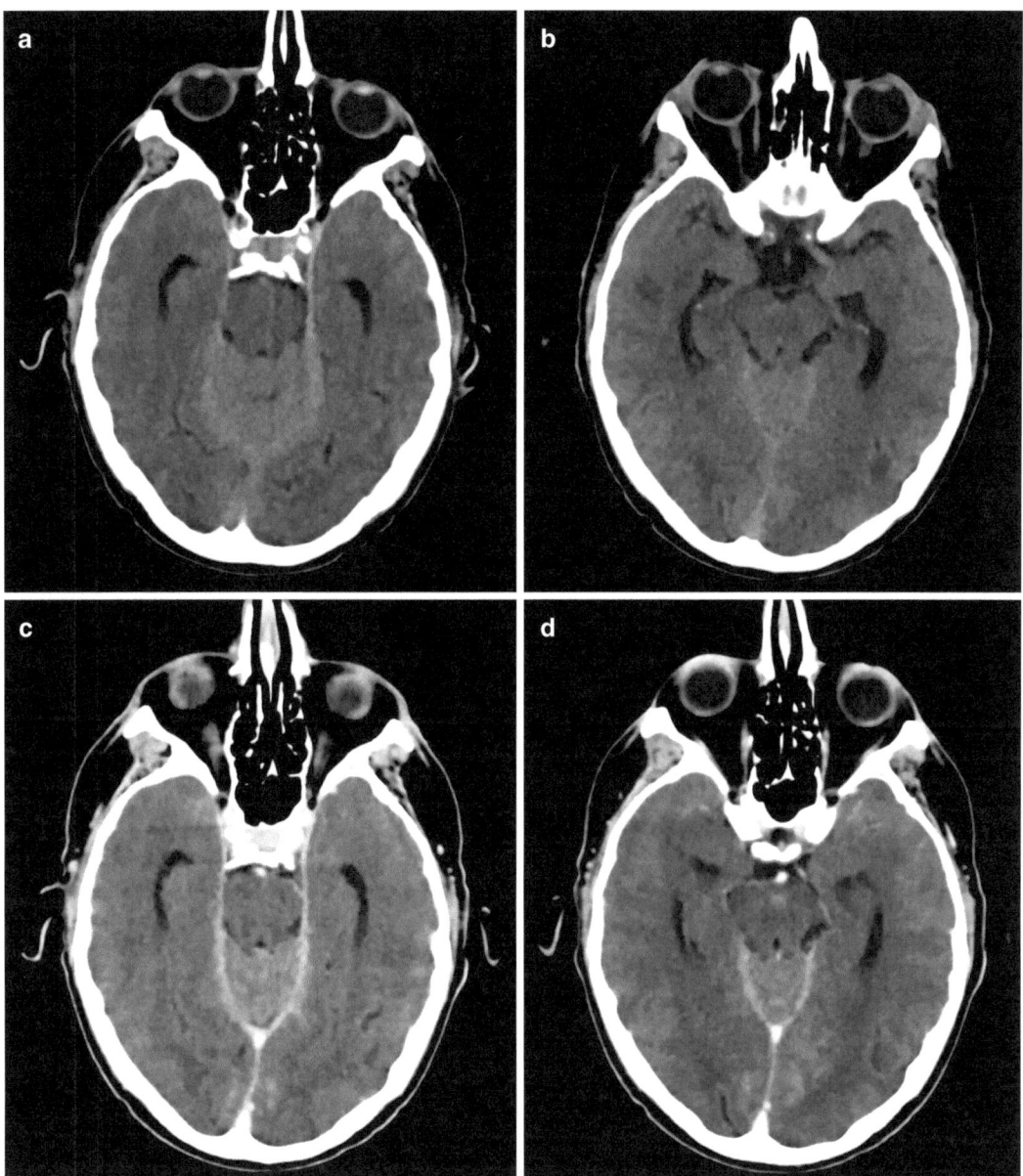

Fig. 1 (**a–d**) Pairs of CT images before (**a, b**) and after (**c, d**) i.v. contrast administration

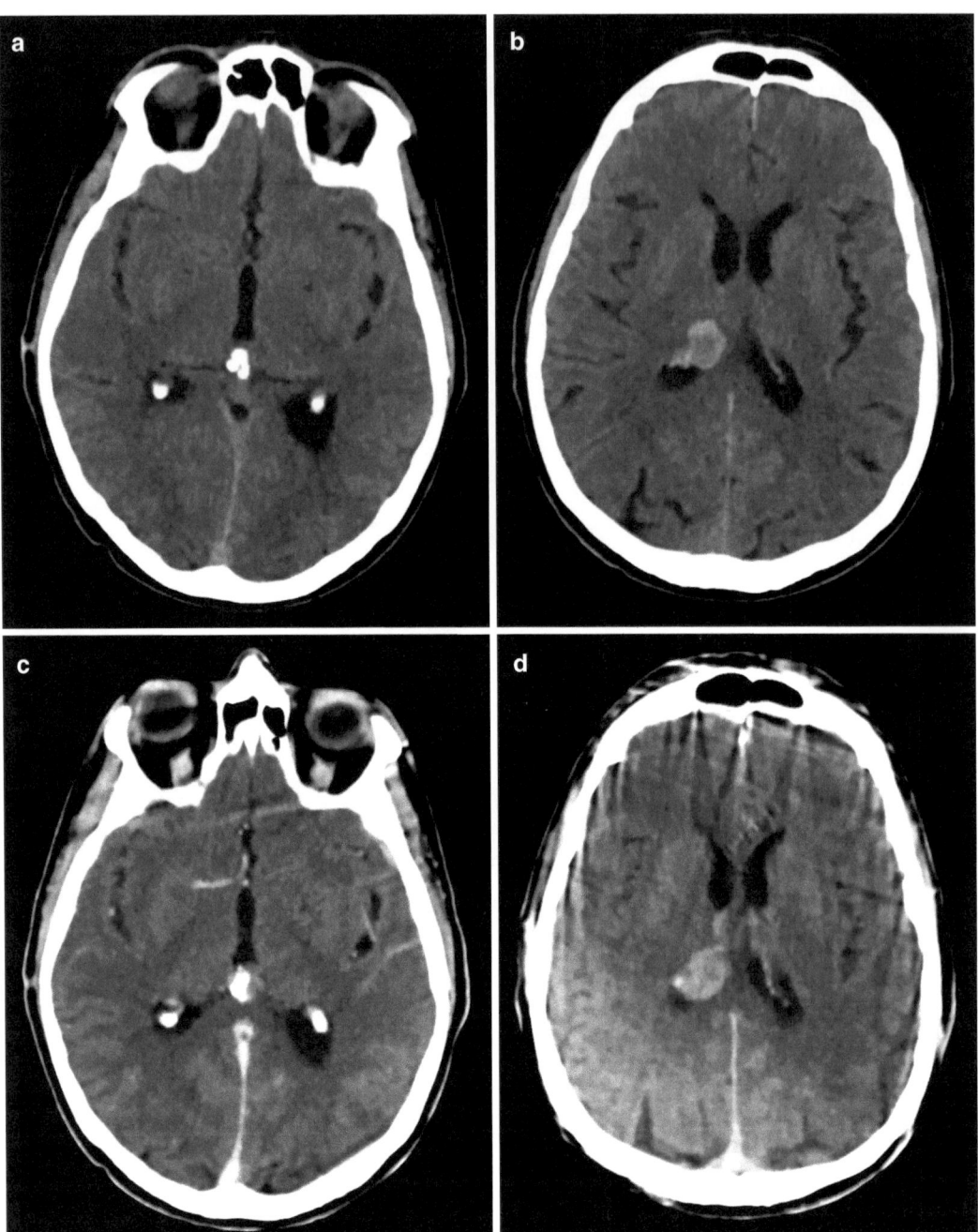

Fig. 2 (**a–d**) Pairs of CT images before (**a**, **b**) and after (**c**, **d**) i.v. contrast administration. Image 2(d) is distorted by artifact

Please record your observations and thoughts on paper before proceeding. Further evaluation was recommended with MRI.

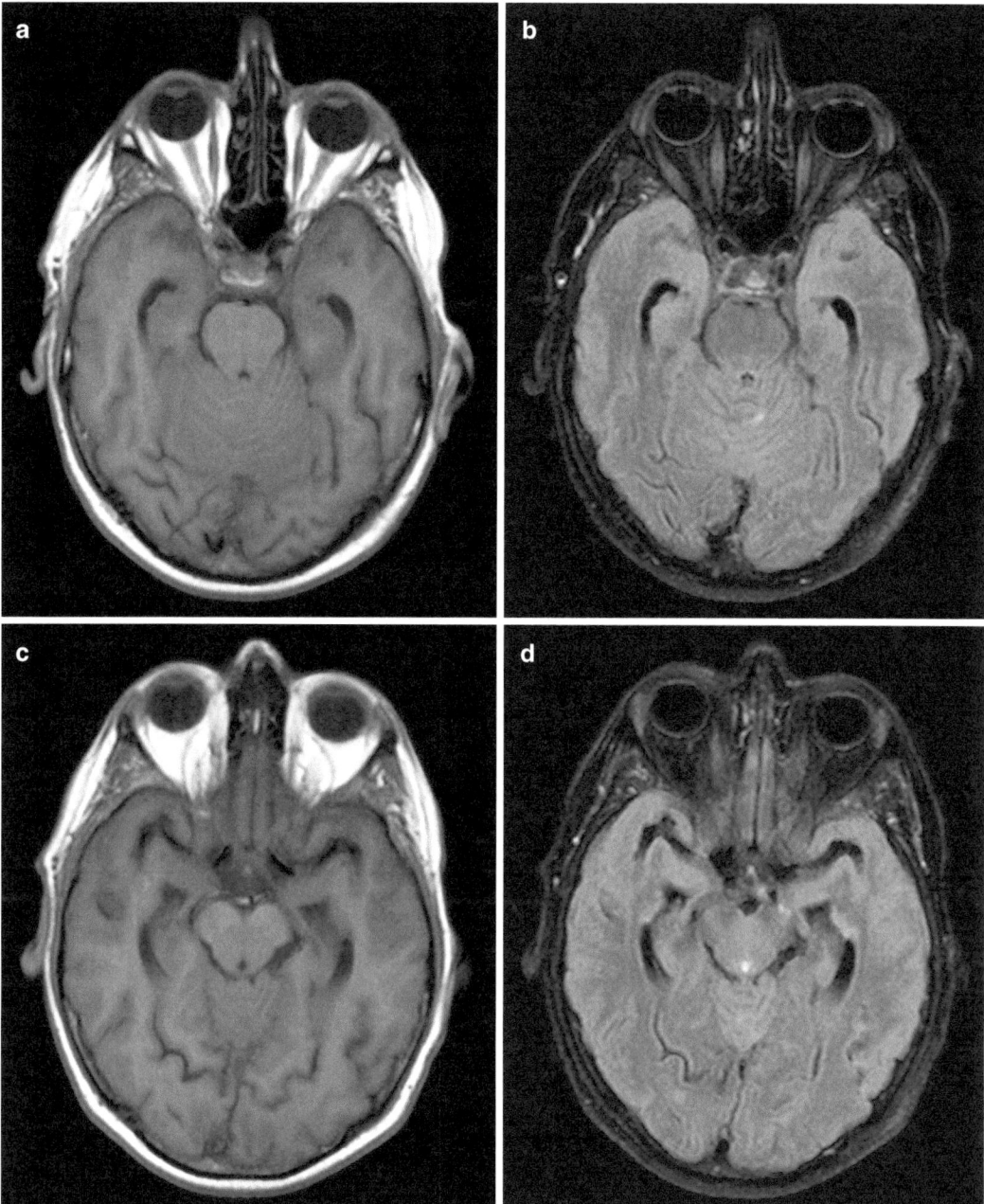

Fig. 3 (**a–d**) Pairs of axial T1 (**a**, **c**) and FLAIR images (**b**, **d**) corresponding to the CT images shown in Fig. 1

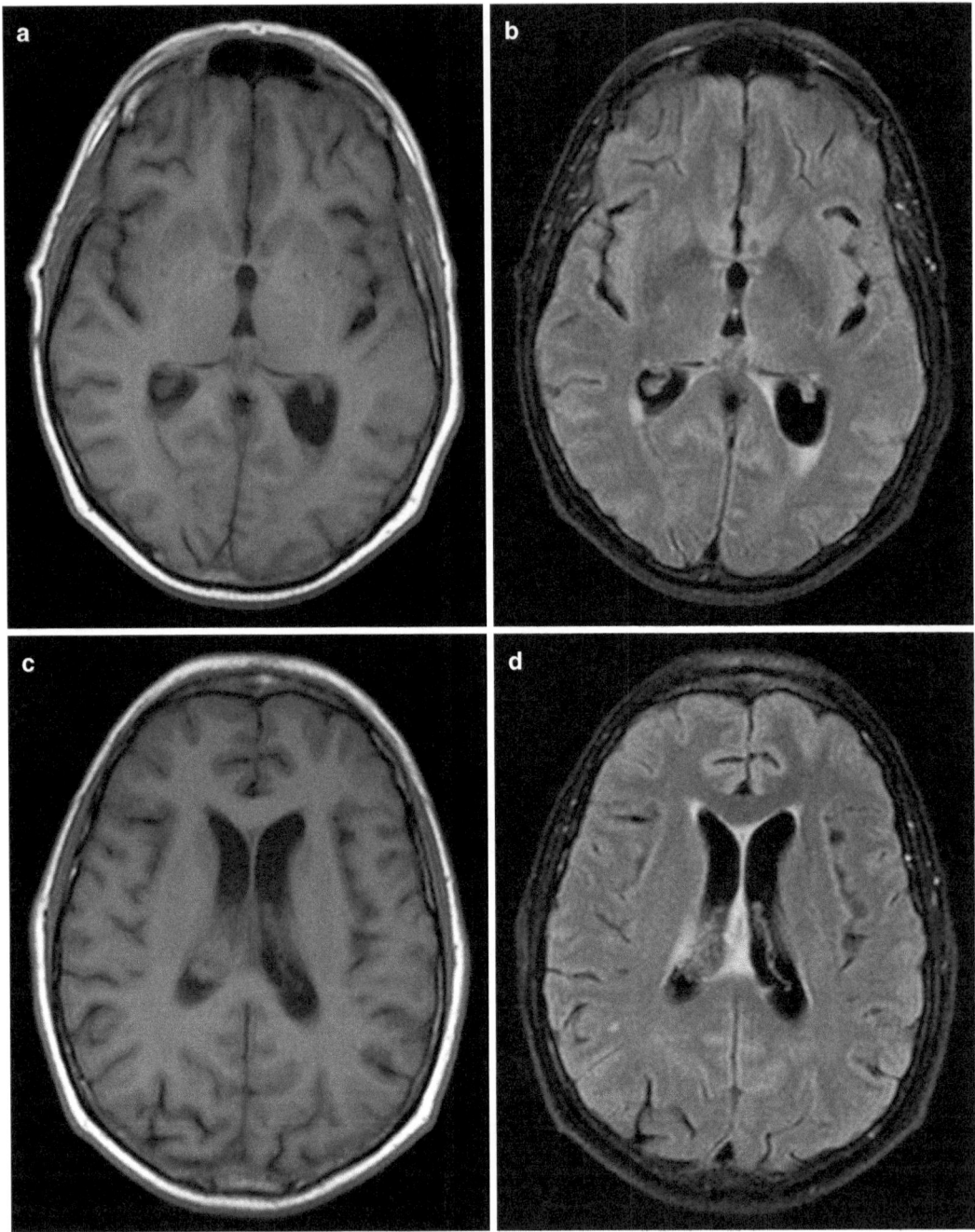

Fig. 4 (**a–d**) Pairs of axial T1 (**a, c**) and FLAIR images (**b, d**) corresponding to the CT images shown in Fig. 2

Please write your observations and thoughts on paper before proceeding to the following set of images.

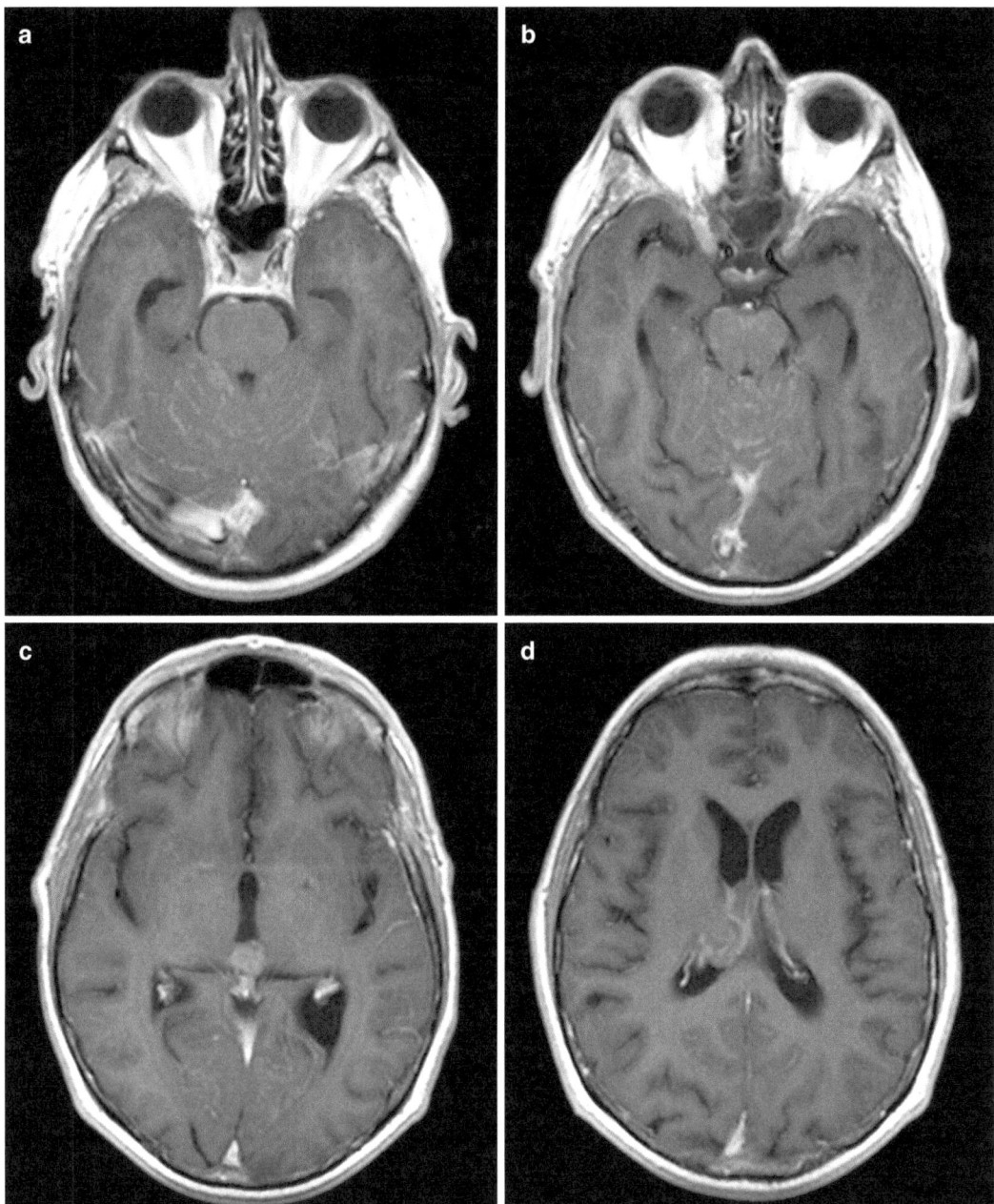

Fig. 5 (**a–d**) The axial T1w images from Figs. 2 and 3 after i.v. gadolinium

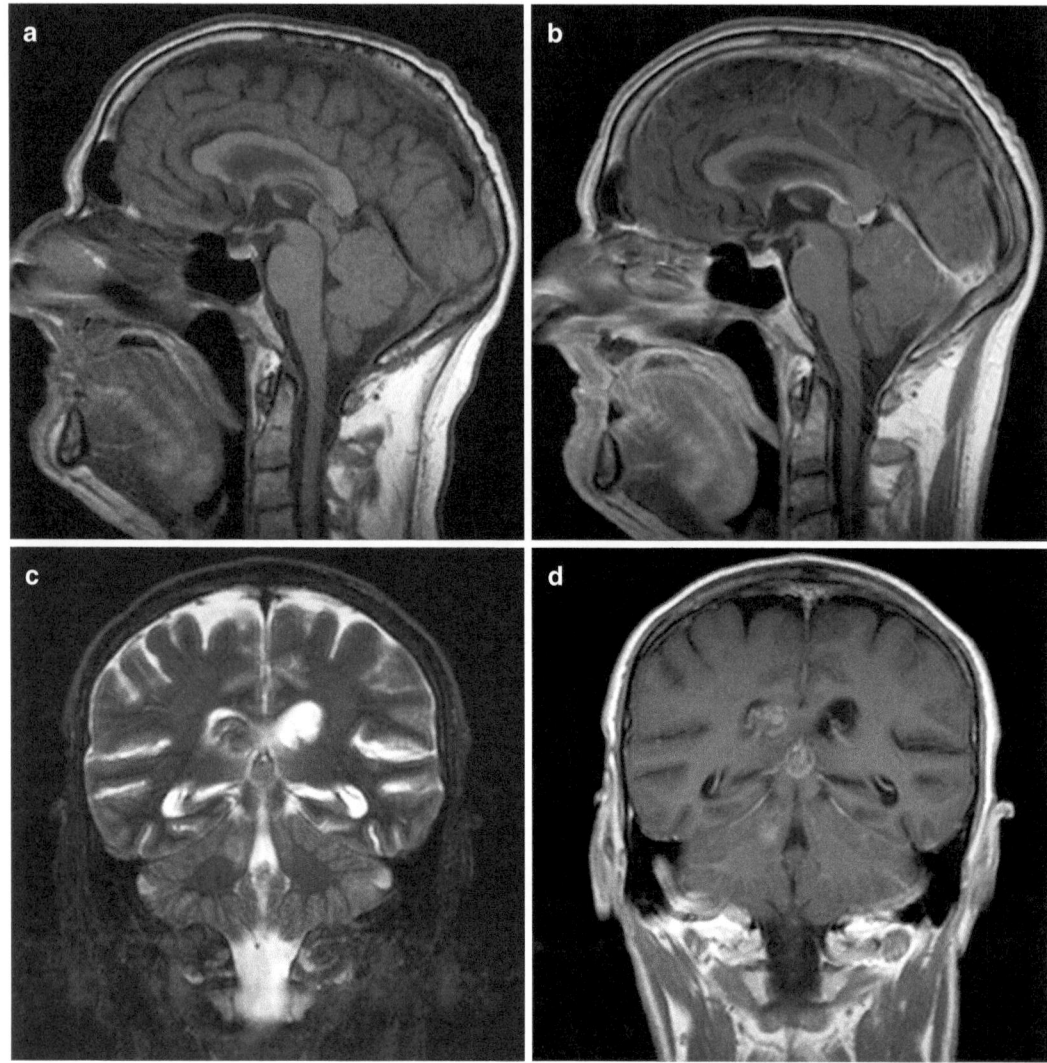

Fig. 6 (**a–d**) Midsagittal T1w pre (**a**), and post (**b**) contrast, coronal STIR (**c**) and coronal T1w post contrast (**d**) images

Please complete and finalize your report before we proceed to the discussion of this case.

Discussion

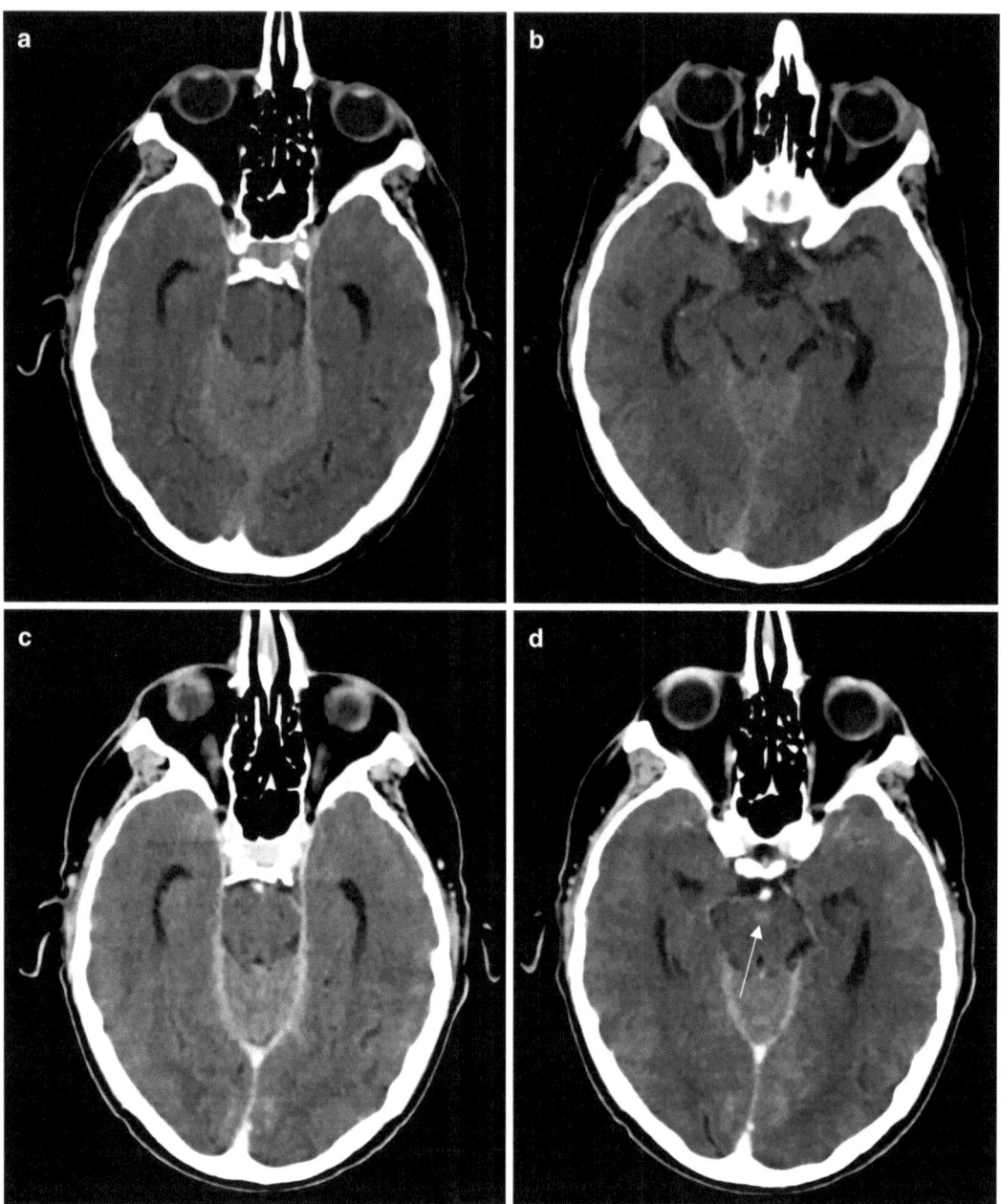

Fig. 7 Same as Figs. 1 and 2

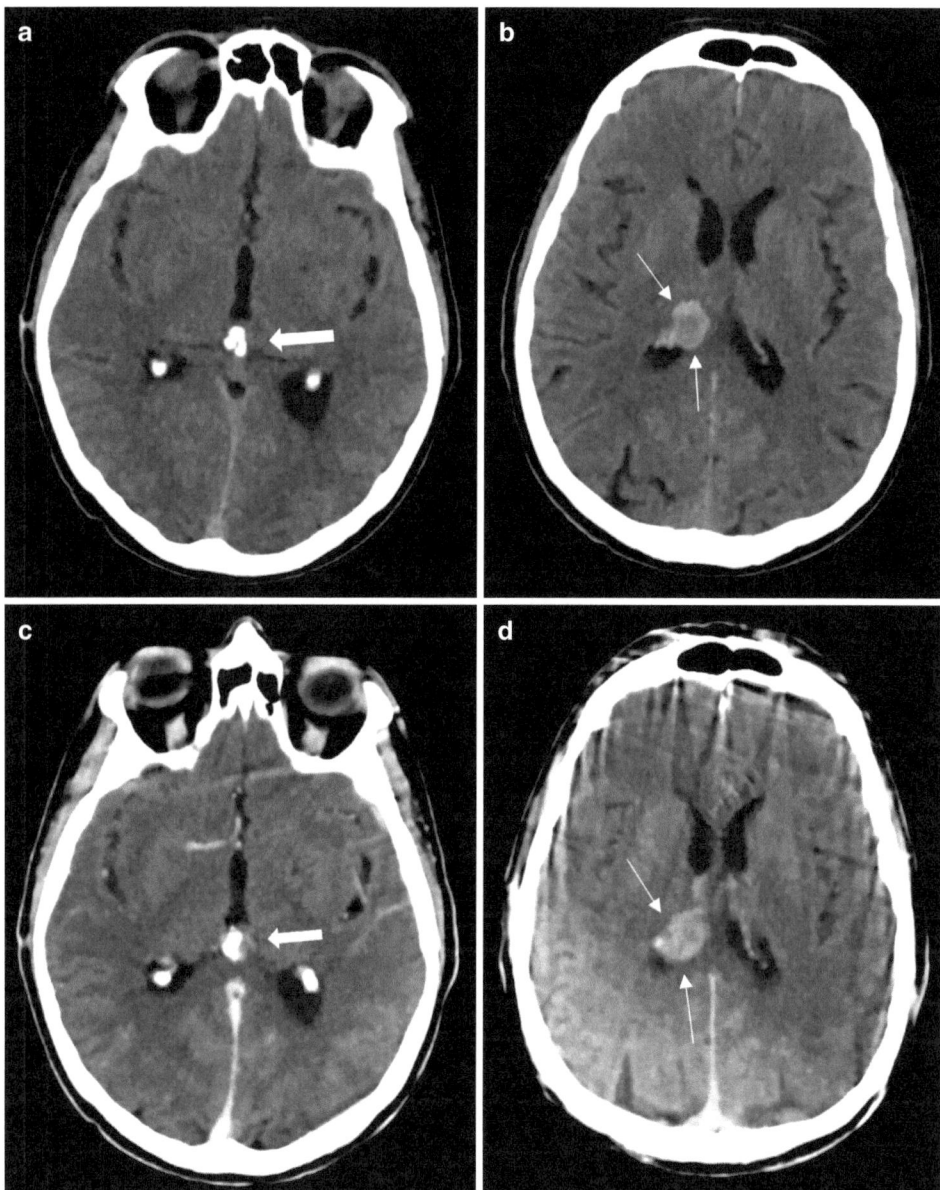

Fig. 8 Same as Figs. 1 and 2

There is mild dilatation of the temporal horns and rounding of the frontal horns, suggesting hydro-cephalus. Note the disproportionate enlargement of the lateral ventricular bodies relative to the sulci and the Sylvian fissures. Partial obscuration of the quadrigeminal plate cistern is a subtle finding. There is also a suggestion of abnormal leptomeningeal enhancement in the interpeduncular cistern (thin arrow in 7d). A soft tissue nodule partially engulfs the calcified pineal gland and protrudes in the 3rd ventricle (thick arrows in Fig. 8). An inhomogeneous, hyperdense mass is centered on the choroid plexus of the right lateral ventricle (thin arrows in Fig. 8) and displays minimal contrast enhancement.

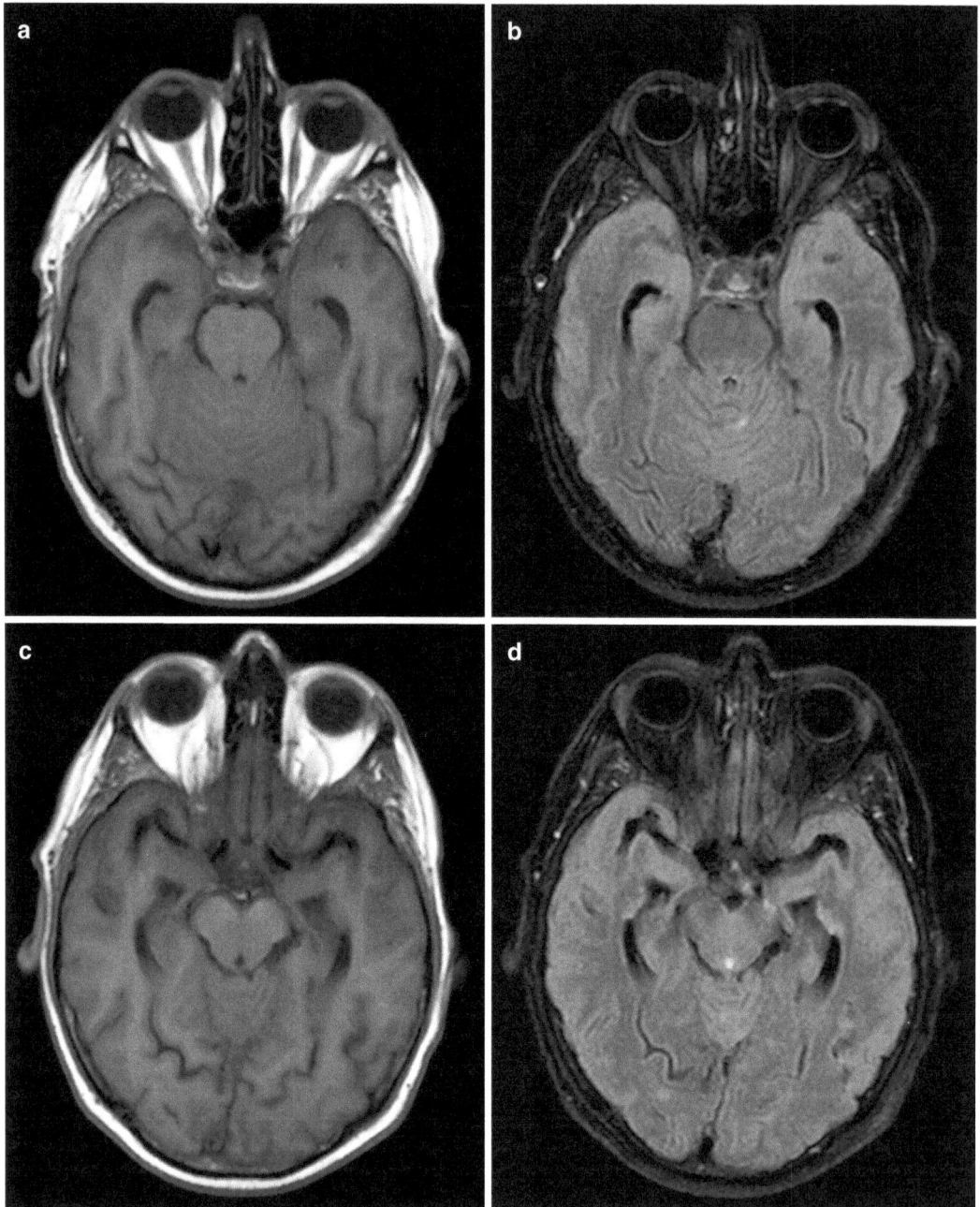

Fig. 9 Same as Fig. 3 (**a–d**) Pairs of T1w and FLAIR images in the infra- and supra-tentorial compartments, without contrast enhancement

Note dilatation of the temporal horns.

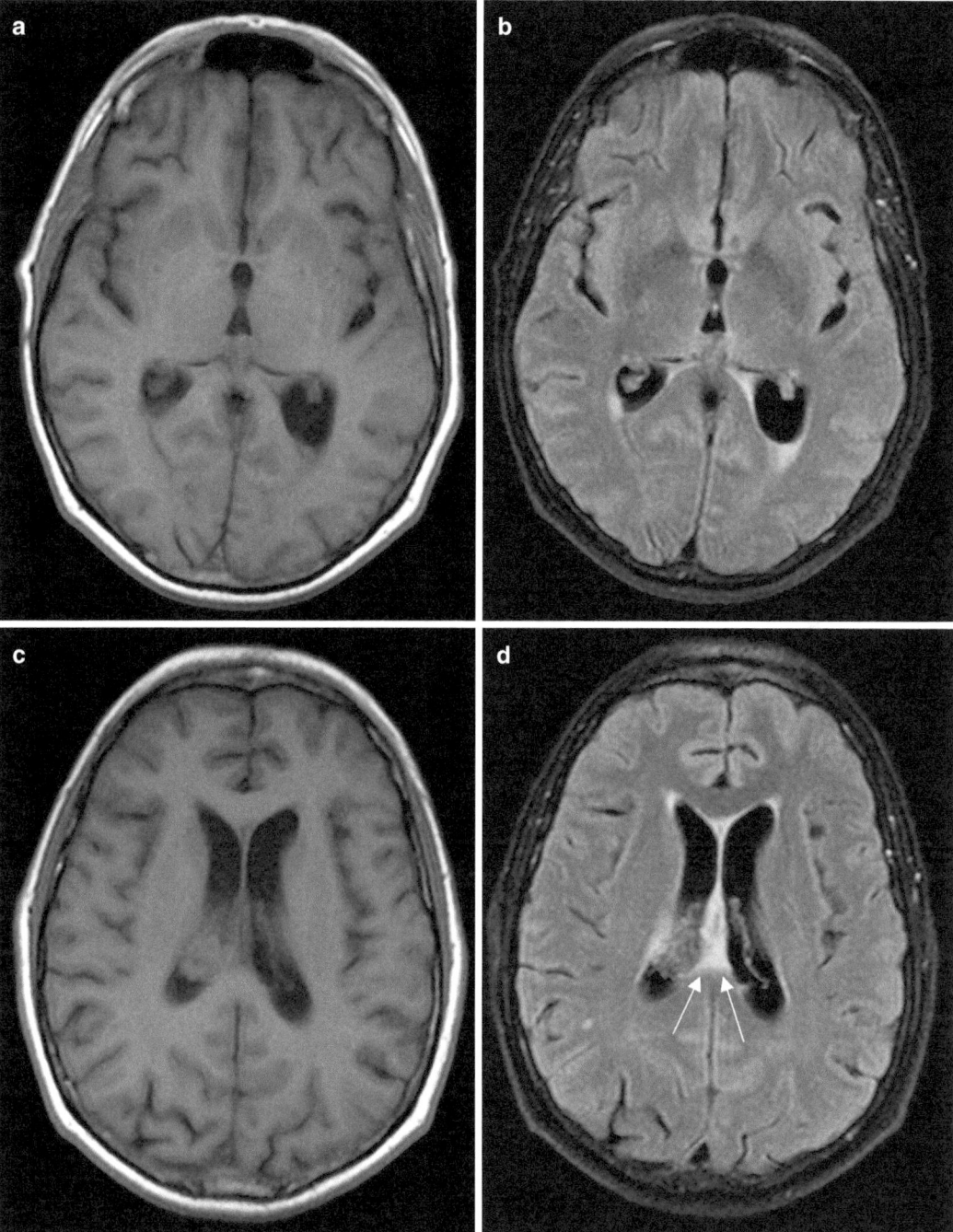

Fig. 10 Same as Fig. 4 (**a–d**) Pairs of T1w and FLAIR images in the infra- and supra-tentorial compartments, without contrast enhancement

Note periventricular edema around the dilated temporal horns. Edema also tracks along the fornix and the callosal-septal interface (arrows).

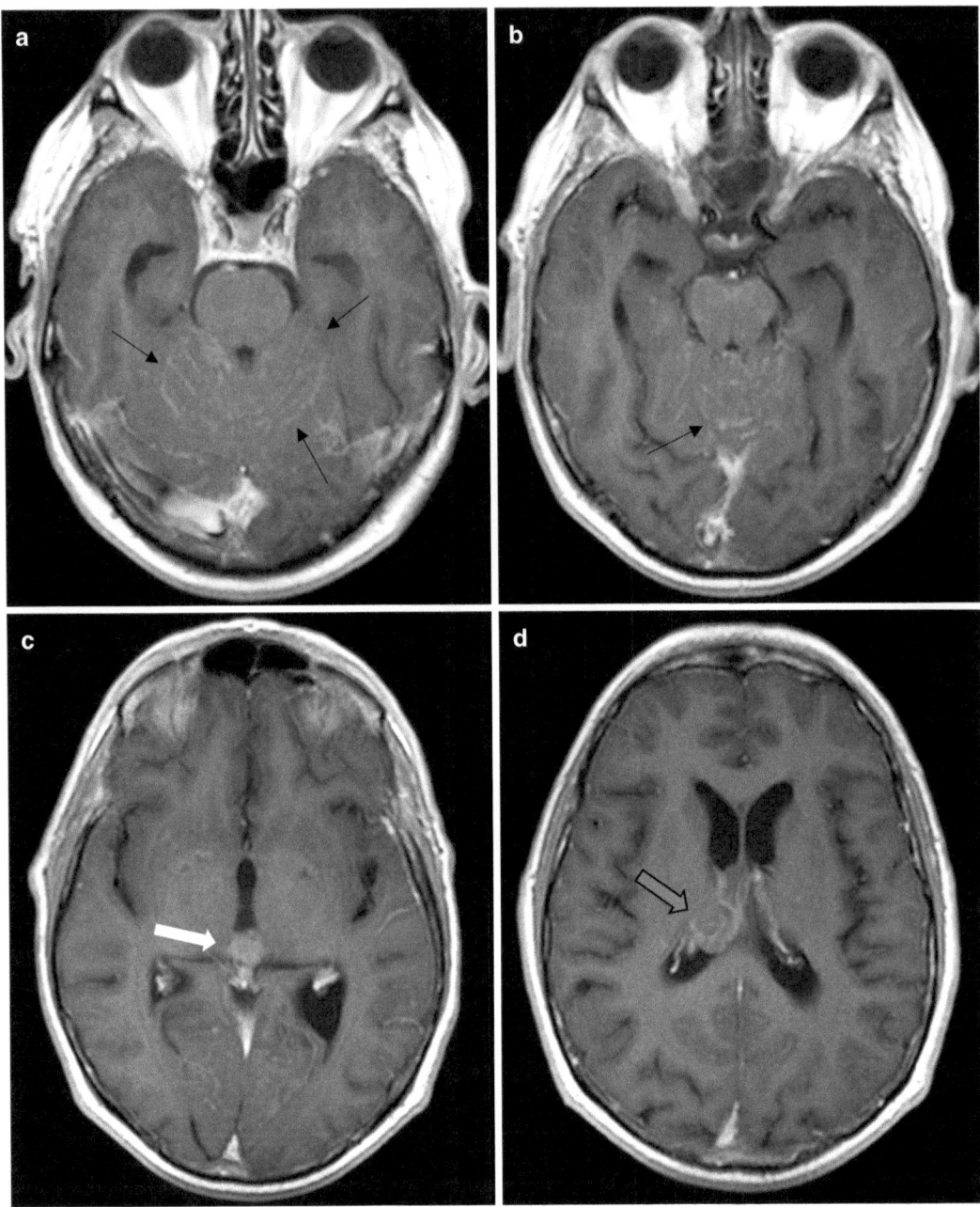

Fig. 11 Same as Fig. 5

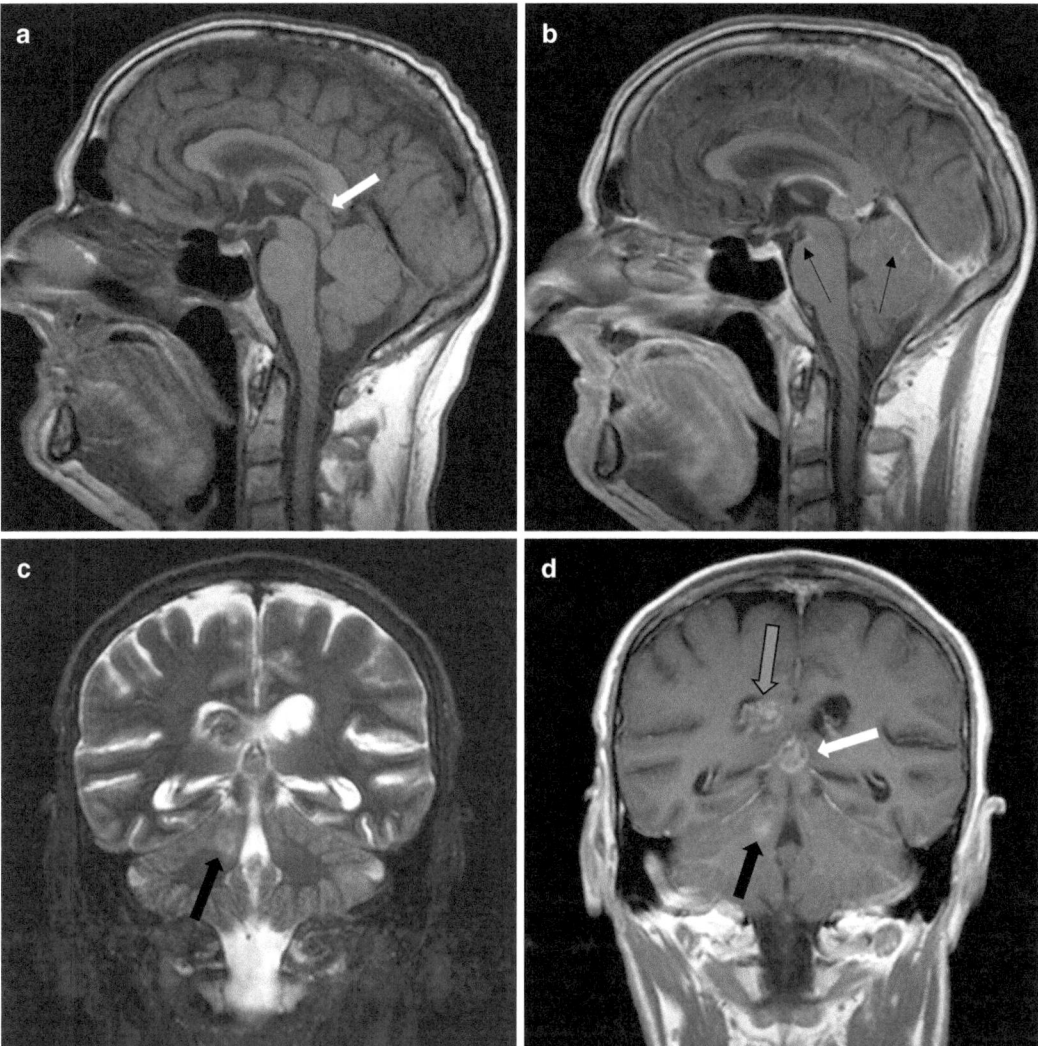

Fig. 12 Same as Fig. 6

Note subtle leptomeningeal seeding of the cerebellar folia and ventral pons (thin black arrows). The pineal metastasis (thick white arrow) is more obvious compared to the CT. There is inhomogeneous enhancement of the plexal metastases (open arrows). The coronal images show an additional metastasis in the right cerebellar hemisphere (solid thick black arrows).

Teaching Point

Midline or bilateral symmetric lesions may escape detection.

Case 16

A 75-year-old female with chronic low back pain. Past medical history was noncontributory. The lumbar spine was evaluated with CT.

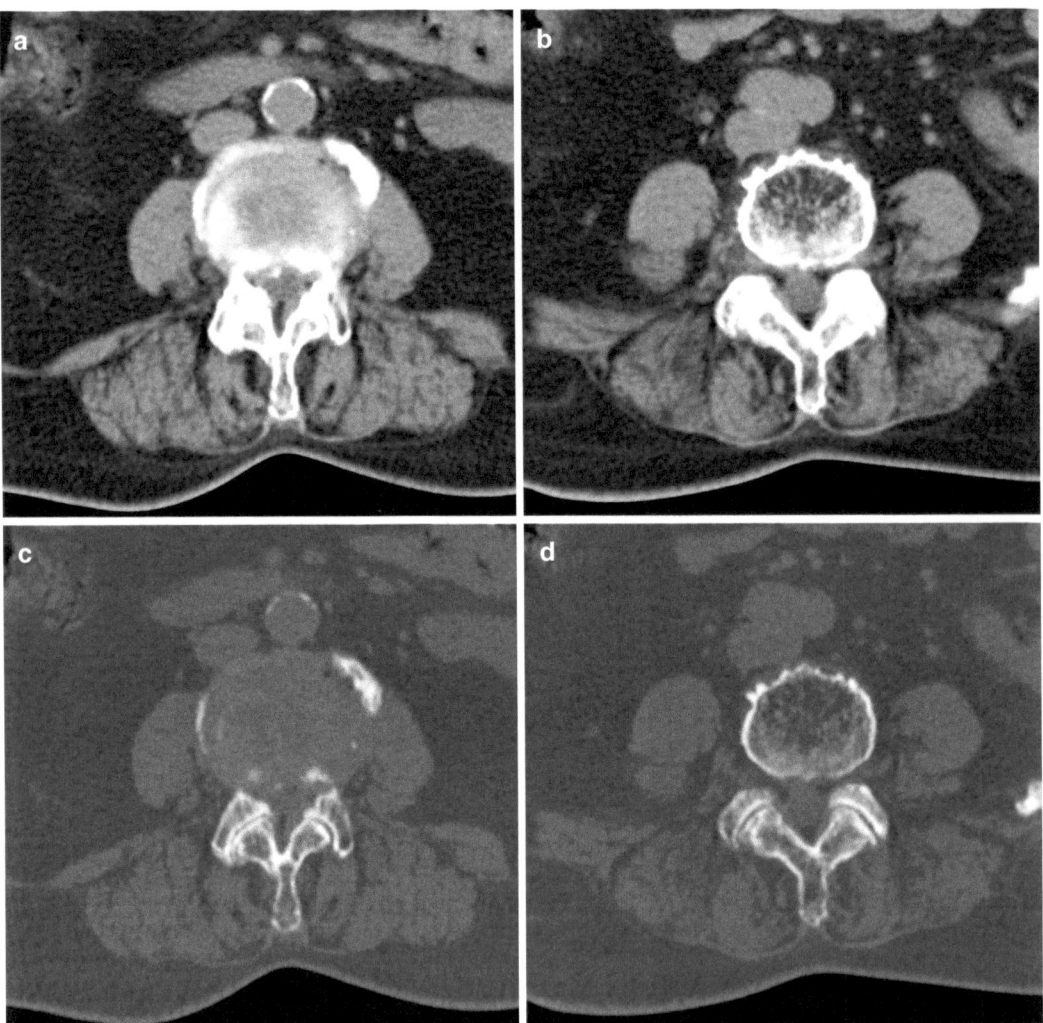

Fig. 1 (**a–d**) Pairs of CT images in soft tissue (**a**, **b**) and bone (**c**, **d**) windows

Please commit your observations and thoughts on paper before proceeding.

Discussion

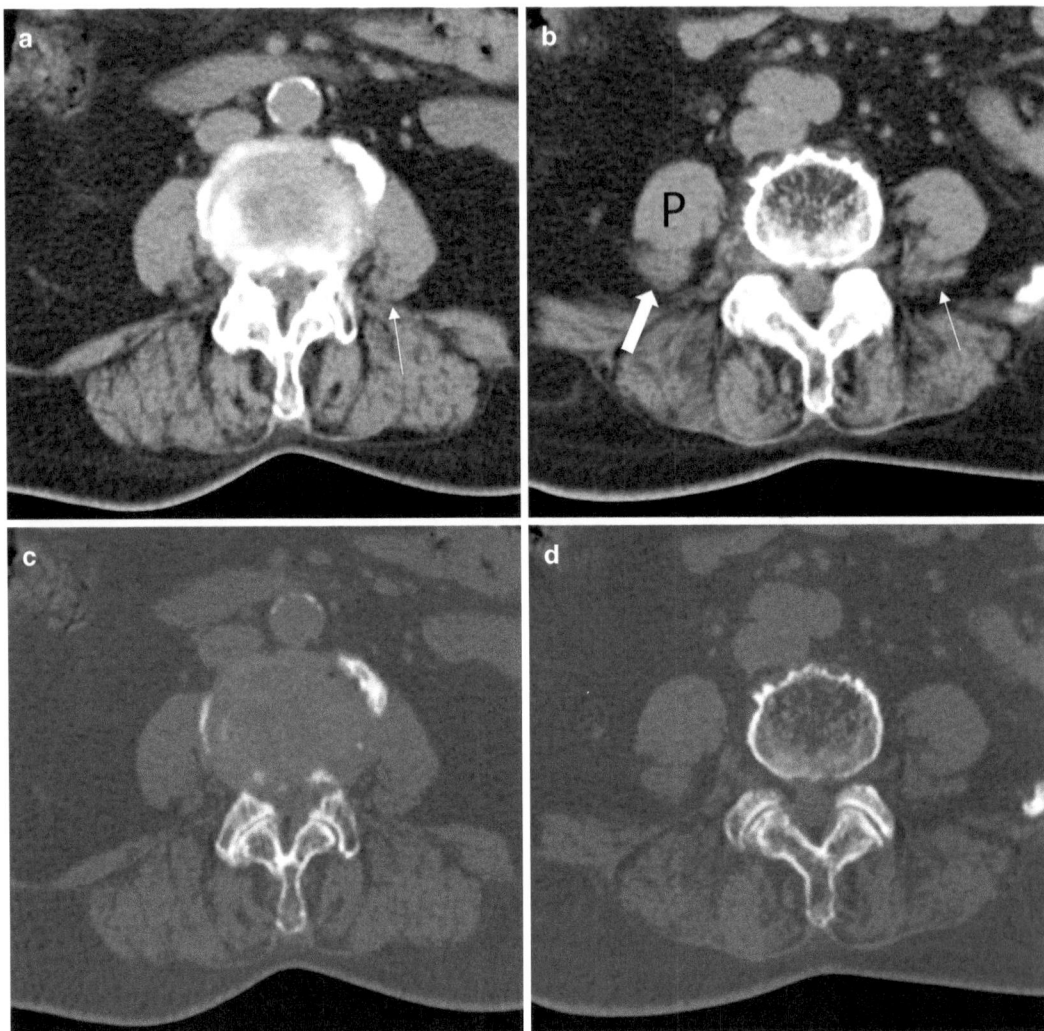

Fig. 2 Same as Fig. 1 (**a–d**) Pairs of CT images in soft tissue and bone windows

There is apparent asymmetry in the size of the psoas muscles, the right (P) being "larger" than the left. This finding is due to a slightly hypodense mass (thick arrow) in the fat compartment dorsal to the right psoas muscle. We may be tempted to call a second, isodense mass is the same location on the left side (thin arrow). This pseudomass represents accessory slips of the left psoas muscle. Confirmation of both the mass and the pseudomass is provided in Fig. 4 of Case 10, since this patient is the same as in Case 10.

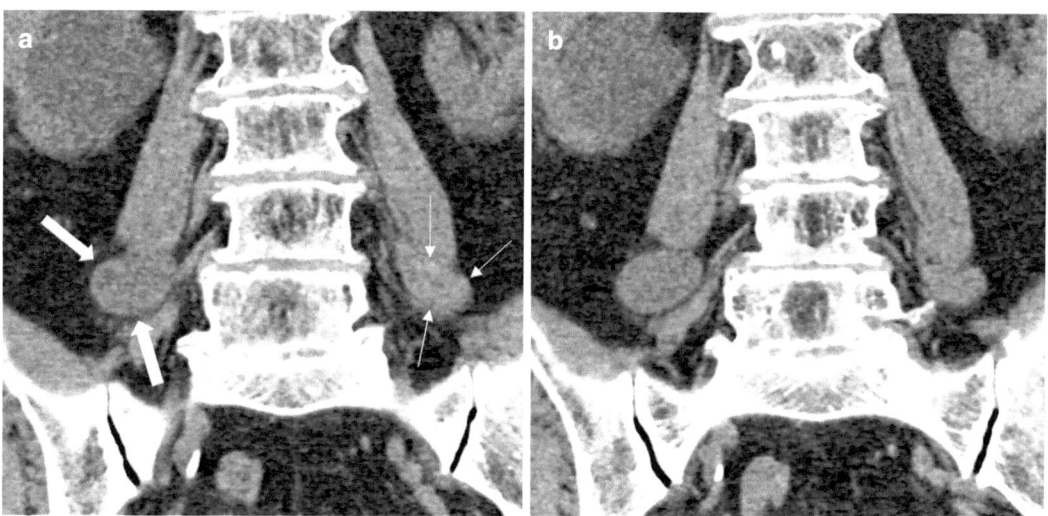

Fig. 3 (**a, b**) Two coronal CT reconstructions in soft tissue window. The schwannoma is indicated with the thick arrows and the pseudomass is indicated with the thin arrows. Note slight difference in CT density between the two

Teaching Point

Obliteration of fat planes and right-left asymmetry may be the only clues of disease.

Case 17

A 69-year-old female with 3 month history of pre- and postprandial vomiting. Associated weight loss was attributed to diminished food intake. A CT scan was requested.

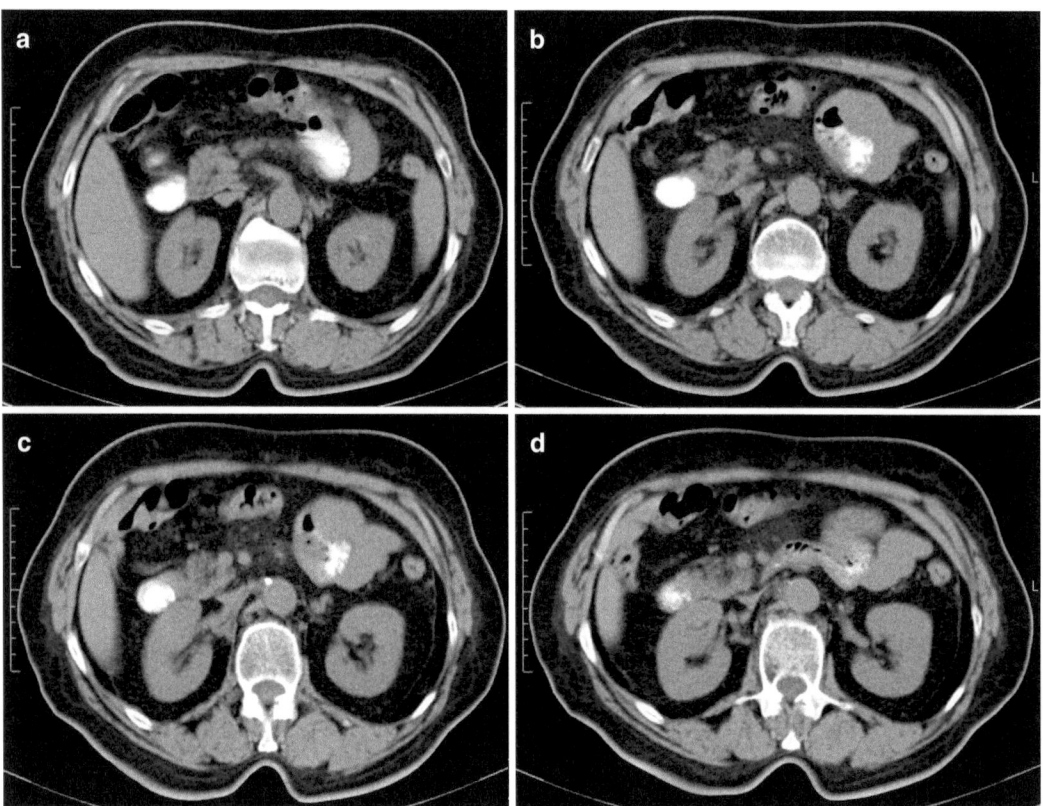

Fig. 1 (**a–d**) Four consecutive CT images after oral, before i.v. contrast

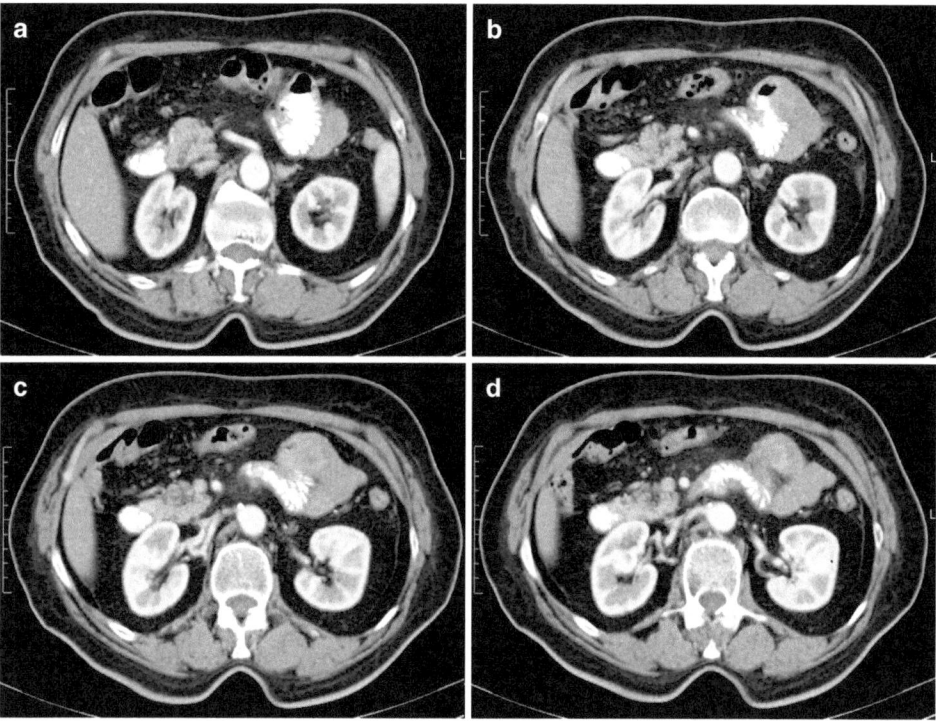

Fig. 2 (**a–d**) Same images as in Fig. 1 after i.v. contrast, arterial phase

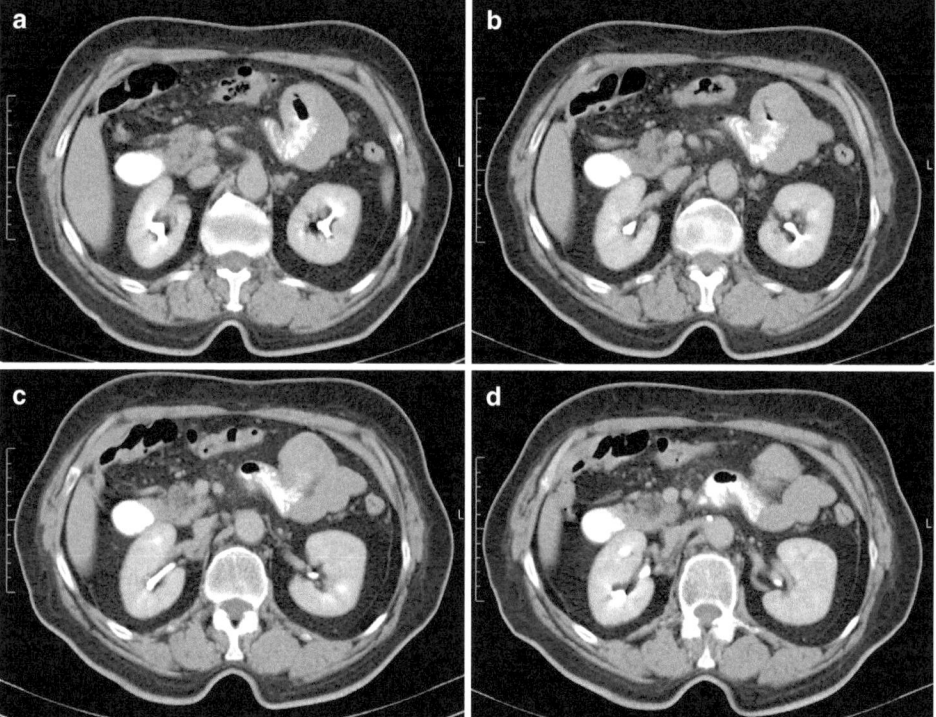

Fig. 3 (**a–d**) Same images as in Fig. 1 after i.v. contrast, equilibrium phase

Please write your observations and thoughts before turning the page.

Please study now the following 4 reconstructions.

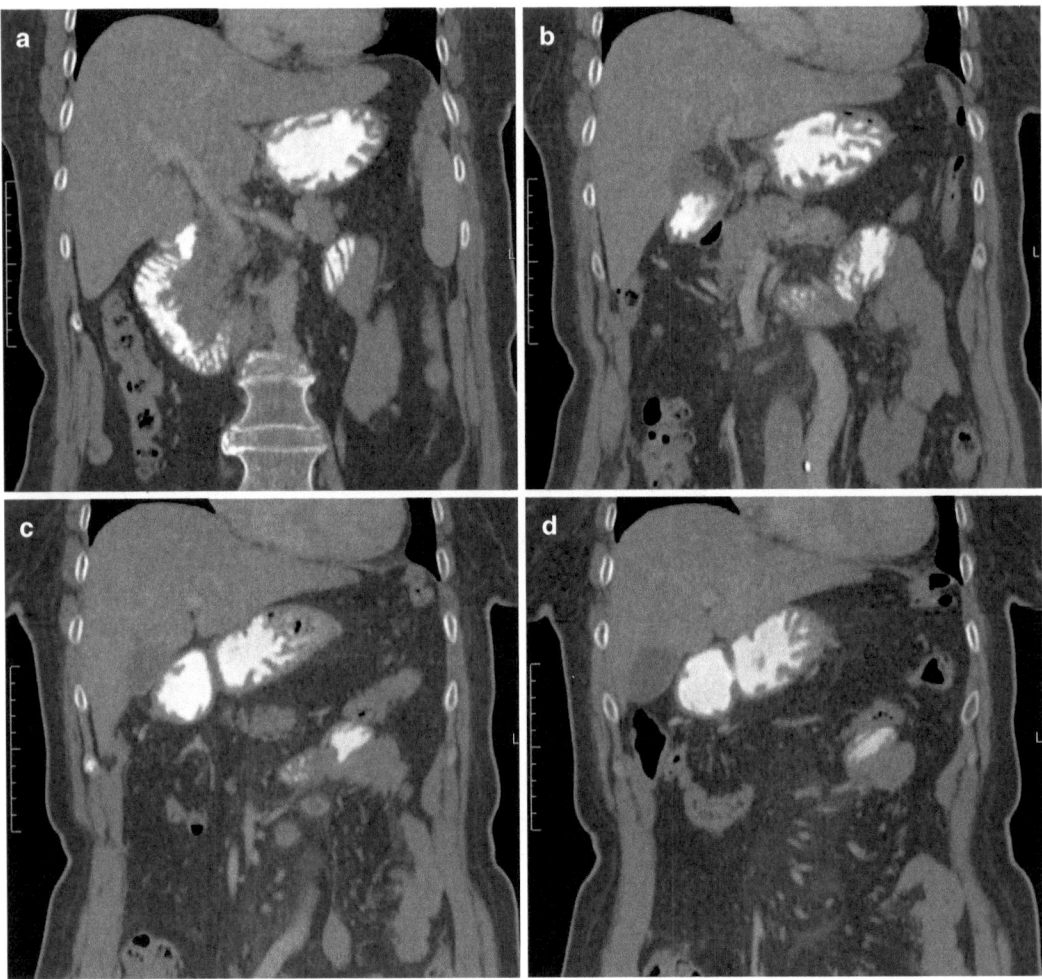

Fig. 4 (**a–d**) Coronal CT reconstructions of the portal phase scan (from dorsal to ventral)

What information do you gain from these reconstructions?

An MR scan was requested for further evaluation.

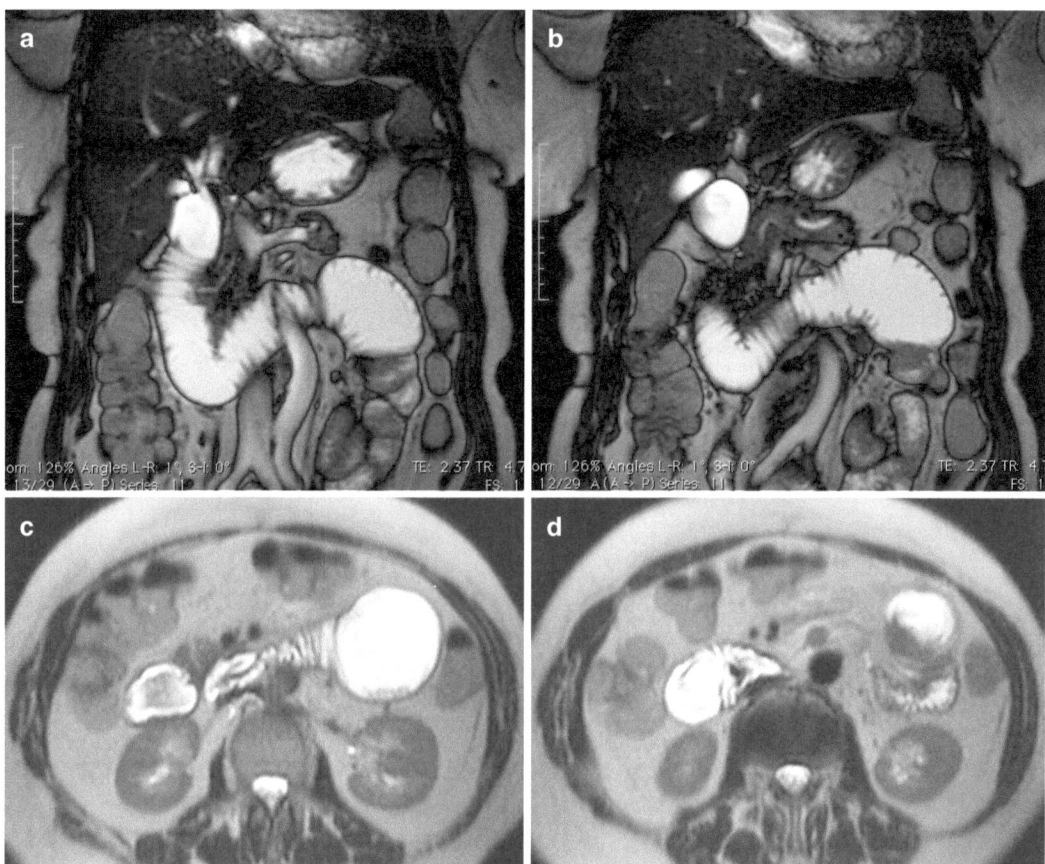

Fig. 5 (**a–d**) Coronal true FISP (**a**, **b**) and axial HASTE (**c**, **d**) images

Do these images confirm the preliminary diagnosis?

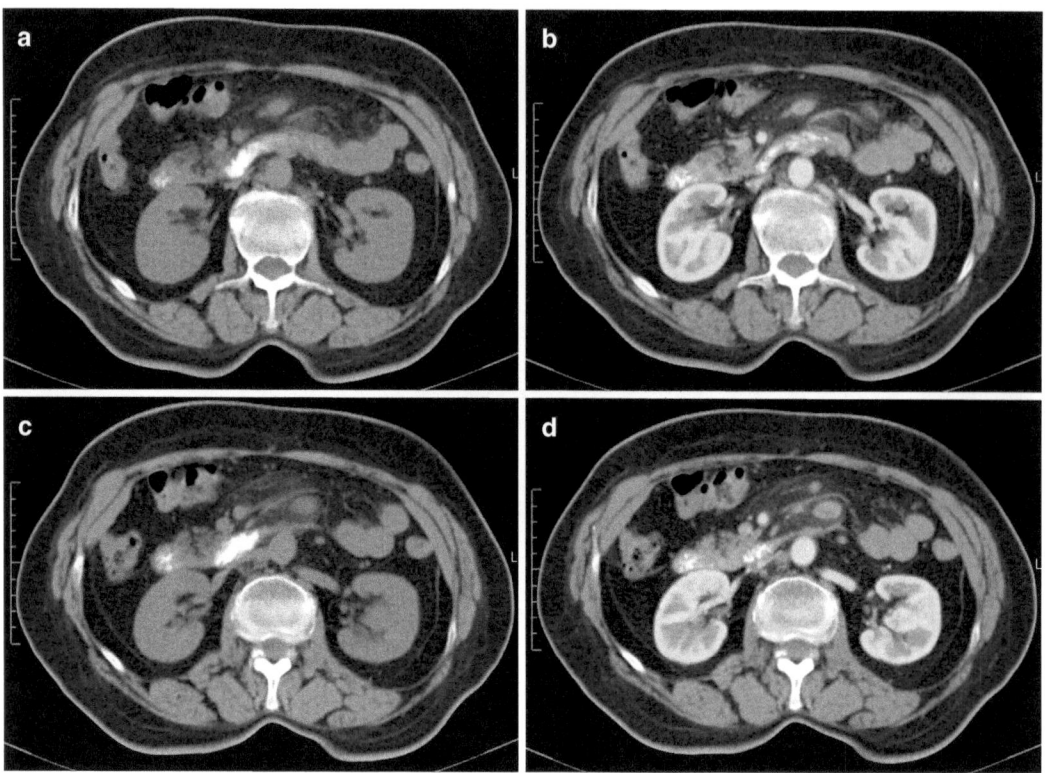

Fig. 6 (**a–d**) Two pairs of CT images, before (**a**, **c**) and after i.v. contrast, (**b**) and (**d**) in the portal phase, at levels more caudal to images in Figs. 1, 2, and 3

What additional information is provided in these images?
   Please formulate your diagnosis or your differential.

Discussion

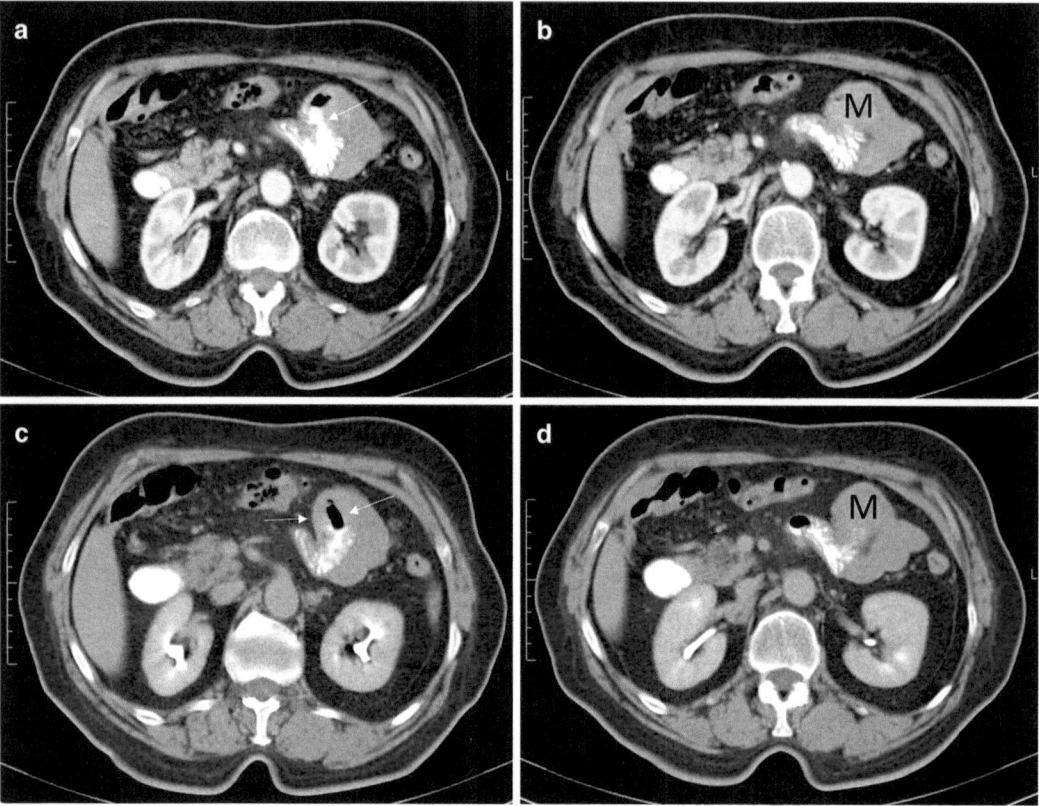

Fig. 7 (**a–d**) Pairs of CT images at arterial and delayed phases, selected from Figs. 2 and 3

Note mild dilatation of proximal jejunum (arrows) and non-advancement of gastrografin beyond that level. The equilibrium phase scan [images (b) and (d) of this figure] was obtained about 8 min after the plain scan (Fig. 1), yet there is no significant difference in the appearance of the proximal small bowel or in the distribution of oral contrast. The abrupt cutoff of the column of gastrografin is caused by a mass (M) that appears to originate in the bowel wall.

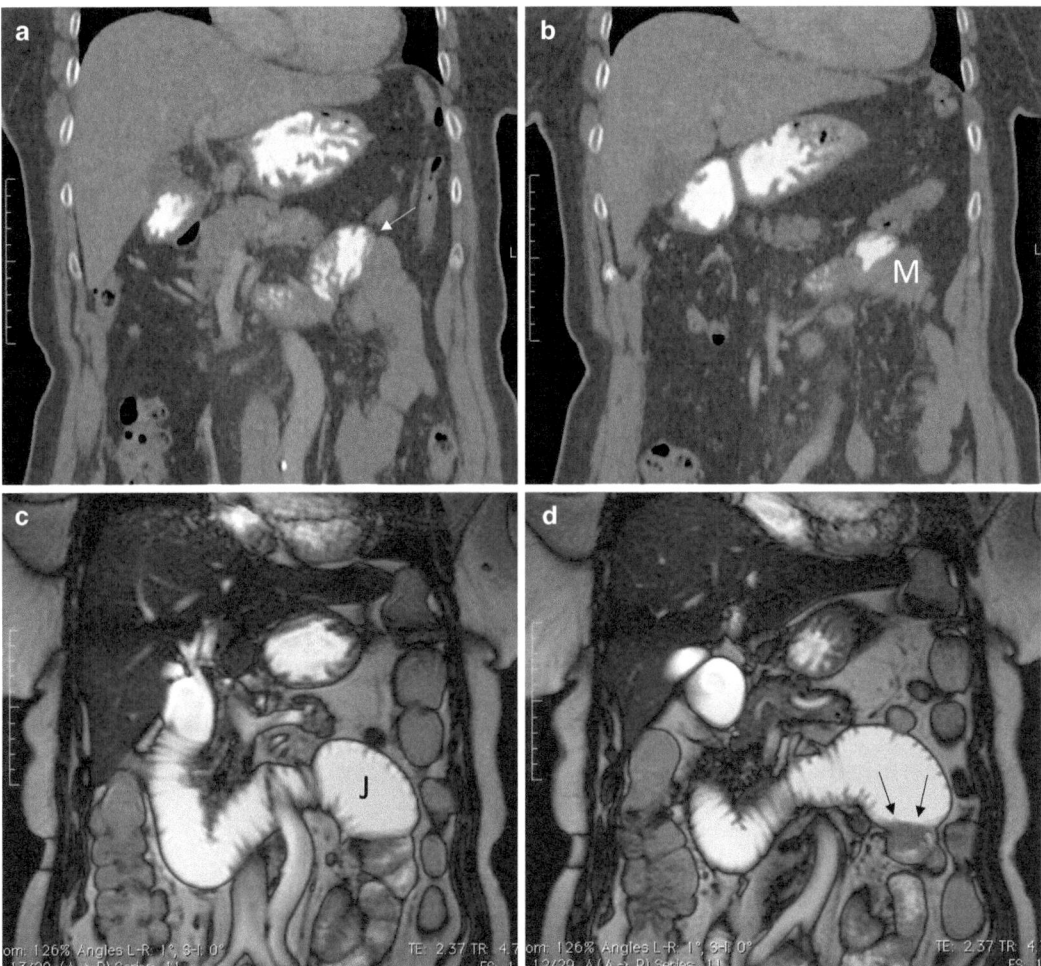

Fig. 8 (**a–d**) Coronal CT reconstructions (**a, c**) and coronal MR (**b, d**) images, also shown in Figs. 4 and 5

The coronal plane in this case is optimal for demonstrating the arrest of the oral contrast (white arrow) due to a bowel wall mass (M).

On MRI we see stasis of fluid and overdistention of the proximal jejunum (J). Thus it is easy to detect a short segment of thickened jejunal wall (black arrows) occluding the lumen.

The findings were confirmed endoscopically. The endoscopist used a colonoscope to reach this far. The biopsies revealed …?

Take a few moments to think about it before proceeding.

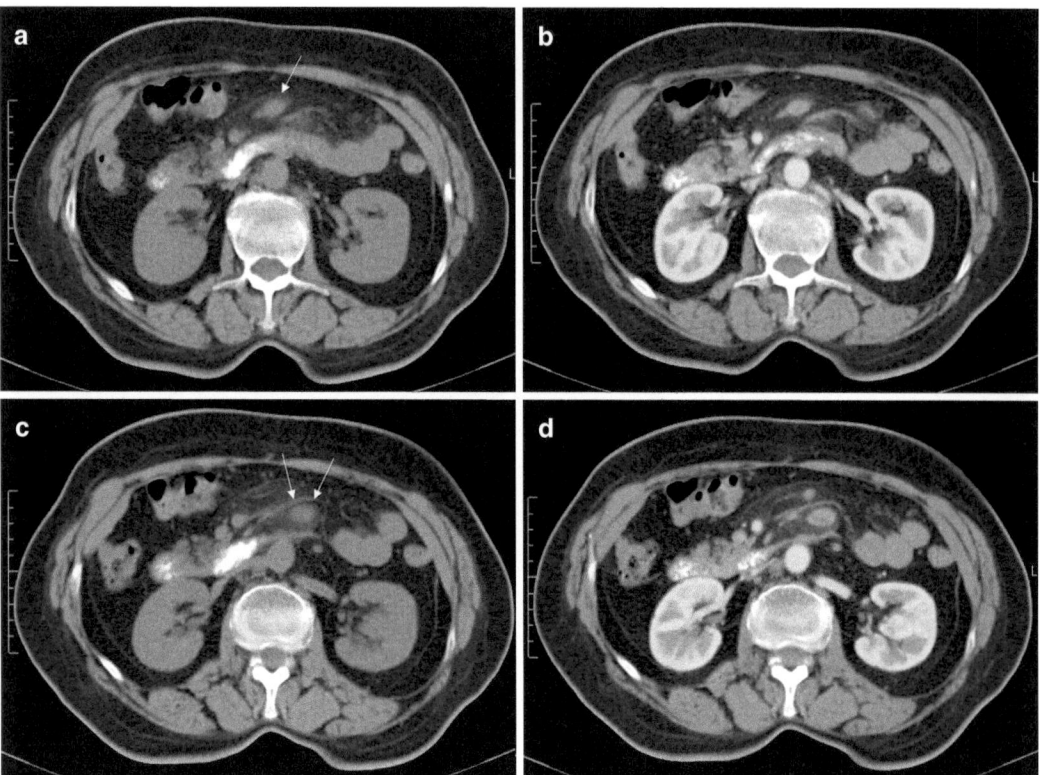

Fig. 9 (**a–d**) Pairs of CT images before and after i.v. contrast (portal phase)

The pertinent findings are: necrotic mesenteric lymph nodes (arrows) and haziness of the mesenteric fat.

What is the final diagnosis?

The patient underwent surgical resection of the thickened bowel wall.

The final histopathologic and clinical diagnosis was *primary adenocarcinoma of the jejunum* [71–73].

Teaching Point

An overlooked element of diagnosis is the anticipated time—dependent changes of structures that possess inherent motility or that can change their position, shape, and size (width) in response to stimuli. The prototype example is, of course, the gastrointestinal tract. Other examples are the ureters and the renal pelvocalyceal systems when challenged with a volume load or an osmotic load. I have seen cases of partial ureteral obstruction with a normal ureteral caliber in the plain scan, developing mild hydronephrosis and hydroureter in the excretory phase.

Case 18

A 68-year-old male status post total nephrectomy 4 years previously, for stage Ia renal cell carcinoma. He has not received chemotherapy or radiation therapy and appears disease free. He presents for follow-up. Preoperative imaging studies or reports are not available; the patient and his current oncologist cannot provide any relevant information. An MRI scan was requested.

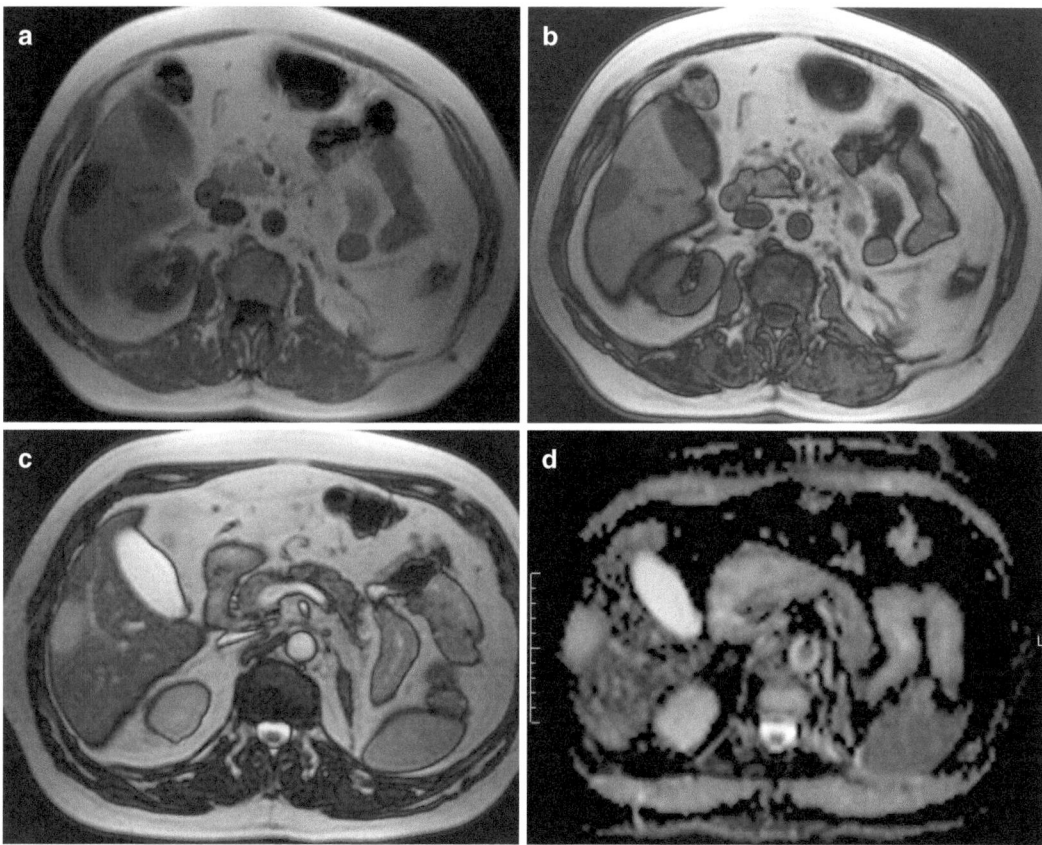

Fig. 1 (**a–d**) Axial T1w in phase (**a**) and opposed phase (**b**) images, true FISP image (**c**) and ADC map (**d**)

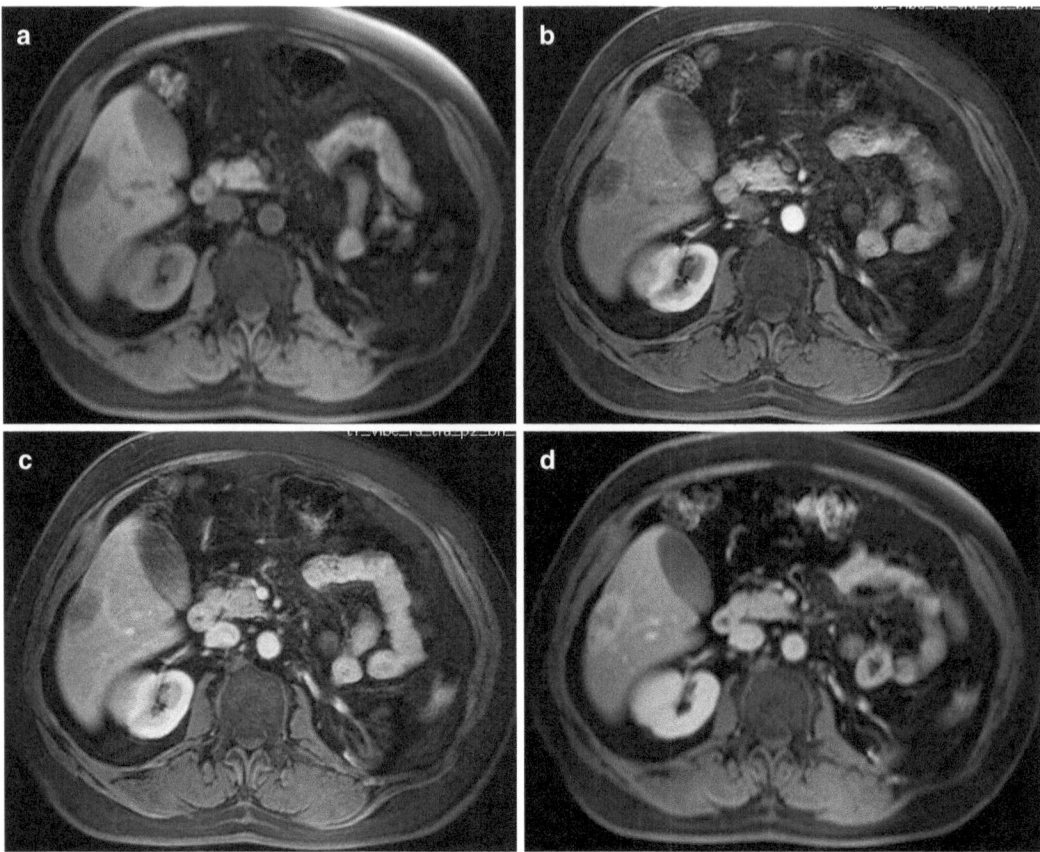

Fig. 2 (**a–d**) Plain T1 gradient echo (GE) with fat suppression (FS) image (**a**), and post injection of gadolinium images (**b–d**): T1 VIBE in arterial (**b**) and portal (**c**) phases and T1 GE FS in equilibrium phase (**d**)

Please write your observations and thoughts before proceeding.

A few days later the patient found a postoperative MR examination that had been obtained 1 year previously. Representative images are shown in Figs. 3 and 4.

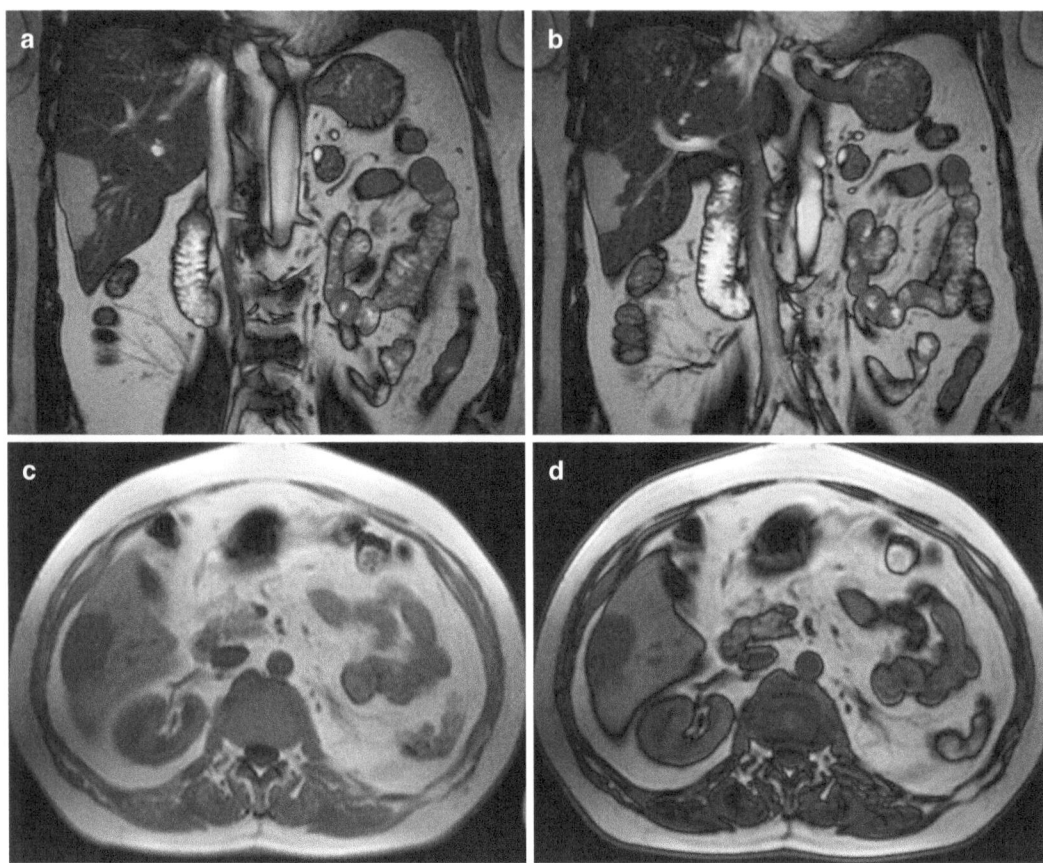

Fig. 3 (**a–d**) Coronal true FISP (**a**, **b**) and axial T1w in (**c**) and opposed phase (**d**) images

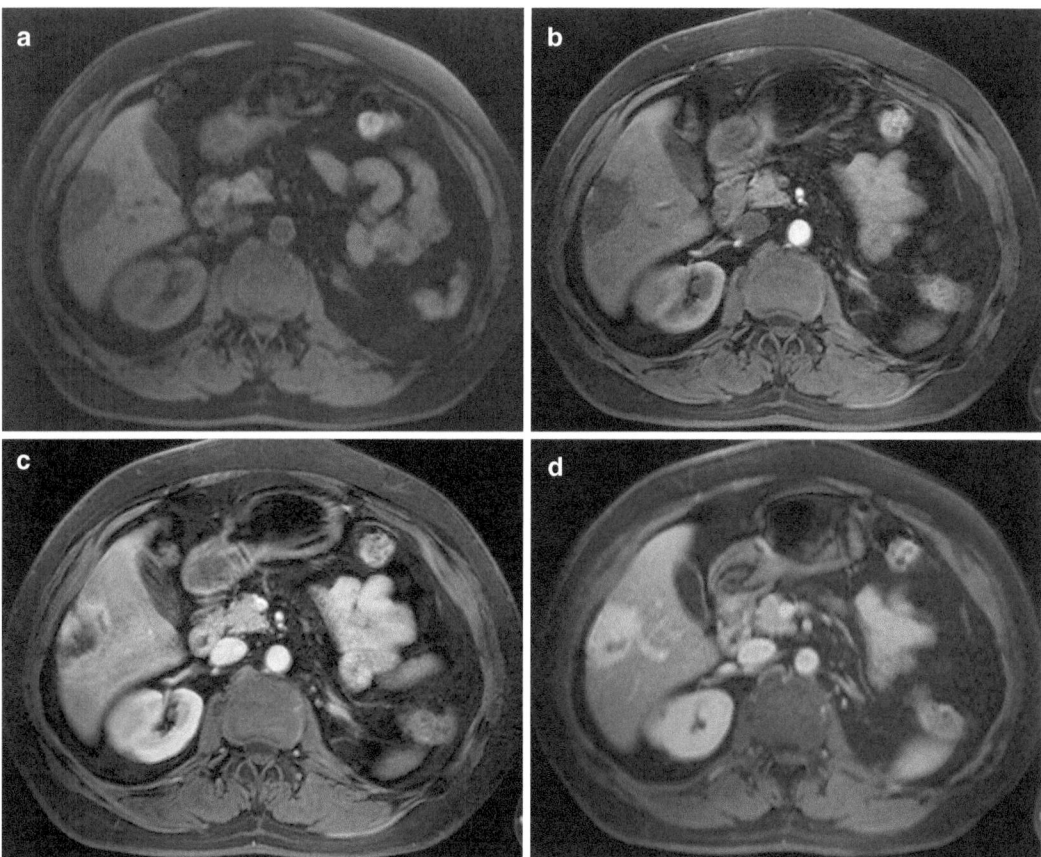

Fig. 4 Plain T1w GE FS image (**a**) and three post contrast images in the arterial, portal (T1 VIBE), (**b**, **c**) and equilibrium (T1 GE FS) phases (**d**)

Please compare the two studies. What is your diagnosis?

Discussion

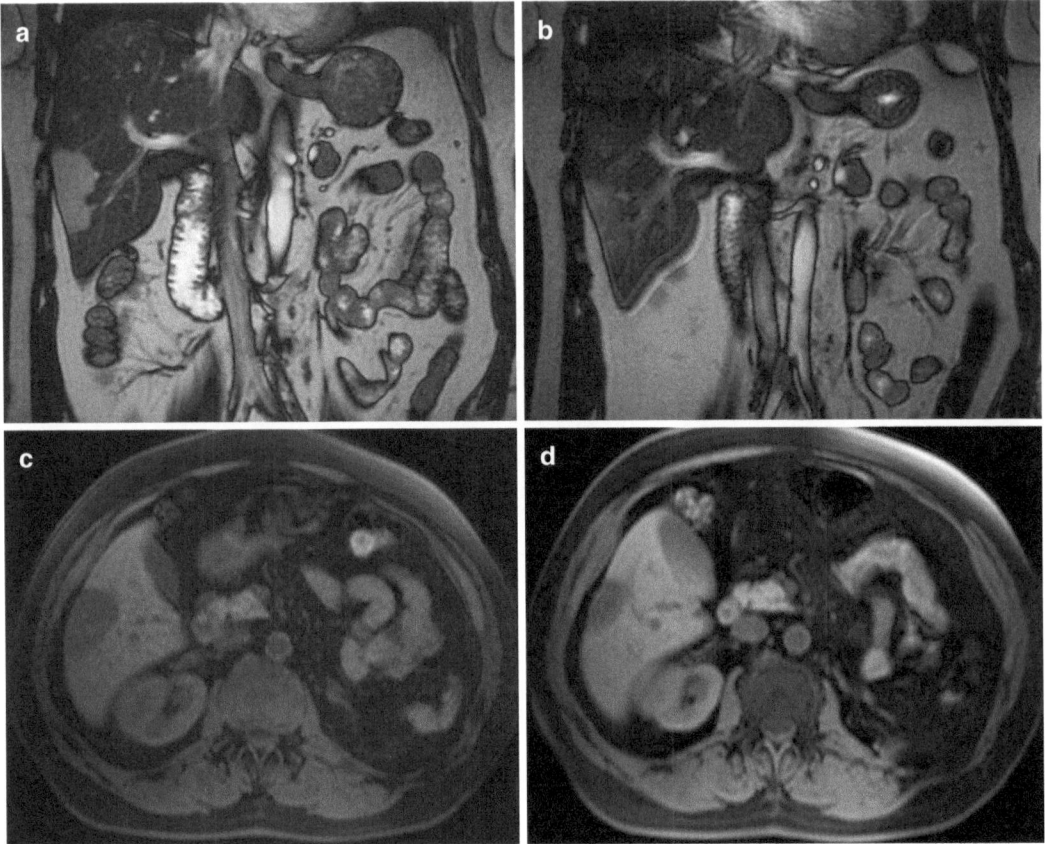

Fig. 5 (**a–d**) Comparison of the two MRI studies, performed 1 year apart, in pairs of Coronal true FISP (**a, b**) and plain axial T1w gradient echo (GE) fat suppressed (FS) images (**c, d**). The most recent study is on the right half of the page (**b, d**)

Let's analyze the case in the sequence in which it was presented, in other words we will start with the most recent MRI, i.e., Figs. 1 and 2.

There is a subcapsular lesion in the right lobe of the liver. Its borders are well defined in the T1w images, but less so in the true FISP image. It has homogeneous, moderately high T2 and moderately low T1 signal intensity compared with normal liver parenchyma. It has neither cystic nor necrotic components. There are no foci of fat or hemorrhage. There is no restriction of diffusion. Contrast enhancement is sluggish, with slow centripetal advancement and incomplete filling.

The pertinent images from the earlier MRI study are displayed in Figs. 3 and 4. In these images the hepatic lesion looks like a typical hemangioma.

Direct comparison of the two MRI studies can be carried out in Figs. 5 and 6.

Comparing the two studies we notice the following, from the earlier to the most recent study:

(a) the lesion has decreased in size in all three orthogonal axes (from 0.5 to 2.0 cm),
(b) its borders have become less sharp in the true FISP images,

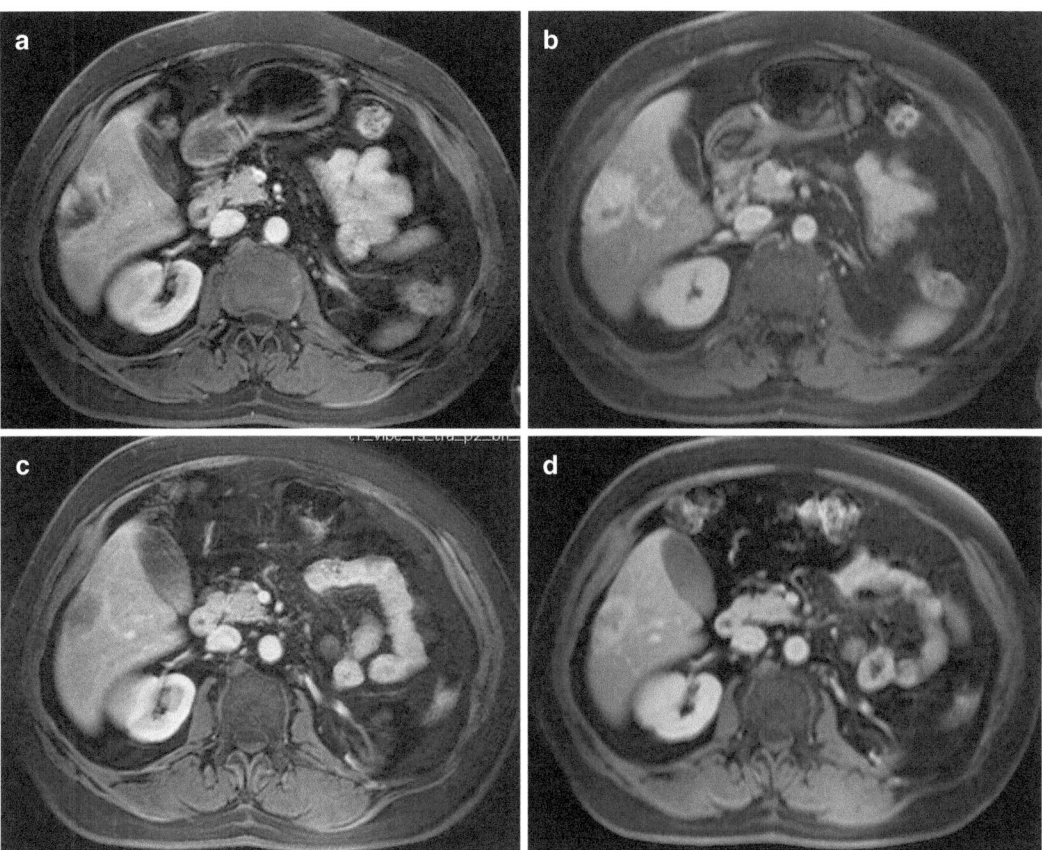

Fig. 6 (**a–d**) Comparison of the two MRI studies, performed 1 year apart, in pairs of post contrast T1w images from the portal phase (**a**, **c**) and equilibrium (**b**, **d**) phases (VIBE and GE FS respectively). The most recent MRI is (**c**) and (**d**)

(c) its signal intensity has diminished in the true FISP sequence,
(d) there is diminished intensity of contrast enhancement and there is slower centripetal "filling."

Looking at the aortic lumen and the rest of the enhancing structures, it is safe to assume that the amount of contrast medium and the speed of injection were about the same between the two examinations. There was no history of an external factor that could be responsible for the interval changes. Thus we have to conclude that the differences we observe are solely due to the natural course of a benign, yet evolving hepatic nodule. Which diagnosis fits this picture? I propose *involuting sclerosing hemangioma* [74, 75].

Teaching Point

Keep in mind the uncommon variants of common diseases. Please revisit Chap. 7, Sect. 7.2.1.4.
Keep in mind that any condition may evolve as part of its natural history. Please cross reference Sect. 7.2.1.7 in Chap. 7.

Case 19

The patient is a 63-year-old female from Albania who speaks only her native language. A relative was able to offer partial information. Thus it was not possible to obtain a complete medical history. She was referred by an internist after a sonogram showed a large, ill-defined, inhomogeneous space occupying lesion in the liver. She complained of progressive abdominal pain, shortness of breath, and weight loss due to loss of appetite, for the past 6 months. She denied fever or chills. She gave no history of prior surgeries.

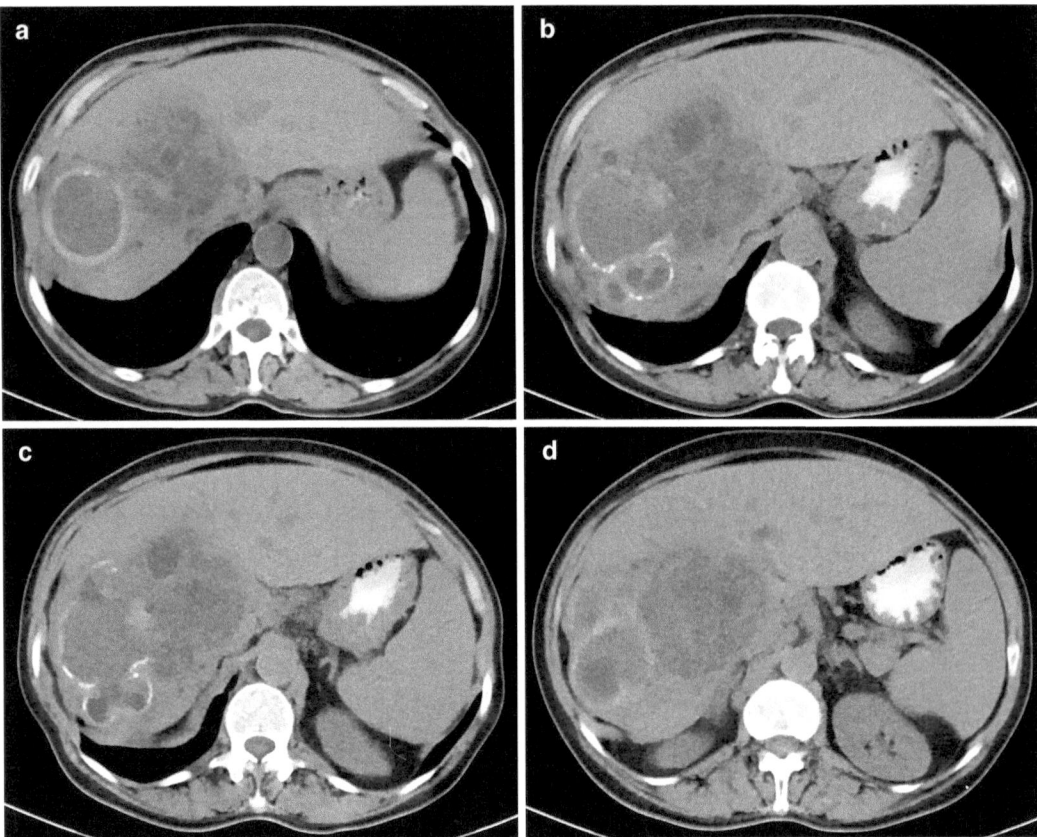

Fig. 1 (**a–d**) Axial CT images through the liver. Intravenous contrast was not administered, because of a history of allergic shock

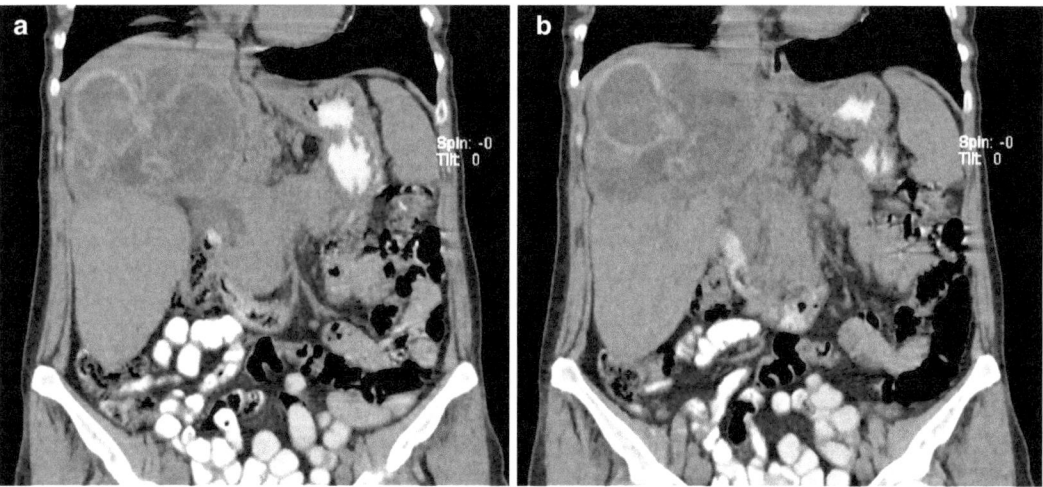

Fig. 2 (**a**, **b**) Coronal CT reconstructions

Please record your observations and your thoughts on paper before proceeding.

A CT scan of the chest was obtained at the same time as the abdominal CT scan.

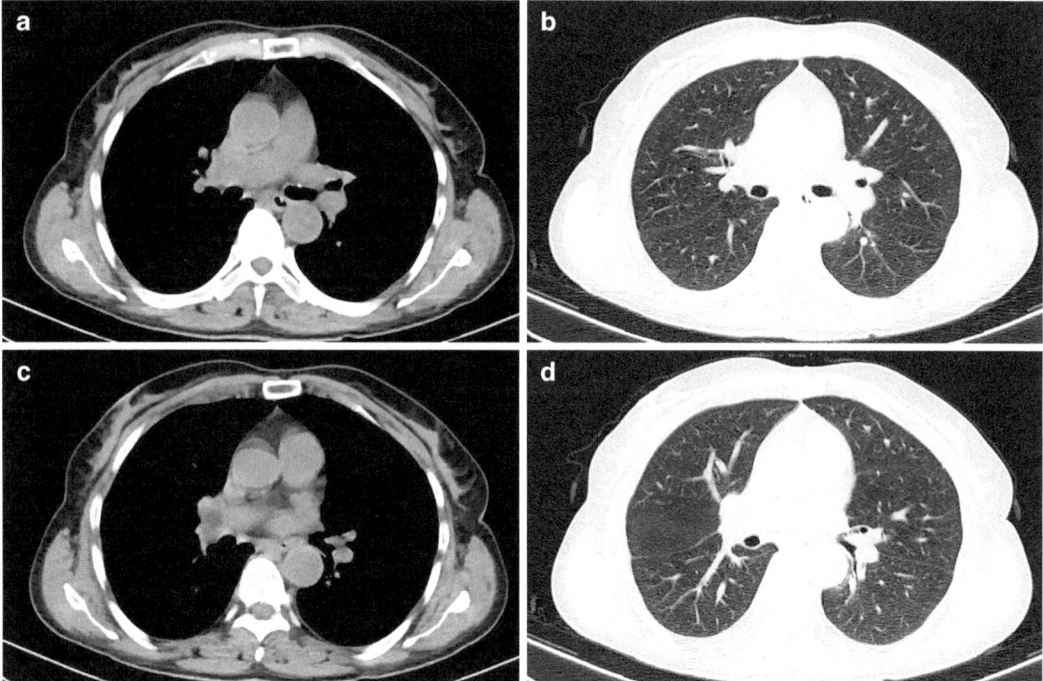

Fig. 3 (**a–d**) Pairs of CT images in mediastinal (**a, c**) and lung (**b, d**) windows

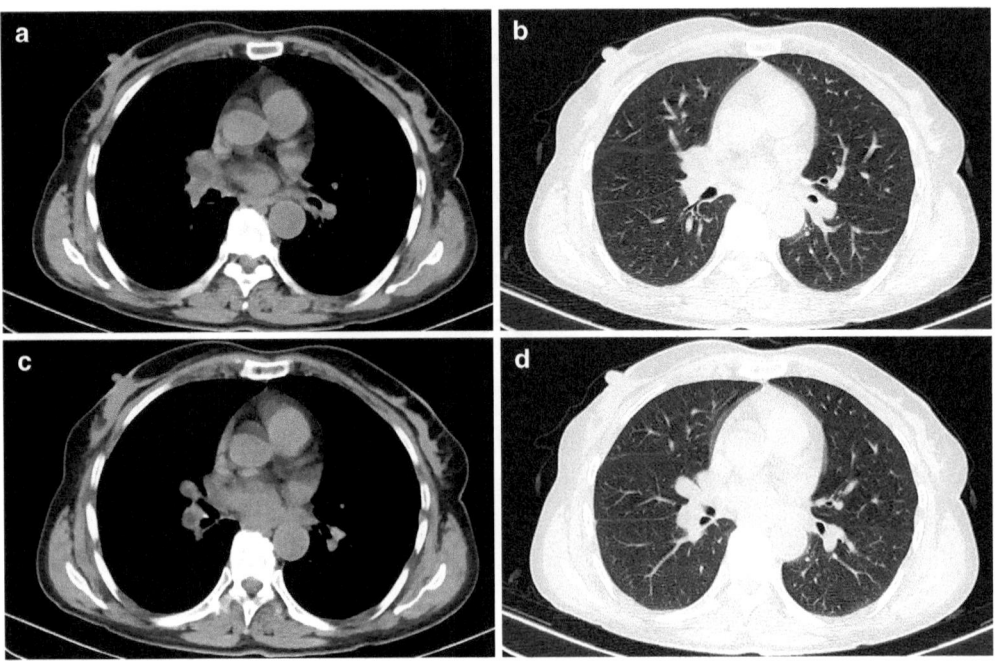

Fig. 4 (**a–d**) Pairs of CT images in mediastinal (**a**, **c**) and lung (**b**, **d**) windows

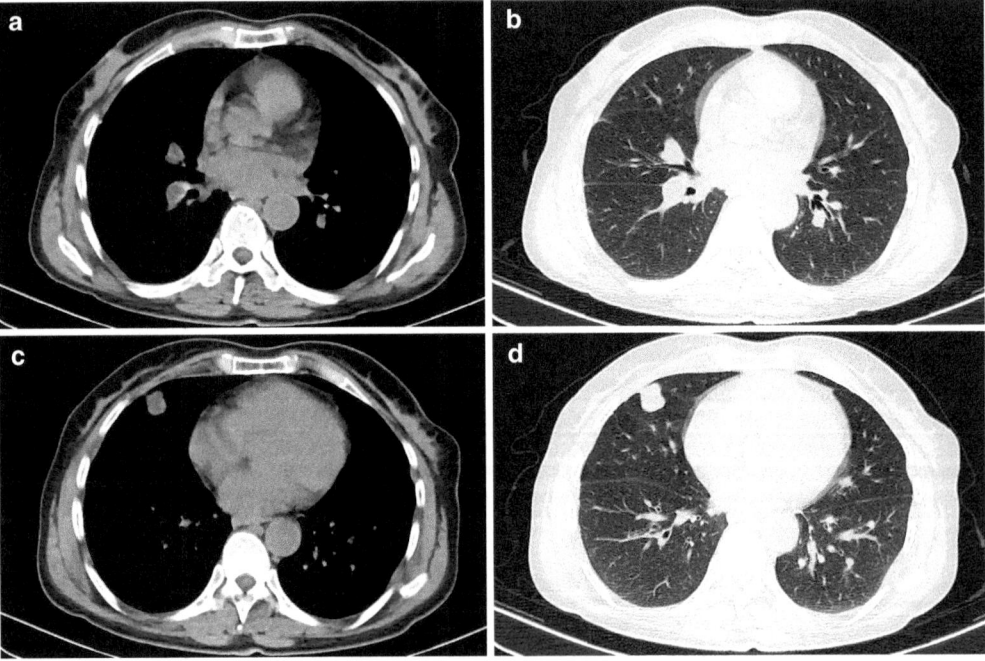

Fig. 5 (**a–d**) Pairs of CT images in mediastinal (**a**, **c**) and lung (**b**, **d**) windows

What abnormalities do you detect?
Can you provide a specific diagnosis or a short differential?

Discussion

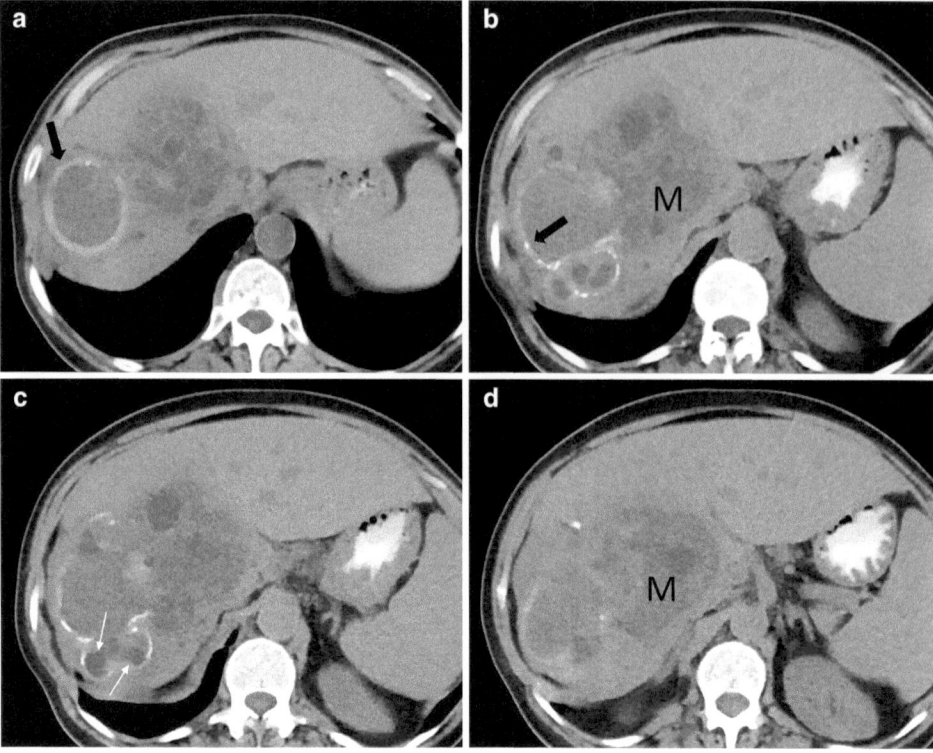

Fig. 6 (**a–d**) Close up views of images though the liver, shown in Fig. 1

This is a complex case. Let's try to put together the pieces of the puzzle.

A large (16 cm), inhomogeneous lesion has replaced a significant part of the right lobe of the liver, extends to the caudate lobe, and has reached the border of the left lobe of the liver. The right and middle hepatic veins are not discernible. Vascular obscuration may be due to compression, invasion, or thrombosis. Let's now look for specific details that may guide us to the correct path. The right half of the lesion consists of multiple lobes with a thin or slightly thick, complete or partial, hyperdense capsule or pseudocapsule (black arrows). These rims also carry dot like and short curvilear calcifications. Within a dorsal lobe of the "mass" we see small "cysts" (white arrows), whose density measurements were in the range of water

So far, so good: does this part of the "mass" make you think of a specific diagnosis? Take your time to think it over, before turning the page.

Answer: how about *echinococcosis* [76–78]?

OK, but how do we deal with the left half of the mass (M)? It does not have capsules, solid calcifications, or water-like cysts. Now, we are presented with a dilemma: are looking at a single lesion or at two different ones?

(a) If it is a single entity, then it displays simultaneously two different phases of its natural history. To be more specific, is it possible that an echinococcal cyst has partially ruptured, and spilled some of its contents? In this case, reactive inflammatory and fibrous tissue would try to contain the advancing front of parasitic infestation. As the parasitic infiltrate expands rapidly, it may leave areas of necrosis in its core. This complex host–parasite interaction could easily explain the appearance of the left half of the lesion (M).

(b) The other possibility is that a preexisting echinococcal cyst is being engulfed partially by another infectious or neoplastic process.

Let's now proceed to the thorax and see if we can choose the correct answer.

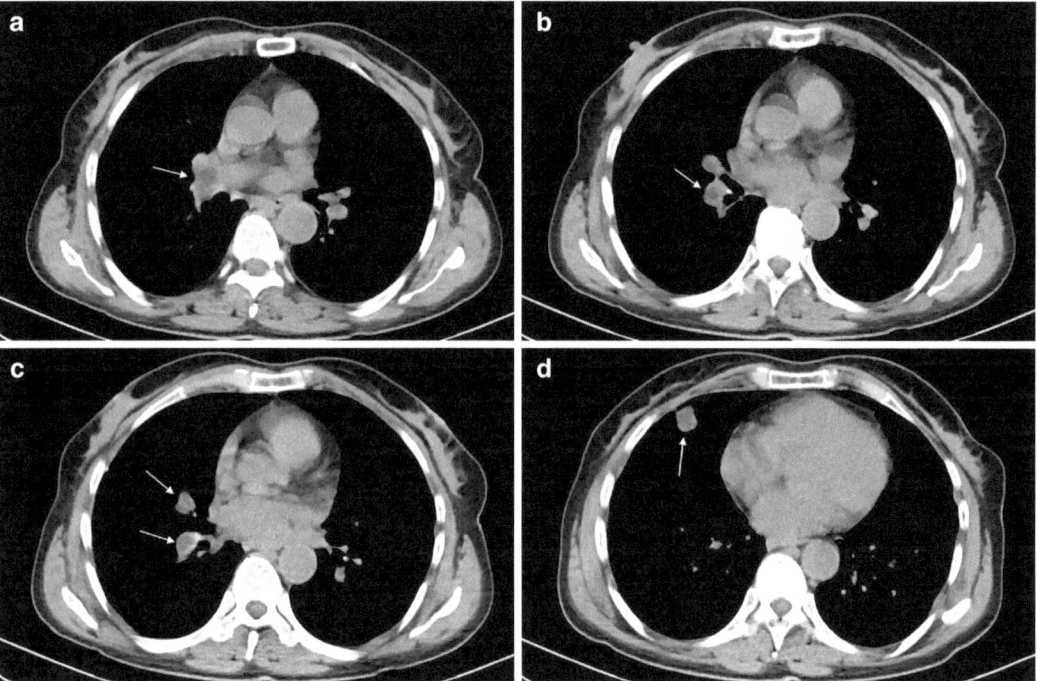

Fig. 7 (**a–d**) Selected images of the chest (mediastinal window) that have been shown in Figs. 3, 4, and 5

The striking feature of these images are the low density and the mild dilatation of the right hilar vessels (thin arrows), and the low density of the right pulmonary nodule (thick arrow). We do not see any calcifications. We see no evidence of perinodular reaction or hemorrhage

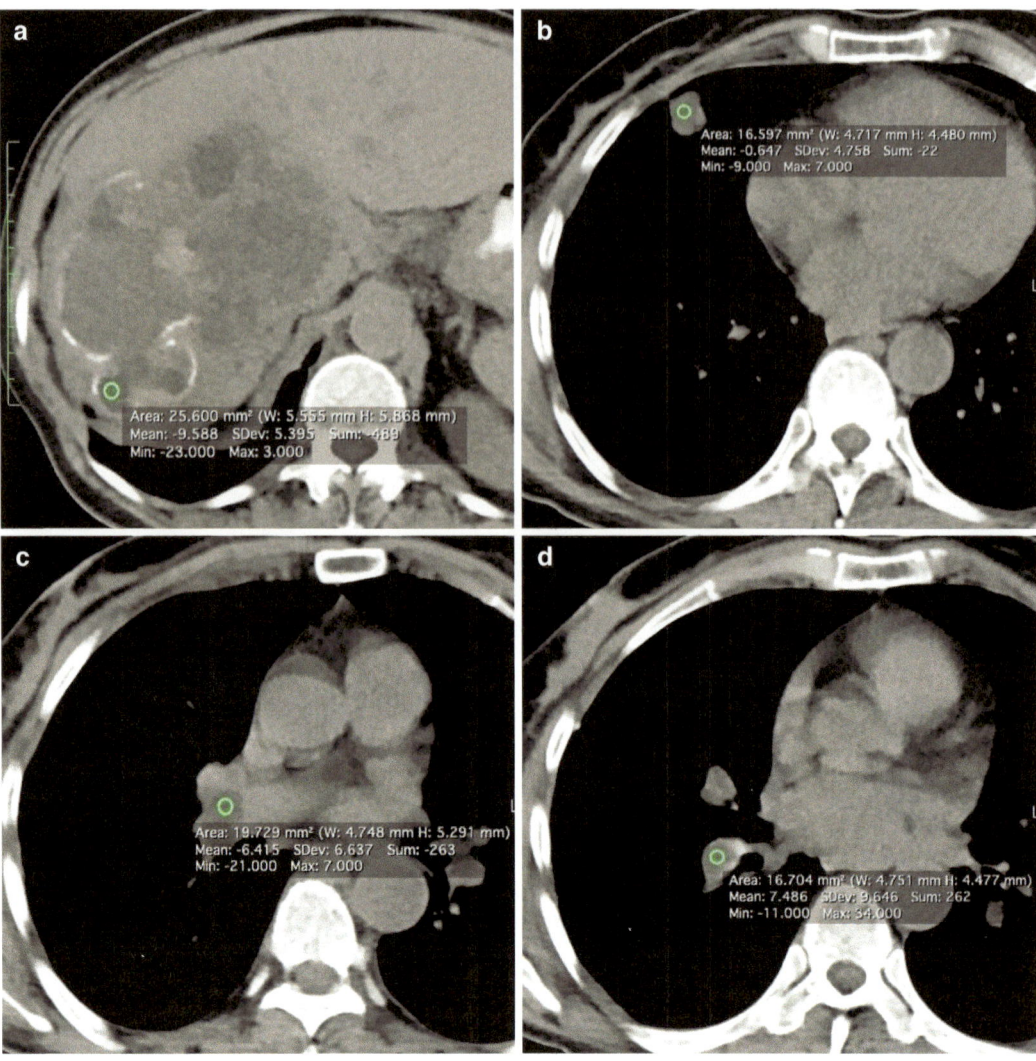

Fig. 8 (**a–d**) Close up views of the right hepatic lobe (**a**), the middle lobe of the right lung (**b**), and the right hilum (**c, d**), with density measurements. These images have been shown already in the prior figures

The mean density of the indicated cyst in the liver is −9.6 HU (SD 5.4 HU), of the lung nodule −0.1 HU (SD 4.8 HU), of the distal right pulmonary arterial trunk −6.4 HU (SD 6.6 HU), and of the descending branch of the right pulmonary artery 7.5 HU (SD 9.6 HU).

Can we make sense of all this information?

Take a few moments to think, before proceeding to the next page.

I propose that the echinococcal infestation of the liver *broke through* its capsule and gained *access* to the *hepatic veins* and subsequently to the *right heart chambers*. Thereafter the echinococcal cysts *embolized* to the *pulmonary arteries*. One of the emboli reached the periphery of the right middle lobe and grew to a pulmonary hydatid cyst.

The patient was lost to follow-up and I do not have confirmation of the presumptive diagnosis.

Teaching Point

Pay meticulous attention to detail.

Strive for a single, unifying diagnosis to encompass multiple findings.

Case 20

A 70-year-old female with endometrial carcinoma, s/p total hysterectomy and chemotherapy. The patient appears disease free and presents for restaging.

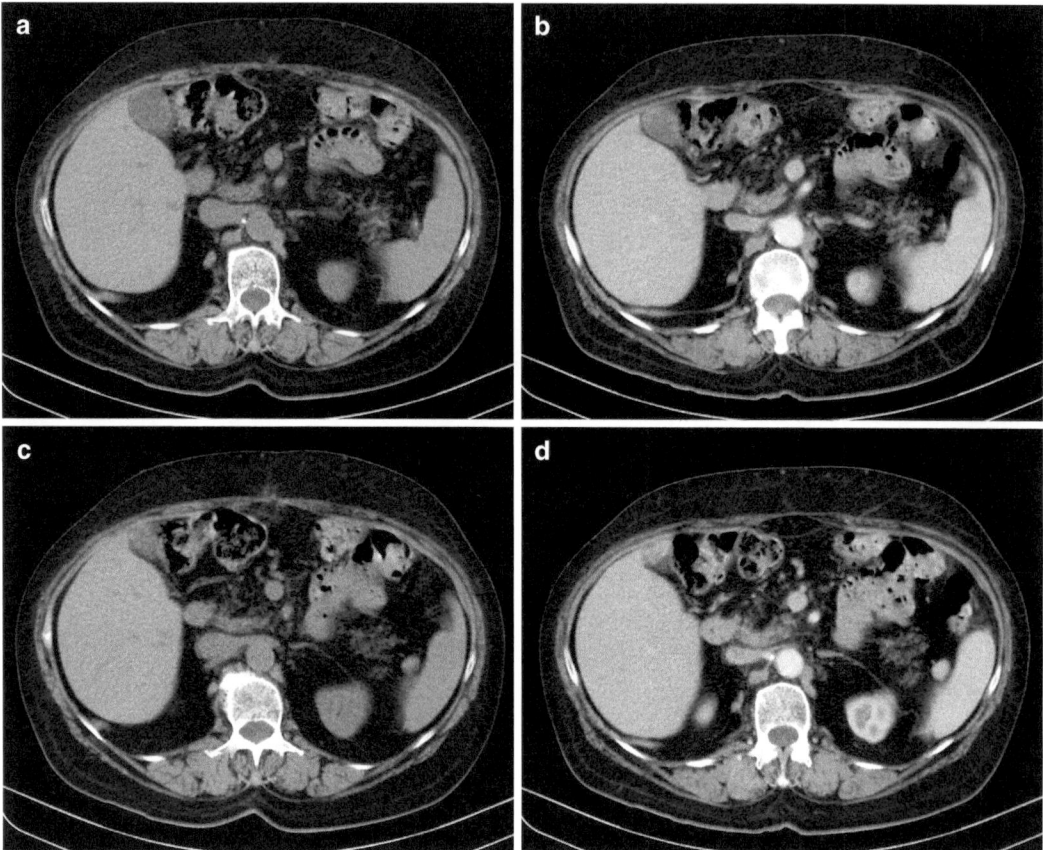

Fig. 1 (**a–d**) Four CT images in pairs through the upper abdomen, before (**a**, **c**) and after (**b**, **d**) i.v. contrast (portal phase)

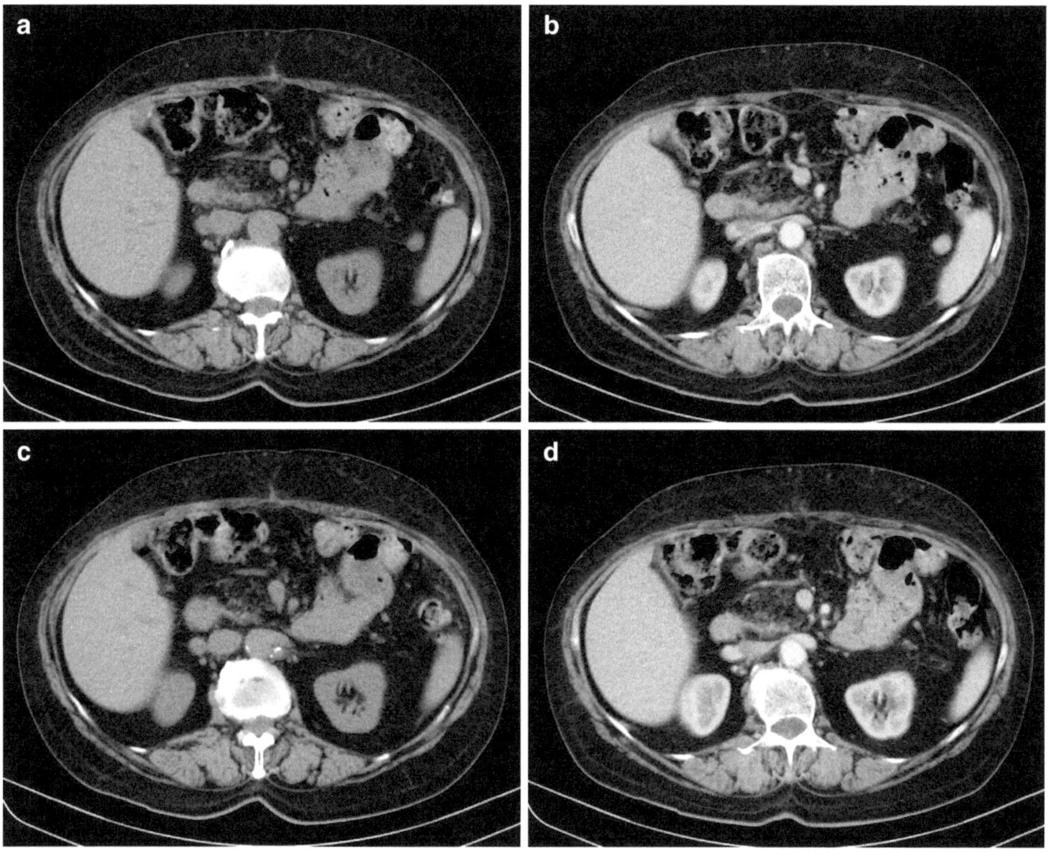

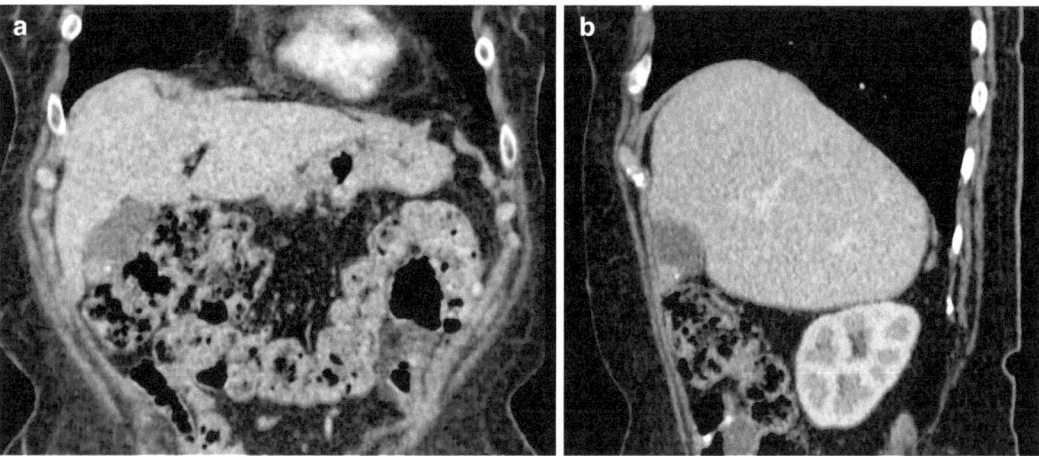

Fig. 2 (**a–d**) Four CT images in pairs through the upper abdomen, before (**a, c**) and after (**b, d**) i.v. contrast (portal phase)

Please describe any findings before proceeding.

Fig. 3 Coronal (**a**) and sagittal (**b**) CT reconstructions

What information can you extract from these images?

An MRI study was performed 2 weeks after the CT scan.

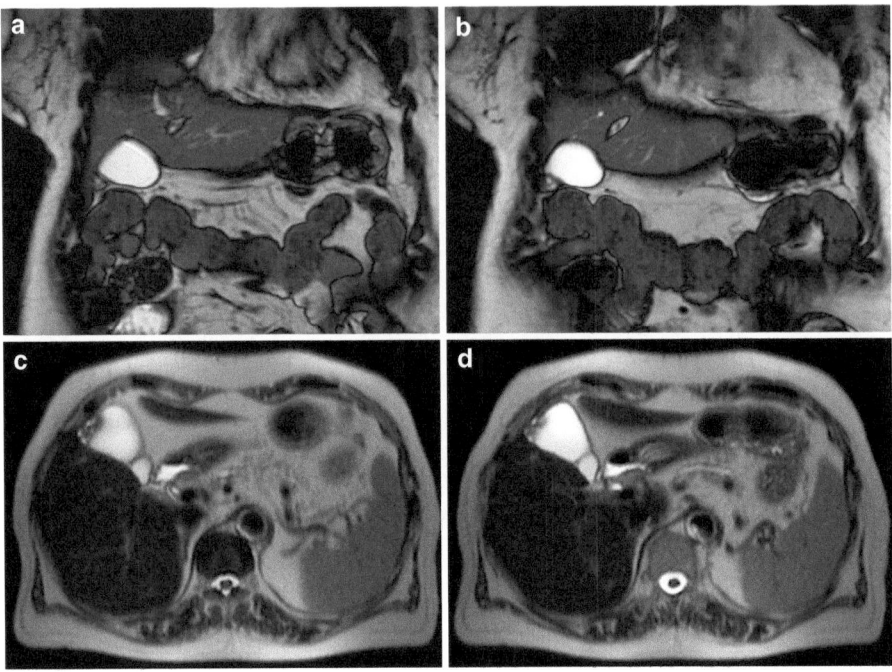

Fig. 4 (**a–d**) Coronal true FISP (**a**, **b**) and axial T2w (**c**, **d**) images through the upper abdomen

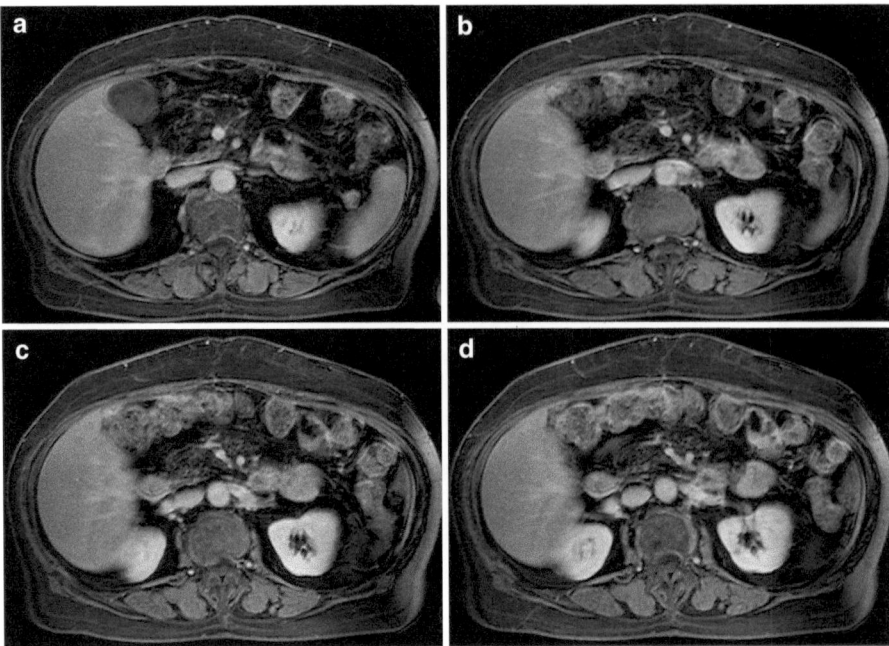

Fig. 5 (**a–d**) Axial VIBE post contrast images (portal phase), corresponding to the CT slices shown in Figs. 1 and 2

What are the findings? What is your diagnosis?

Discussion

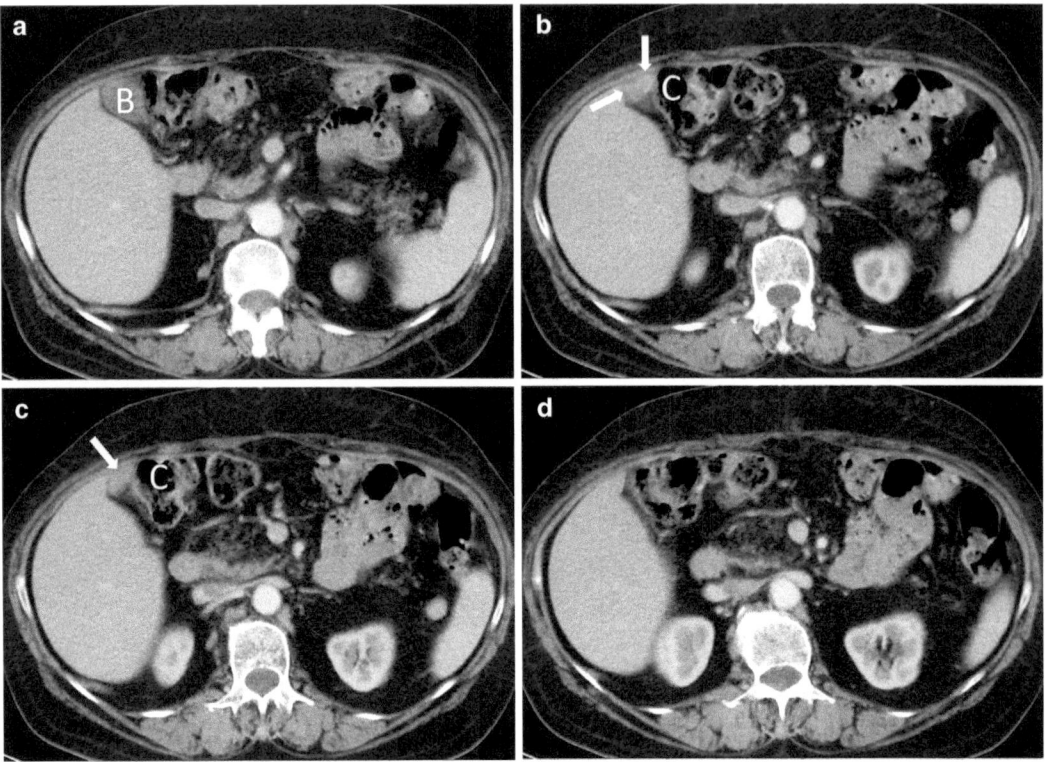

Fig. 6 (**a–d**) Four contrast enhanced CT images (portal phase), selected from Figs. 1 and 2

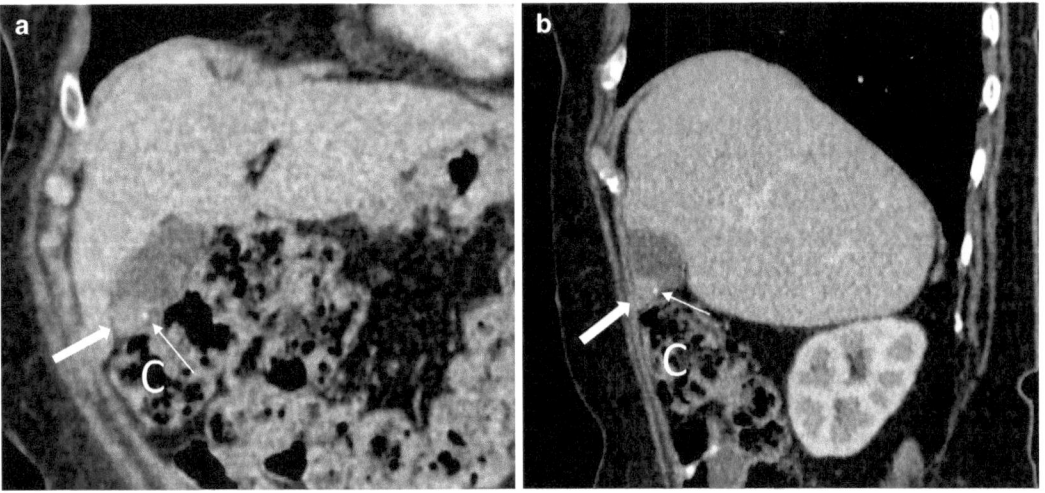

Fig. 7 (**a, b**) Coronal and sagittal CT reconstructions, same as in Fig. 3

A nodule with mild nearly homogeneous contrast enhancement (thick arrows) occupies the region of the fundus of the gallbladder (G). It has a tiny focus of calcification or it has enclosed a tiny calculus (thin arrows) It abuts the stool filled colon (C). Its detection in the axial images is difficult, because the adjacent colic flexure is filled with stool, its contrast enhancement is not pronounced, and it is located in the caudal end of the gallbladder. To ensure that the lesion is not missed one should inspect carefully all images through the gallbladder, and evaluate meticulously the coronal and sagittal reconstructions.

The major diagnostic considerations were adenomyomatosis vs. carcinoma of the gallbladder [79, 80]. There were no findings of recurrent or metastatic disease of the patient's gynecologic malignancy. Thus further evaluation was recommended with an MRI scan.

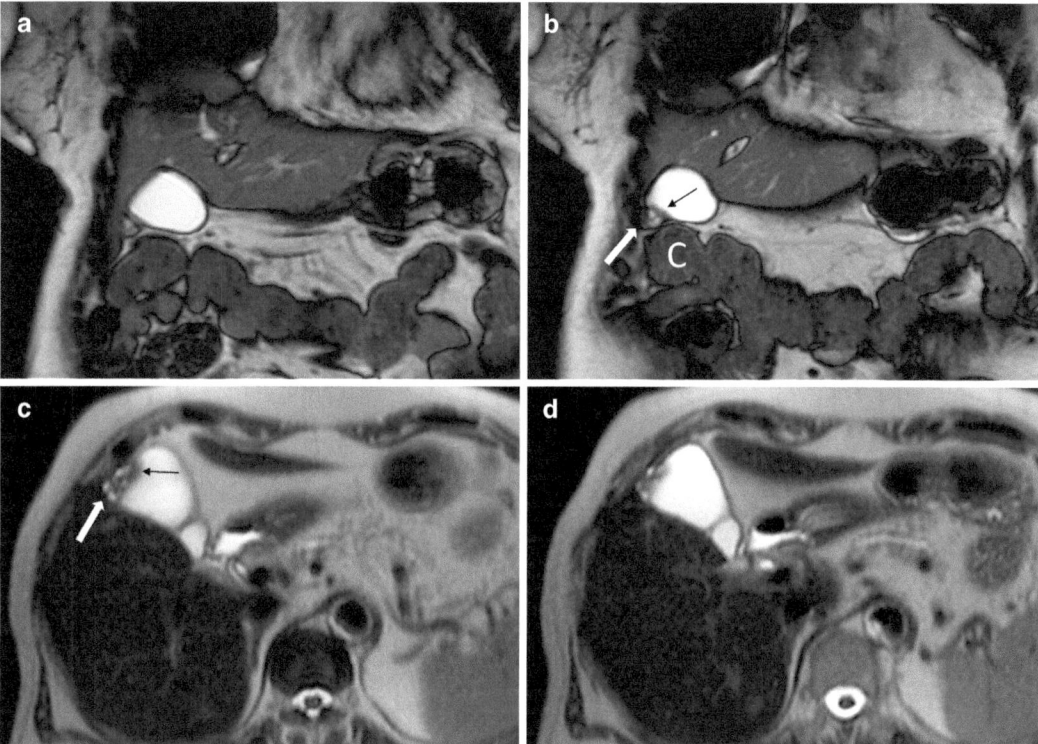

Fig. 8 Coronal true FISP (**a**, **b**) and axial T2w (**c**, **d**) images, same as in Fig. 4, slightly magnified

The nodule appears as multiple tiny cysts (solid arrows) with thin walls. This appearance has been called the "pearl necklace sign." The entire cyst complex is separated from the remainder of the gallbladder by a band like septum or plate like wall thickening (thin arrows)

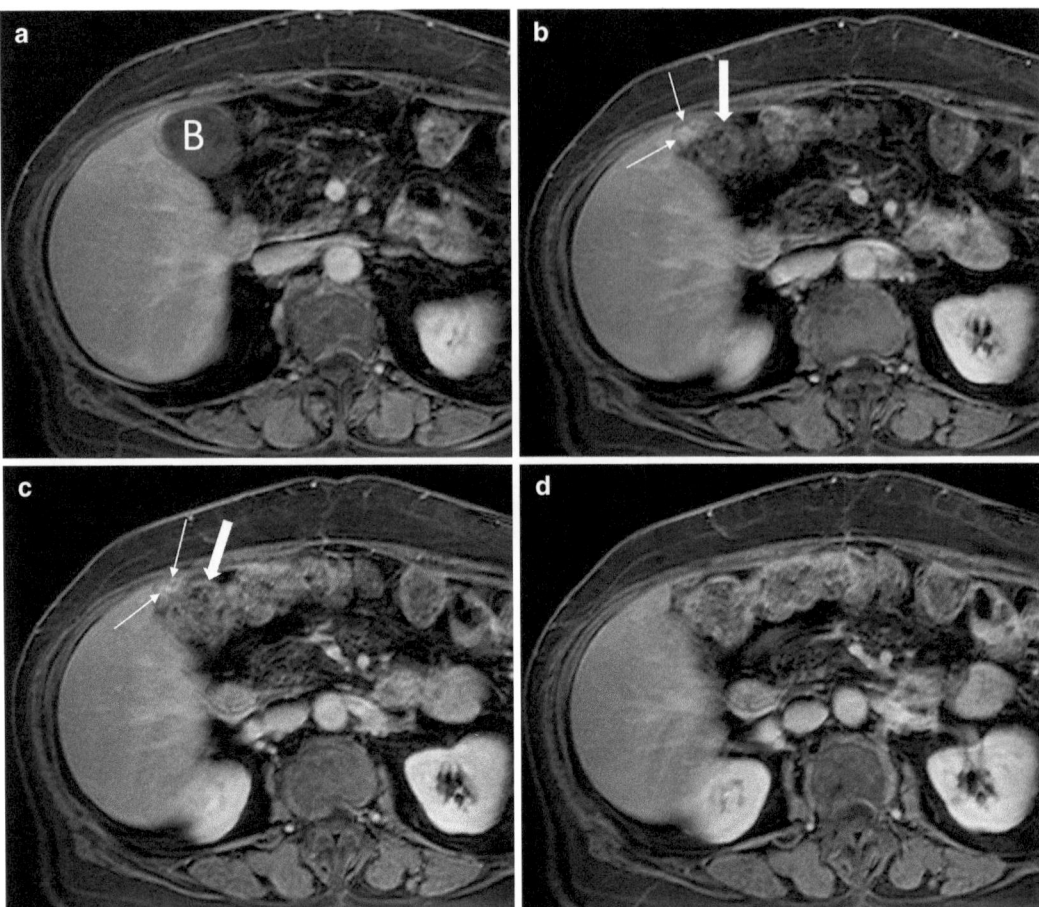

Fig. 9 (**a–d**) Axial VIBE images post i.v. contrast in the portal phase, same as in Fig. 5 (slightly magnified)

There is moderate, inhomogeneous enhancement of the lesion (thin arrows) in the fundus of the gall-bladder (G). Its true nature is easier to appreciate by MRI compared to CT. The nodule is wedged between the liver and the stool filled colon (thick arrows). The intensity of contrast enhancement of the liver and the lesion are similar, thus the lesion does not "stand out" in the VIBE images

Final diagnosis: *adenomyomatosis* of the gallbladder. There were no changes in follow-up CT scans at 6 and 12 months.

Teaching Point

This case is a very good example of the potential "entry" or "exit" slice pitfall; please revisit Chap. 5, "Loading and unloading" bias, Sect. 5.2.2.3.

Case 21

A 67-year-old male s/p resection of a rectal adenocarcinoma, with an end-to-end bowel anastomosis. Subsequently the patient developed two metastases in the left lobe of the liver. The patient presents 1 month after surgical resection of the liver metastases with dull abdominal and pelvic pain. A CT scan was performed. Prior examinations were not available.

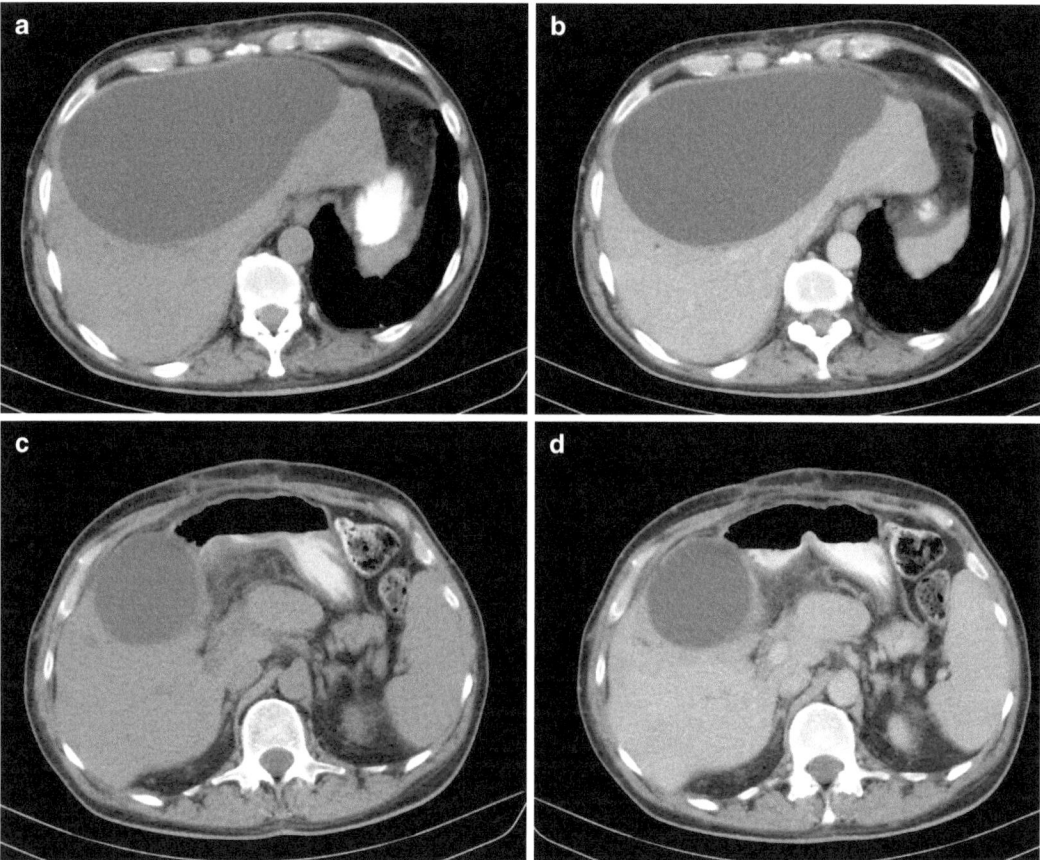

Fig. 1 Selected CT images through the abdomen, in pairs, before (**a**, **c**) and after (**b**, **d**) i.v. contrast. Oral contrast was also administered

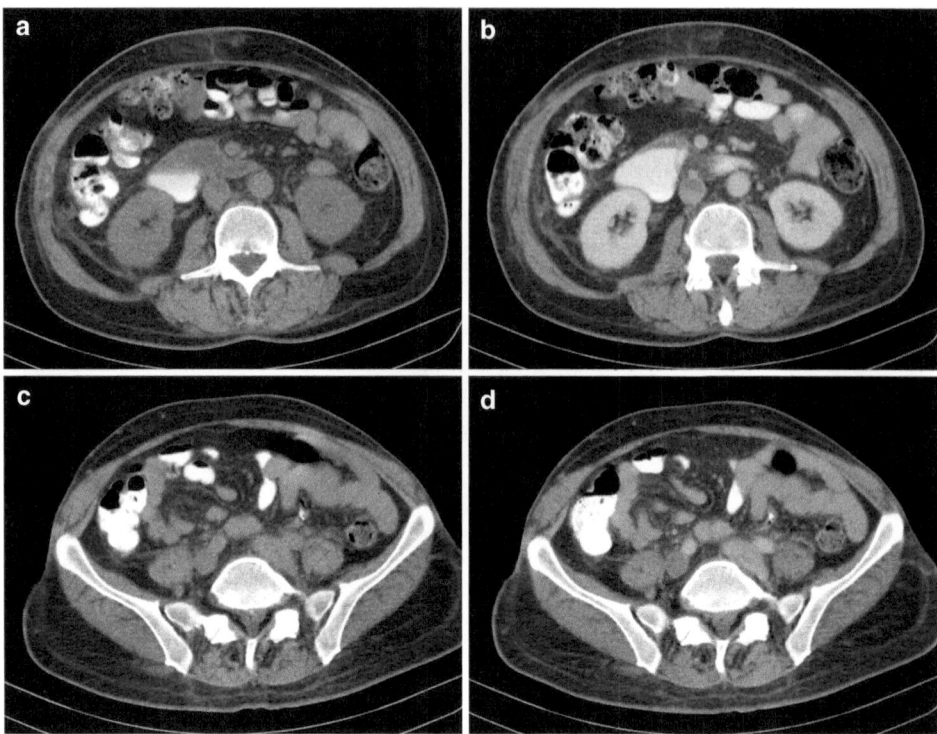

Fig. 2 Selected CT images through the abdomen and pelvis, in pairs, before (**a**, **c**) and after (**b**, **d**) i.v. contrast. Oral contrast was also administered

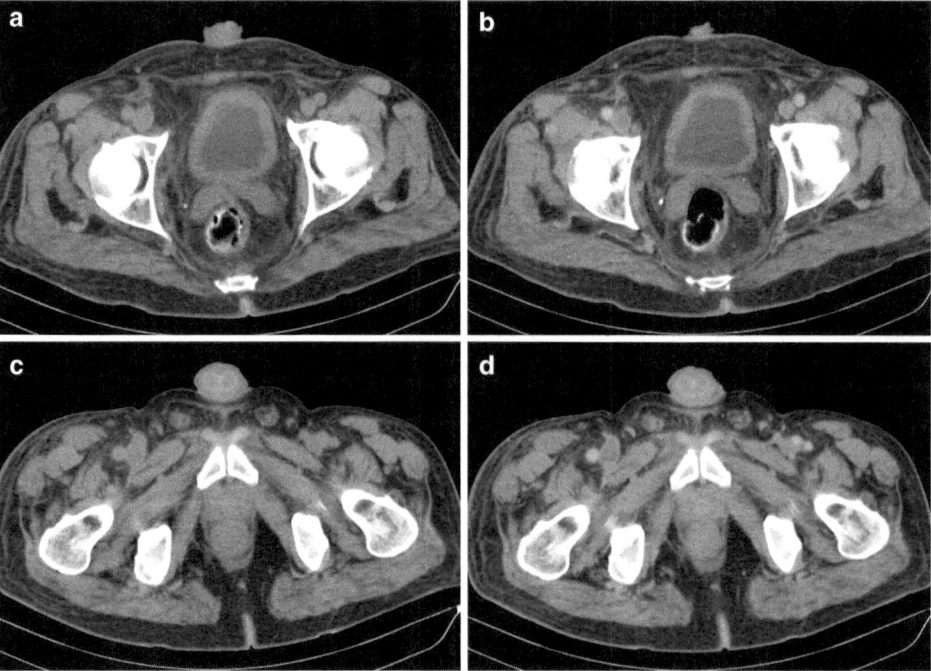

Fig. 3 Selected CT images through the pelvis, in pairs, before (**a**, **c**) and after (**b**, **d**) i.v. contrast. Oral contrast was also administered

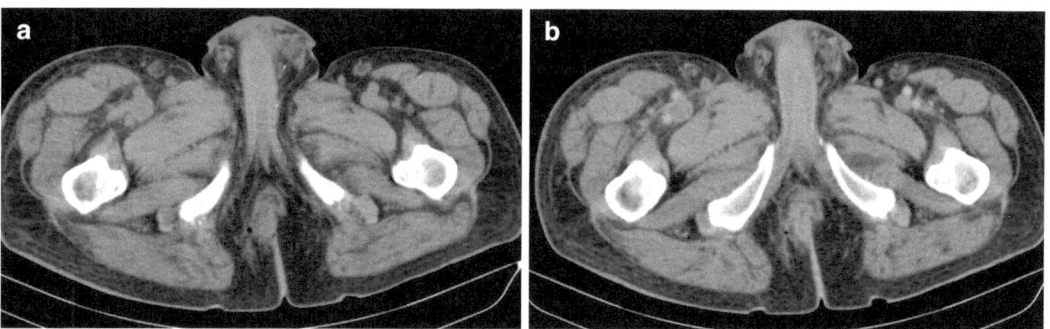

Fig. 4 CT images through the perineum, before (**a**) and after (**b**) i.v. contrast

Please record your observations before proceeding.

Discussion

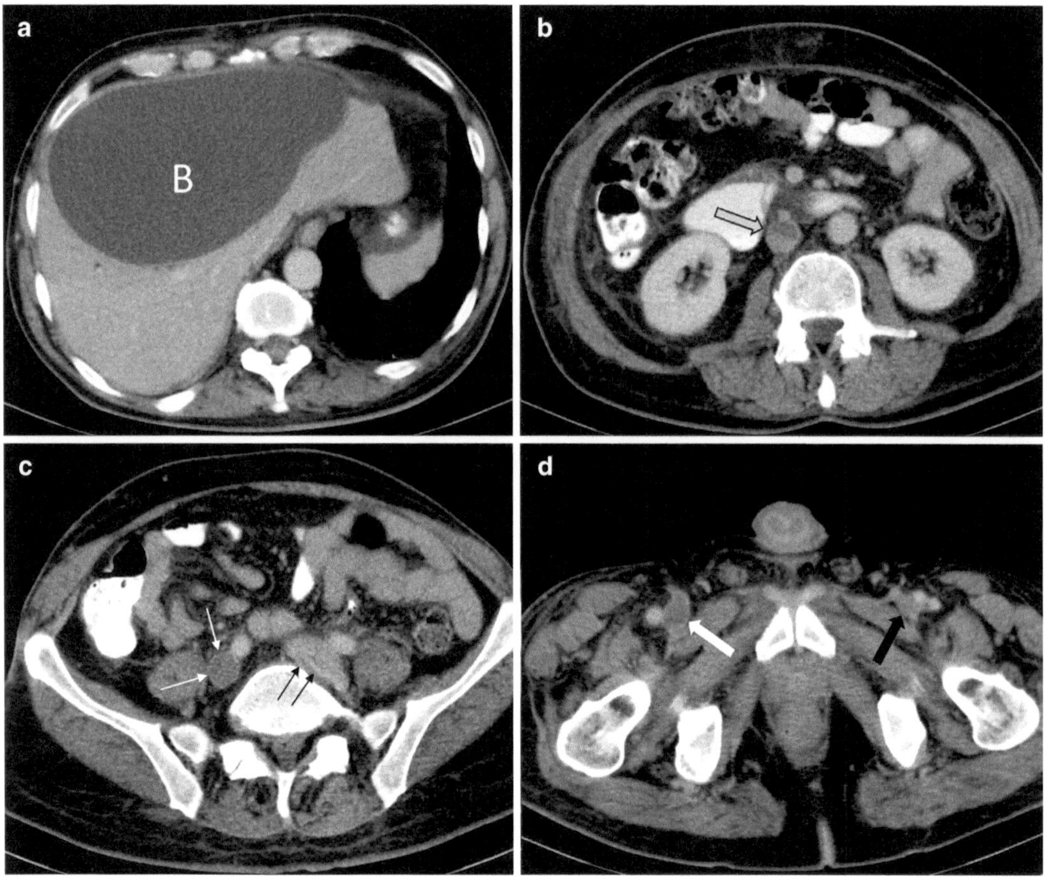

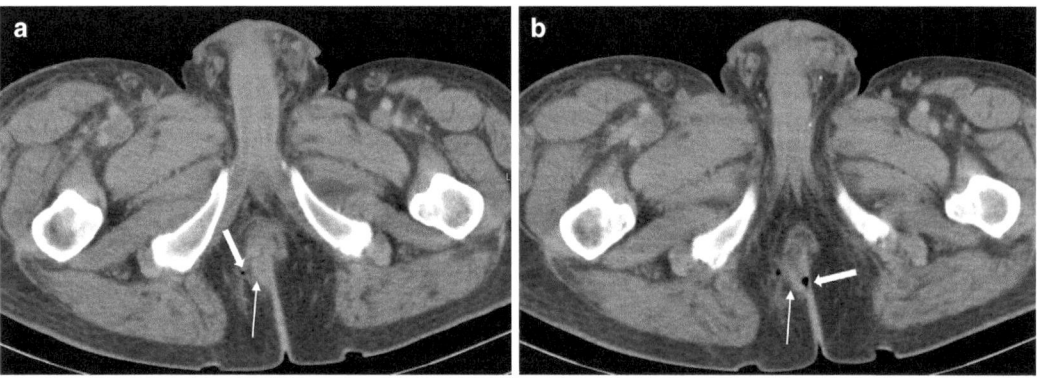

Fig. 5 (**a–d**) Post i.v. contrast images selected from Figs. 1, 2, and 3, photographed with slightly different window settings: WW 75 and WL 340. The default settings in Figs. 1, 2, and 3 were WW 60 and WL 400

Fig. 6 (**a, b**) Same two images as in Fig. 4, photographed with slightly different settings, WW 75 WL 500, compared to the default settings of WW 60 WL 400

Fig. 5: A large subcapsular fluid collection (B) deforms the liver. It was a biloma due to surgical trauma to the biliary tree.

Note inhomogeneous enhancement of the lumen of the infrarenal vena cava (open arrow). There is no enhancement of the lumen of the right common iliac vein (thin white arrows); compare with the contralateral side (thin black arrows). Clot fills and expands the lumen of the right common femoral vein (thick white arrow); compare with the left side (thick black arrow).

The extensive venous thrombosis was confirmed with color-duplex sonography. Inferiorly the clot extended to the tibial veins.

Fig. 6: Note perirectal fistula (thin arrows) with air bubbles (thick arrows) and fat stranding.

Teaching Point

Beware of the satisfaction of search bias. The obvious finding, the large biloma, may hinder the detection of the extensive venous thrombosis. The phlebothrombosis may in turn distract us from noticing the perirectal fistula. Please revisit Chap. 3, "Blind Spots", Sect. 3.4 and Chap. 5, "Satisfaction of Search", Sect. 5.2.2.3.

Case 22

A 77-year-old female with breast carcinoma, s/p right mastectomy, and axillary lymphadenectomy. There was no evidence of spread beyond the right axillary lymph nodes. The patient presents for a routine follow-up CT scan of the chest, abdomen, and pelvis. Currently there is no clinical or laboratory evidence of recurrence or metastases.

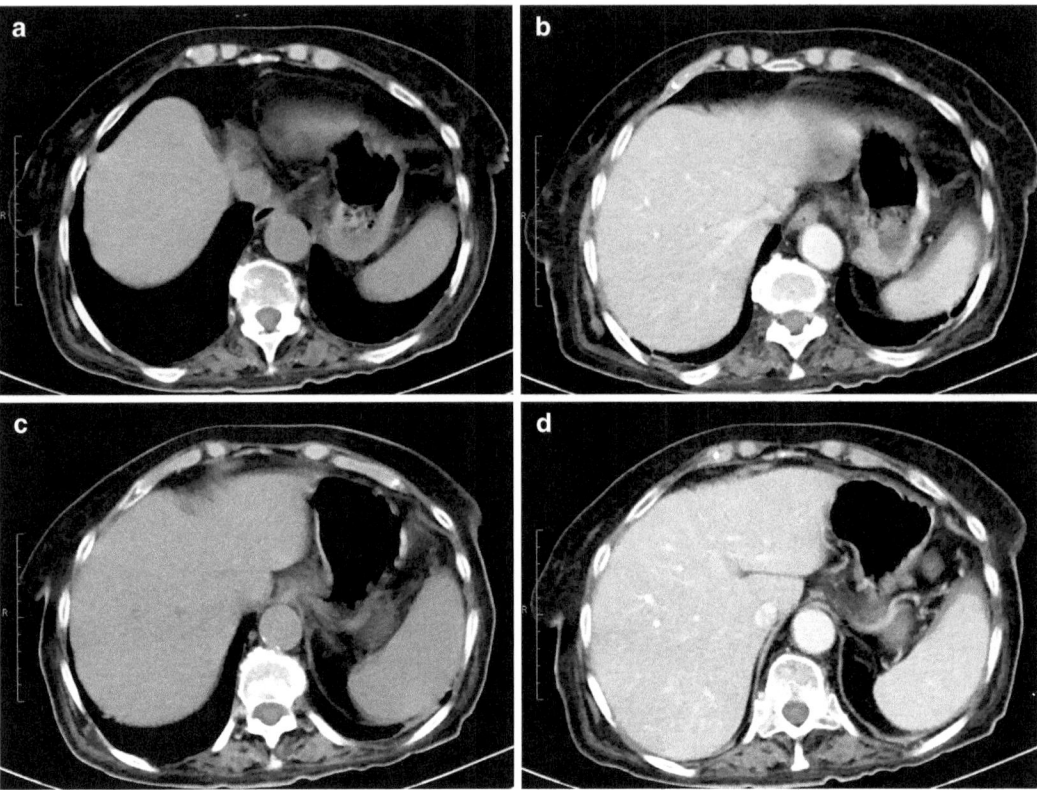

Fig. 1 Pairs of CT slices through the upper abdomen, before (**a**, **c**) and after i.v. contrast (**b**, **d**), portal phase

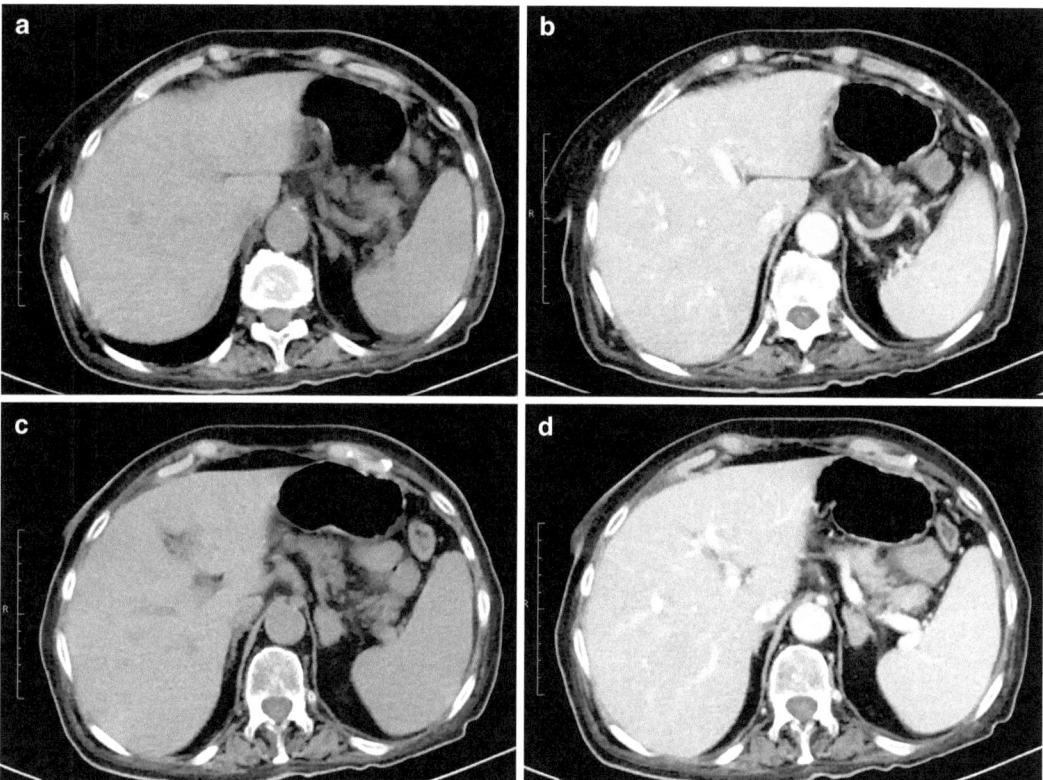

Fig. 2 Pairs of CT slices through the upper abdomen, before (**a**, **c**) and after i.v. contrast (**b**, **d**), portal phase

Please record your observations and your diagnosis before proceeding.

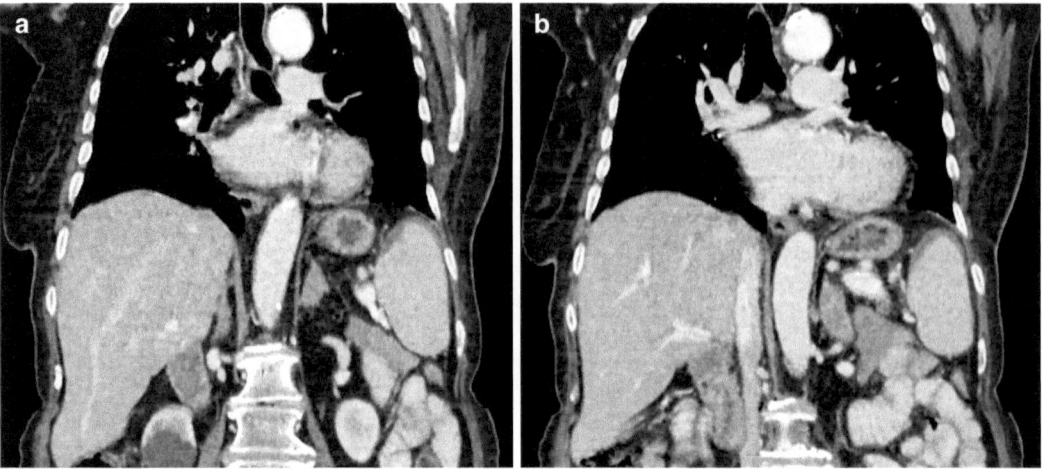

Fig. 3 (**a, b**) Two coronal CT reconstructions, post i.v. contrast

Can you confirm your preliminary diagnosis?

Discussion

A thin film of fluid tracks the upper surface of the spleen. The patient upon questioning revealed that she fell on her left side from a flight of stairs a week prior, but did not pay attention to it. That time interval was enough for the subcapsular hematoma to reach isodensity to spleen in the pre-contrast scan.

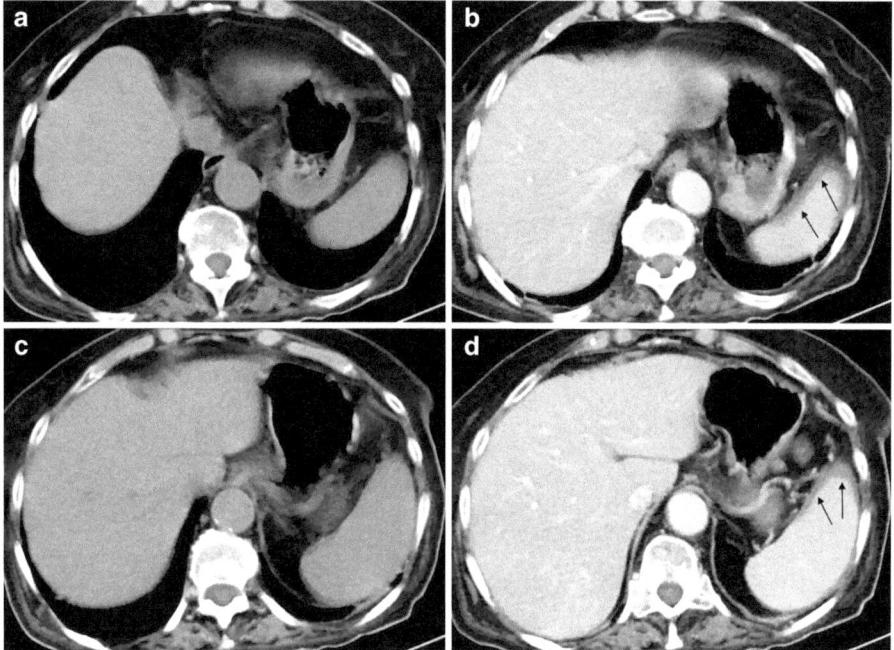

Fig. 4 (a–d) Same images as in Fig. 1, slightly magnified

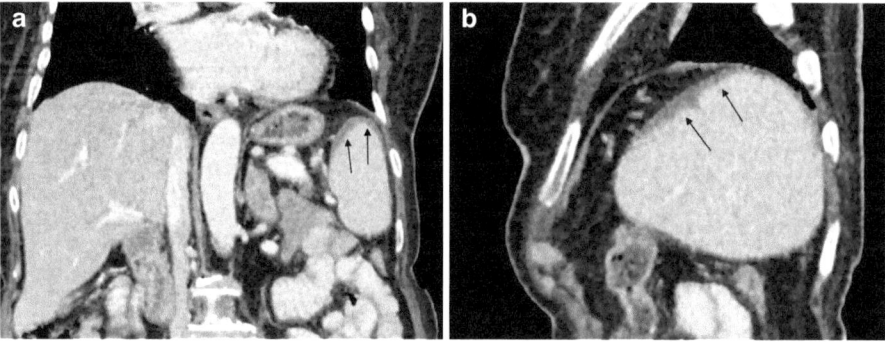

Fig. 5 (a, b) Coronal and sagittal CT reconstructions post i.v. contrast

Teaching Point

Did you have any difficulty processing the findings because you were unduly restricted by the history of breast carcinoma? The history of trauma was evoked after the scan.

Keep an open mind, and consider reading some examinations before you look up the patient's history. Please revisit Sect. 5.2.2.3 in Chap. 5 and Sect. 7.2.1.1 in Chap. 7.

Glossary

ACGME Accreditation Council for Graduate Medical Education

Algorithm A fixed, predetermined set of rules one follows for problem solving. It employs the simple formula "if X, then Y," in order to avoid hesitation and overthinking about reaching a conclusion or executing a desired action

AARS American Roentgen Ray Society

Bias One or more flaws in how we process data and reach conclusions

CanMEDS The Canadian Medical Education Directives for Specialists

Debiasing Questions or strategies to expose our cognitive biases so that we can override them

Deductive reasoning The cognitive process of reaching a true conclusion given a set of premises (conditions), following the rules of logic. In our terms, starting with a set of imaging findings we arrive at the correct diagnosis or at a short differential list that includes the correct diagnosis

ECR European Congress of Radiology

ESR European Society of Radiology

Gestalt German word, meaning shape or form. For our purposes it means the fast detection of a constellation of imaging findings as a unity (shape or form), in other words it means quick pattern recognition

Heuristics Cognitive shortcuts to reach a good enough solution if we are restricted in time or other resources. In medicine and radiology the usual shortcuts are an undue reliance on statistics and on the outcomes of similar cases we have encountered; however, the most probable diagnosis is not necessarily the correct one. Shortcuts may bypass critical findings or evidence that would lead us to the correct diagnosis, instead of the most probable one

Metacognition The processes and methods of assessing one's understanding (knowledge) and performance (skills). In other words, metacognition is a "postmortem" on one's knowledge, thoughts, and cognitive patterns. Metacognition is a valuable learning and adaptive tool, since one can uncover and bring to full awareness his (or her) strengths, weaknesses, and limitations. From this starting point, one can seek and explore ways to expand his (her) knowledge and abilities

RCR Royal College of Radiologists

RANZCR Royal Australian and New Zealand College of Radiologists

© Springer Nature Switzerland AG 2020
H. Chryssikopoulos, *Errors in Imaging*, https://doi.org/10.1007/978-3-030-21103-5

References

1. Epstein RM. Mindful practice. JAMA. 1999;282:833–9.
2. Papa J. Learning sciences principles that can inform the construction of new approaches to diagnostic training. Diagnosis (Berl). 2014;1:125–9.
3. Fish D, de Cossart L. Thinking outside the (tick) box: rescuing professionalism and professional judgment. Med Educ. 2006;40:403–4.
4. Nyhsen CM, Steinberg LJ, O'Connell JE. Undergraduate radiology teaching from the student's perspective. Insights Imaging. 2013;4:103–9.
5. Gutmark R, Halsted MJ, Perry L, Gold G. Use of computer databases to reduce radiograph reading errors. J Am Coll Radiol. 2007;4:65–8.
6. Davis D, O'Brien MA, Freemantle N, Wolf F, Mazmanian P, Taylor-Vaisey A. Impact of formal continuing medical education: do conferences, workshops, rounds, and other traditional continuing education activities change physician behavior or health care outcomes? JAMA. 1999;282:867–74.
7. Rodriguez-Paz JM, Kennedy M, Salas AW, et al. Beyond "see one, do one, teach one,": toward a different training paradigm. Qual Saf Health Care. 2009;18:63–8.
8. ten Cate O. What is a 21st-century doctor? Rethinking the significance of the medical degree. Acad Med. 2014;89:966–9.
9. Levenson R, Atkinson S, Shepherd S. The 21st century doctor: understanding the doctors of tomorrow. General Medical Council (GB). https://www.gmc-uk.org/static/documents/content/The_21st_Century_Doctor_-Understanding_the_doctors_of_tomorrow_2010.pdf. Accessed 15 Dec 2017.
10. Leung A. Resident case review: working smarter to optimize the learning experience. In: Van Deven T, Hibbert KM, Cchem RK, editors. The practice of radiology education: challenges and trends. Heidelberg: Springer; 2010. p. 111–8.
11. Wang SC. Competencies and experiential requirements in radiology training. In: Hibbert KM, Cchem RK, Van deven T, Wang SC, editors. Radiology education: the evaluation and assessment of clinical competence. Heidelberg: Springer; 2012. p. 55–66.
12. Wang SC. Assessment and evaluation in a transnational radiodiagnosis training program. In: Hibbert KM, Cchem RK, Van deven T, Wang SC, editors. Radiology education: the evaluation and assessment of clinical competence. Heidelberg: Springer; 2012. p. 83–100.
13. Fitzgerald R. Radiological error: analysis, standard setting, targeted instruction and teamworking. Eur Radiol. 2005;15:1760–7.
14. Fitzgerald R. Error in radiology. Clin Radiol. 2001;56:938–46.
15. Stanley RJ. How good does it get? AJR. 2004;183:1.
16. Education is not the learning of facts, but the training of the mind to think. Quote Investigator. 2016 May 28. https://quoteinvestigator.com/2016/05/28/not-facts/. Accessed 4 Dec 2015.
17. Richard Feynman: the difference between knowing the name of something and knowing something. Farnam Street Blog. 2015 Jan 05. https://www.farnamstreet-blog.com/205/01/richard-feynman-knowing-something. Accessed 4 Dec 2016.
18. LeadershipNow remembers Peter F. Drucker. 2005. www.leadershipnow.com/druckerremembered.html. Accessed 4 Dec 2016.
19. Fahey L, Prusak L. The eleven deadliest sins of knowledge management. Calif Manag Rev. 1998;40:265–76.
20. Gunderman R, Chan S. Knowledge sharing in radiology. Radiology. 2003;229:314–7.
21. Duke University Radiology Residency. https://radiology.duke.edu/education/residency/. Accessed 16 Dec 2017.
22. Peninsula Radiology Academy. http://www.penra.org.uk/. Accessed 16 Dec 2017.
23. Norwich Radiology Academy. http://norwichradiologyacademy.co.uk/#. Accessed 16 Dec 2017.
24. Graber M. Introduction to diagnostic error. The Society to Improve Diagnosis in Medicine. Diagnostic error resources. Video presentation. www.improvediagnosis.org/page/Education. Accessed 24 Oct 2016.
25. Penn curriculum in cognitive bias and diagnostic error for medical residents. Society to Improve Diagnosis in Medicine. Clinical reasoning toolkit: education. www.improvediagnosis.org/?ClinicalEducation. Accessed 6 Dec 2016.
26. Goodman TR, Kelleher M. Improving novice radiology trainees' perception using fine art. J Am Coll Radiol. 2017;14:1337–40.

H. Chrysikopoulos, *Errors in Imaging*, https://doi.org/10.1007/978-3-030-21103-5

27. Sarkany DS, Shenoy-Bhangle AS, Catanzano TM, Fineberg TA, Eisenberg RL, Slanetz PJ. Running a radiology residency program: strategies for success. Radiographics. 2018;38:1729–43.

28. Goldfarb S, Morrison G. The 3-year medical school-change or shortchange? NEJM. 2013;369:1087–9.

29. Raymond JR Sr, Kerschner JE, Hueston WJ, Maurana CA. The merits and challenges of three-year medical school curricula: time for an evidence-based discussion. Acad Med. 2015;90:1318–23.

30. The American Medical Association accelerating change in medical education initiative. https://www.ama-assn.org/sites/default/files/media-browser/public/about-ama/ace-monograph-interactive_0.pdf. Accessed 16 Dec 2017.

31. Gunderman B. Achieving excellence in medical education. 2nd ed. Heidelberg: Springer; 2011.

32. Drucker PF. Managing oneself. Boston: Harvard Business Review; 1999.

33. Ebuoma LO, Severs FJ, Sedgwick EL, et al. Benefits of professional coaching for radiologists. J Am Coll Radiol. 2017;14:976–9.

34. Pink DH. Drive: the surprising truth about what motivates us. New York: Penguin Random House LLC; 2009.

35. Itri JN, Yacob S, Mithqal A. Teaching communication skills to radiology residents. Curr Probl Diagn Radiol. 2017;46:377–81.

36. Bhargava P. Quick tips for getting back to peak productivity. Curr Probl Diagn Radiol. 2016;45:355.

37. Bhargava P. Extreme Pareto: the one thing. Curr Probl Diagn Radiol. 2017;46:85.

38. Bhargava P. Deep work: a productivity superpower. Curr Probl Diagn Radiol. 2017;46:1–2.

39. Bhargava P. What is all the fuss about productivity? Should you care? Curr Probl Diagn Radiol. 2014;43:233–4.

40. Kostrubiak DE, Kwon M, Lee J, et al. Mentorship in radiology. Curr Probl Diagn Radiol. 2017;46:385–90.

41. Gunderman B. Leadership in healthcare. Heidelberg: Springer; 2009.

42. Houpt JL, Gilkey RW, Erhinghaus SH. Learning to lead in the Academic Medical Center. Heidelberg: Springer; 2015.

43. Bhargava P, Mohammed TLH. Three simple strategies for effective leadership. Curr Probl Diagn Radiol. 2016;45:1.

44. Itri JN, Lawson LM. Ineffective leadership. J Am Coll Radiol. 2016;13:849–55.

45. Heitkamp DE, Kerridge WD, Ballenger ZE, Tawadros AM, Gunderman RB. A leadership development program for radiology residents. J Am Coll Radiol. 2017;16:1468–70.

46. Arnander F. We are all leaders: leadership is not a position, it's a mindset. Chichester: Wiley; 2013.

47. Sharma R. The leader who had no title: a modern fable on real success in business and in life. New York: Simon and Schuster; 2010.

48. Matalon SA, Howard SA, Gaviola GC, et al. Customized residency leadership tracks: a review of what works, what we're doing and ideas for the future. Curr Probl Diagn Radiol. 2018;47:359–63.

49. Davenport MS, Dunnick NR. Lessons on leadership. Radiographics. 2018;38:1688–93.

50. Norman G, Eva KW. Diagnostic error and clinical reasoning. Med Educ. 2010;44:94–100.

51. Holsgrove GJ. Guide to postgraduate exams: multiple-choice questions. Br J Hosp Med. 1992;48:757–61.

52. Veloski JJ, Rabinowitz HK, Robeson MR, Young PR. Patients don't present with five choices: an alternative to multiple-choice tests in assessing physicians' competence. Acad Med. 1999;74:539–46.

53. AMA Wire. University of Michigan changes med school curriculum to improve physician training. 2017 Mar 7. https://wire.ama-assn.org/education/university-michigan-changes-med-school-curriculum-improve-physician-training. Accessed 17 Dec 2017.

54. AMA Wire. 9 challenges medical educators want to solve right now. 2015 Oct 8. https://wire.ama-assn.org/education/9-challenges-medical-educators-want-solve-right-now. Accessed 17 Dec 2017.

55. AMA Wire. Creating the impossible: key innovations, solutions in med ed. 2017 Oct 5. https://wire.ama-assn.org/education/creating-impossible-key-innovations-solutions-med-ed. Accessed 17 Dec 2017.

56. AMA Wire. 21 more schools tapped to transform physician training. 2015 Nov 4. https://wire.ama-assn.org/education/21-more-schools-tapped-transform-physician-training. Accessed 17 Dec 2017.

57. AMA Wire. 6 students discuss creating the med school of the future. 2017 Mar 6. https://wire.ama-assn.org/education/6-students-discuss-creating-med-school-future. Accessed 17 Dec 2017.

58. Burk-Rafel J, Jones RL, Farlow JL. Engaging learners to advance medical education. Acad Med. 2017;92:437–40.

59. Hardman RL, Lopera JE, Cardan RA, Trimmer CK, Josephs SC. Common and rare collateral pathways in aortoiliac occlusive disease: a pictorial essay. AJR. 2011;197:W519–24.

60. Krishnan A, Shirkoda A, Tehrazandeh J, Armin AR, Irwin R, Les K. Primary bone lymphoma: radiographic-MR imaging correlation. RadioGraphics. 2003;23:1371–83.

61. Lim CY, Ong KO. Imaging of musculoskeletal lymphoma. Cancer Imaging. 2013;13:448–57.

62. Slone HW, Blake JJ, Shah R, Guttikonda S, Bourekas EC. CT and MRI findings of intracranial lymphoma. AJR. 2005;184:1679–85.

63. Haldorsen IS, Espeland A, Larsson E-M. Central nervous system lymphoma: characteristic findings on traditional and advanced imaging. AJNR. 2011;32:984–92.

64. Partovi S, Karimi S, Lyo JK, Esmaeili A, Tan J, Deangelis LM. Multimodality imaging of primary CNS lymphoma in immunocompetent patients. Br J Radiol. 2014;87(1036):20130684. https://doi.org/10.1259/bjr.20130684.

65. George AE, Russell EJ, Kricheff II. White matter buckling: CT sign of extraaxial mass. AJR. 1980;135:1031–6.

66. Parker EA. Analysis of mass effect. In: Naidich TP, Castillo M, Cha S, Smirniotopoulos JG, editors. Imaging of the brain. Expert radiology series. Philadelphia: Elsevier Saunders; 2013. p. 68–9.
67. Chee DWY, Peh WCG. Pictorial essay: Imaging of peripheral nerve sheath tumors. J Can Assoc Radiol. 2011;62:176–82.
68. Kakkar C, Shetty CM, Koteshwara P, Bajpai S. Telltale signs of peripheral neurogenic tumors on magnetic resonance imaging. Indian J Radiol Imaging. 2015;25:453–8.
69. Paddock M, Robson N. The curious case of the disappearing IVC: a case report and review of the aetiology of inferior vena cava agenesis. J Radiol Case Rep. 2014;8:38–47.
70. Bass JE, Redwine MD, Kramer LA, Huynh PT, Harris J Jr. Spectrum of congenital anomalies of the inferior vena cava: cross-sectional imaging findings. Radiographics. 2000;20:639–52.
71. Ugurlu MM, Asoglu O, Potter DD, Barnes SA, Harmsen WS, Donohue JH. Adenocarcinomas of the jejunum and ileum: a 25-year experience. J Gastrointest Surg. 2005;9:1182–8.
72. Li J, Wang Z, Liu N, Hao J, Xu X. Small bowel adenocarcinoma of the jejunum: a case report and literature review. World J Surg Oncol. 2016;14:177.
73. Sailer J, Zacherl J, Schima W. MDCT of small bowel tumours. Cancer Imaging. 2005;7:224–33.
74. Doyle DJ, Khalili K, Guindi M, Atri M. Imaging features of sclerosed hemangioma. AJR. 2007;189:67–72.
75. Behbahani S, Hoffman JC, Stonebridge R, Mahboob S. Clinical case report: sclerosing hemangioma of the liver, a rare but great mimicker. Radiol Case Rep. 2016;11:58–61.
76. Kantarci M, Bayraktutan U, Karabulut N, et al. Alveolar echinococcosis: spectrum of findings at cross-sectional imaging. RadioGraphics. 2012;32:2053–70.
77. Salem R, Zrig A, Trimech T, et al. Pulmonary embolism in echinococcosis: two case reports and literature review. Ann Trop Med Parasitol. 2011;105:85–9.
78. Poyraz N, Demirbas S, Korkmaz C, Uzun K. Pulmonary embolism originating from a hepatic hydatid cyst ruptured in the inferior vena cava: CT and MRI findings. Case Rep Radiol. 2016;2016:3589812. https://doi.org/10.1155/2016/3589812.
79. Bang SH, Lee JY, Woo H, et al. Differentiating between adenomyomatosis and gallbladder cancer: revisiting a comparative study of high-resolution ultrasound, multidetector CT, and MR imaging. Korean J Radiol. 2014;15:226–34.
80. Ching BH, Yeh BM, Westphalen AC, Joe BN, Qayyum A, Coakley FV. CT differentiation of adenomyomatosis and gallbladder cancer. AJR. 2007;189:62–6.

Suggested Reading

1. Gladwell M. Outliers: the story of success. New York: Little Brown and Company; 2008.
2. Dacher JN, Charlin B, Bergeron D, Tardif J. Consultation skills in radiology: a qualitative study. Can Assoc Radiol J. 1998;3:167–71.
3. Peterson C. Factors associated with success or failure in radiological interpretation: diagnostic thinking approaches. Med Educ. 1999;33:251–9.
4. Robinson PJ. Radiology's Achilles' heel: error and variation in the interpretation of the Roentgen image. Br J Radiol. 1997;70:1085–98.
5. Gunderman RB, Nyce JM. The tyranny of accuracy in radiologic education. Radiology. 2002;222:297–300.
6. Itri JN, Tappouni RR, McEachern RO, Pesch RO, Patel SH. Fundamentals of diagnostic error in imaging. RadioGraphics. 2018;38:1845–65.
7. Schiff GD. Minimizing diagnostic error: the importance of follow-up and feedback. Am J Med. 2008;121(5 suppl):S38–42.
8. Brook OR, O'Connell AM, Thornton E, Eisenberg RL, Mendiratta-Lala M, Kruskal JB. Quality initiatives: anatomy and pathophysiology of errors occurring in clinical radiology practice. RadioGraphics. 2010;30:1401–10.
9. Graber ML. Taking steps toward a safer future: measures to promote timely and accurate medical diagnosis. Am J Med. 2008;121(suppl 5):S43–6.
10. Kelly AM. Basic definitions. In: Abujudeh HH, Bruno MA, editors. Quality and safety in radiology. Oxford: Oxford University Press; 2012. p. 3–11.
11. Roddie ME. Approach to characterizing radiological errors. In: Peh WCG, editor. Pitfalls in diagnostic radiology. Heidelberg: Springer; 2015. p. 133–42.
12. Kahlben CL, Yetter EM, Olson MC, Posniak HV, Aranha GV. Assessing the resectability of pancreatic carcinoma: the value of re-interpreting abdominal CT performed at other institutions. AJR. 1998;171:1571–6.
13. Berlin L. Malpractice and radiologists in Cook County IL: trends in 20 years of litigation. AJR. 1995;165:781–8.
14. Berlin L. Defending the "missed" radiographic diagnosis. AJR. 2001;176:317–22.
15. Berlin L. Medicolegal-malpractice and ethical issues in radiology: reporting the missed radiologic diagnosis. AJR. 2013;201:W516.
16. Berlin L. To disclose or not to disclose radiologic errors: should patient-first supersede radiologist self-interest? Radiology. 2013;268:4–7.
17. Berlin L. To whom is the radiologist responsible? AJR. 2012;198:W191.
18. Berlin L. Medicolegal-malpractice and ethical issues in radiology. Who supervises the CT scan protocol? AJR. 2016;207:W1–2.
19. Berlin L. Medicolegal-malpractice and ethical issues in radiology. Interpreting large FOV versus limited FOV images. AJR. 2016;207:W19.
20. Berlin L. Medicolegal-malpractice and ethical issues in radiology. Should the name of a colleague who was asked to offer an informal consultation be included in the final report of a radsiologic examination? AJR. 2016;206:W41.
21. Berlin L. Medicolegal-malpractice and ethical issues in radiology. Judging the competency of a radiologist colleague. AJR. 2016;206:W29.
22. Berlin L. Medicolegal-malpractice and ethical issues in radiology. What is reasonable conduct? AJR. 2015;205:W565.
23. Berlin L. Medicolegal-malpractice and ethical issues in radiology. Reporting agreement or disagreement when overreading outside radiology examinations. AJR. 2015;205:W382.
24. Berlin L. Medicolegal-malpractice and ethical issues in radiology. CT examination performed on the wrong patient. AJR. 2015;205:W224.
25. Berlin L. Medicolegal-malpractice and ethical issues in radiology. Pejorative comments on radiology reports. AJR. 2015;204:W605.
26. Berlin L. Medicolegal-malpractice and ethical issues in radiology. Role of the expert witness. AJR. 2015;204:W371.
27. Berlin L. Radiologic errors and malpractice: a blurry distinction. AJR. 2007;189:517–22.
28. Berlin L. Who should notify an emergency department patient when a preliminary radiologic reading is found to be incorrect? AJR. 2012;199:W654.

29. Berlin L. Medicolegal-malpractice and ethical issues in radiology. CT scout views and standard of care. AJR. 2014;203:W741.
30. Berlin L. Medicolegal-malpractice and ethical issues in radiology. Overdiagnosis, false-positive findings, and malpractice. AJR. 2014;203:W549.
31. Berlin L. Is there a difference between "standard of care" and "standard of practice"? AJR. 2012;199:W655.
32. Berlin L, Murphy DR, Singh H. Breakdowns in communication of radiological findings: an ethical and medico-legal conundrum. Diagnosis (Berlin L). 2014;1:263–8.
33. Berlin L. Medicolegal-malpractice and ethical issues in radiology. Combined CT examinations: should they be interpreted by the same Radiologist or split? AJR. 2014;203:W337.
34. Berlin L. Medicolegal-malpractice and ethical issues in radiology. Electronic health records and malpractice litigation: malpractice pitfalls. AJR. 2014;203:W447–8.
35. Berlin L. Communicate all actionable findings now, not later. J Am Coll Radiol. 2014;11:924–5.
36. Berlin L. Medicolegal-malpractice and ethical issues in radiology. Liability for reaction to contrast media administration. AJR. 2014;202:W597.
37. Berlin L. Point: mammography, breast cancer and overdiagnosis: the truth versus the whole truth versus nothing but the truth. J Am Coll Radiol. 2014;11:642–7.
38. Berlin L. Medicolegal-malpractice and ethical issues in radiology. Routine comparison radiography of the extremities: should it be ordered and if so, how should it be billed? AJR. 2014;202:W182.
39. Berlin L. Liability of radiologist for ordering contrast medium. AJR. 2012;199:W524.
40. Berlin L. Medicolegal-malpractice and ethical issues in radiology. Disclaimers on reports. AJR. 2013;201:W657.
41. Berlin L. Medicolegal-malpractice and ethical issues in radiology. Recommending additional and follow-up radiologic examinations. AJR. 2013;201:W656.
42. Berlin L. Screening for early detection of breast cancer: overdiagnosis versus public education. Radiology. 2014;270:310–1.
43. Berlin L. Is there a difference between "standard of. care" and "standard of practice"? AJR. 2012;199:W655.
44. Berlin L. Medicolegal-malpractice and ethical issues in radiology. What is "reasonable assurance of receipt?". AJR. 2013;201:W159.
45. Berlin L. Professionalism and disclosing errors. AJR. 2012;198:W315.
46. Berlin L. Medicolegal-malpractice and ethical issues in radiology. Proofreading radiology reports. AJR. 2013;200:W691–2.
47. Berlin L. Medicolegal-malpractice and ethical issues in radiology. Adding to a referring physician's order without permission. AJR. 2013;200:W216.
48. Berlin L. Medicolegal-malpractice and ethical issues in radiology: the incidentaloma. AJR. 2013;200:W91.
49. Berlin L. Malpractice issues in radiology. Perceptual errors. AJR. 1996;167:587–90.
50. Berlin L, Hendrix RW. Perceptual errors and negligence. AJR. 1998;170:863–7.
51. Berlin L. Errors of omission. AJR. 2005;185:1416–21.
52. Berlin L. Medicolegal-malpractice and ethical issues in radiology. Reordering incorrect radiologic examinations. AJR. 2017;208:W54–5.
53. Whang JS, Baker SR, Patel R, Luk L, Castro A III. The causes of medical malpractice suits against radiologists in the United States. Radiology. 2013;266:548–54.
54. West RW. Radiology malpractice in the emergency room setting. Emerg Radiol. 2000;7:14–8.
55. Won E, Rosenkrantz AB. Informal consultations between radiologists and referring physicians, as identified through an electronic medical record search. AJR. 2017;209:1–4.
56. Busardo FP, Frati P, Santurro A, Zaami S, Fineschi V. Errors and malpractice lawsuits in radiology: what the radiologist needs to know. Radiol Med. 2015;120:779–84.
57. Raskin MM. Survival strategies for radiology: some practical tips on how to reduce the risk of being sued and losing. J Am Coll Radiol. 2006;3:689–93.
58. Fileni A, Magnavita N, Mirk P, et al. Radiologic malpractice litigation in Italy: an observational study over a 14-year period. AJR. 2010;194:1040–6.
59. Waite S, Scott JM, Legasto A, Kolla S, Gale B, Krupinski EA. Systemic error in radiology. AJR. 2017;209:629–39.
60. Sheng AY, Castro A, Lewiss RE. Awareness, utilization, and education of the ACR appropriateness criteria: a review and future directions. J Am Coll Radiol. 2016;13:131–6.